"A remarkable contribution to the growing field of pandemic studies, *Viral World* tracks forms of relations constitutive of COVID-19 pandemic. 'Viral worlding' is the conceptual frame that illuminates interlaced relationalities, in a book that bridges international politics, theories of global society, and interdisciplinary studies of media."

Bishnupriya Ghosh, *Professor of English and Global Studies, University of California, Santa Barbara, USA, and author of* The Virus Touch: Theorizing Epidemic Media *(2023)*

"Rather than present a linear narrative of the pandemic or case studies cropped around national borders, Long T. Bui's *Viral World* performs the looping disjointed sense of time emblematic of this crisis. The book ambitiously traverses the world and jumps scales like the coronavirus itself. It is a daring holistic effort that aims to capture the multiple dimensions of COVID-19."

Li Zhang, *Assistant Professor of Sociology and Environmental Studies, Amherst College, USA, and author of* The Origins of COVID-19: China and Global Capitalism *(2021)*

T0256299

VIRAL WORLD

This book argues that the catastrophe of COVID-19 provided a momentous time for groups, institutions, and states to reassess their worldviews and relationship to the entire world. Following multiple case studies across dozens of countries throughout the course of the pandemic, this book is a timely contribution to cultural knowledge about the pandemic and the viral politics at the heart of it.

Mapping the various forms of global consciousness and connectivity engendered by the crisis, the book offers the framework of "viral worlding," defined as viral forms of relationality, becoming, and communication. It demonstrates how worlding or world-making processes accelerated with the novel coronavirus. New emergent forms of being global "went viral" to address conditions of inequality as well as forge possibilities for societal transformation. Considering the tumult wrought by the pandemic, Bui analyzes progressive movements for democracy, abolition, feminism, environmentalism, and socialism against the world-shattering forces of capitalism, authoritarianism, racism, and militarism. Focusing on ways the pandemic disproportionately impacted marginalized communities, particularly in the Global South, this book juxtaposes the closing of their lifeworlds and social worlds by hegemonic global actors with increased collective demands for freedom, mobility, and justice by vulnerable people.

The breadth and depth of the book thus provide students, scholars, and general readers with critical insights to understanding the world(s) of COVID-19 and collective efforts to build better new ones.

Long T. Bui is Associate Professor of Global and International Studies at the University of California, Irvine, USA. His research explores digital media and popular culture, global Asias, Asian American studies, cultural geography, critical education studies, critical refugee studies, history and memory, race, gender, and sexuality. He is the author of *Returns of War: South Vietnam and the Price of Refugee Memory* (2018) and *Model Machines: A History of the Asian as Automaton* (2021).

The COVID-19 Pandemic Series

This series examines the impact of the COVID-19 pandemic on individuals, communities, countries, and the larger global society from a social scientific perspective. It represents a timely and critical advance in knowledge related to what many believe to be the greatest threat to global ways of being in more than a century. It is imperative that academics take their rightful place alongside medical professionals as the world attempts to figure out how to deal with the current global pandemic, and how society might move forward in the future. This series represents a response to that imperative.

Series Editor: J. Michael Ryan

Titles in this Series:

Transformations in Social Science Research Methods during the COVID-19 Pandemic
Edited by J. Michael Ryan, Valerie Visanich and Gaspar Brändle

Social Structure Adaptation to COVID-19
Impact on Humanity
Edited by Suresh Nanwani and William Loxley

Viral World
Global Relations During the COVID-19 Pandemic
Long T. Bui

VIRAL WORLD

Global Relations During the COVID-19 Pandemic

Long T. Bui

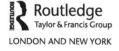

Routledge
Taylor & Francis Group

LONDON AND NEW YORK

Designed cover image: Long T. Bui

First published 2024
by Routledge
4 Park Square, Milton Park, Abingdon, Oxon OX14 4RN

and by Routledge
605 Third Avenue, New York, NY 10158

Routledge is an imprint of the Taylor & Francis Group, an informa business

British Library Cataloguing-in-Publication Data
A catalogue record for this book is available from the British Library

ISBN: 978-1-032-69451-1 (hbk)
ISBN: 978-1-032-69452-8 (pbk)
ISBN: 978-1-032-69453-5 (ebk)

DOI: 10.4324/9781032694535

Typeset in Sabon
by Newgen Publishing UK

CONTENTS

FIGURES

FOREWORD

When the World Health Organization first declared COVID-19 to be a global pandemic on March 11, 2020, few were prepared for what would follow in the coming months (and years). Ongoing debates about globalization were given fodder as the SARS-CoV-2 virus spread, and did so seemingly without concern for artificial humanly created constructs like national borders, racial categories, and the like. But as the virus wore on, it didn't take long to realize the importance of those seemingly "artificial" human constructs. Minority groups and impoverished nations largely bore the brunt of infections and deaths, while the global elite sheltered in place and enjoyed the privilege of privilege.

The COVID-19 pandemic not only (re)presented a (not so) new crisis to an increasingly global community of both humans and nonhuman denizens of the planet, it also highlighted the multiple forms of social and ecological crises that had already long been plaguing our shared social and physical spaces. Perhaps the truly "novel" aspect of the COVID-19 pandemic has been that it has both highlighted our shared singular world and the multiple ways in which that world is inhabited by multiple other worlds.

Bui has recognized all of the above by deploying the concept of "viral worlds." In this way, he recognizes not only the empirical reality of an increasing global connectivity but also the equal reality of a growing desire for a change in business as usual. This volume not only documents the "realities" of the COVID-19 pandemic but also their spirit. Inequalities abound, but so do possibilities.

One of the most dreaded impacts of a COVID-19 world, and of viral worlds more generally, is the potential of the spread of disease, loneliness, and a wide range of -isms and -phobias to overpower the potentials of awareness, activism, and a genuine humanism. Bui's work not only documents this dread but also does much to help mitigate it by offering a deeper understanding of the ways in which the COVID-19 pandemic has been both novel (including in opportunities) as well as a little bit of history repeating (including in politics trumping possibilities). At base, Bui demonstrates the importance of combining historical understandings (and ones we have often been so quick to discard or forget) with contemporary realities (we really are more interconnected as a species and as multiple species).

Viral Worlds skillfully combines the hook of an autoethnographic narrative with the bait of meticulously researched data to deliver the capture of a piece of truly (to echo the alliterative nature of the book's subtitles) informative, insightful, and innovative scholarship.

J. Michael Ryan
Series Editor, *The COVID-19 Pandemic Series*
December 2023

ACKNOWLEDGMENTS

I wrote this book to process and make sense of the COVID-19 pandemic, while being moored in the United States, a center of gravity for the crisis. My big-picture account of this moment comes out of the angst of spatial confinement due to quarantine, which coincided with my career worries as a professor up for tenure in early 2020, which I got in January—the same month the novel coronavirus was discovered in the country. Showing no major signs of infection at first, some of my best friends eventually became "long haulers" unable to do their work or get out of bed. I consider myself lucky as I watch them struggle to do work. My mind drifted toward two centenarian grandparents who suddenly passed away, possibly from the novel coronavirus. My mother had just come out of the hospital for an unknown ailment. She was covered by the Affordable Care Act, which the Donald Trump administration proceeded to strip away. Such contemptible actions made little sense with a looming pandemic.

While billions went under seclusion, COVID-19 allowed people to also step into previously closed-off parts of the world, giving room to share and enter the lives of others. This is what is meant by a viral world, where we infect each other with love, hope, and understanding to create a better world. I thank everyone for teaching me a fair bit about myself within the macrocosm of a raging pandemic. From social media to the creative arts and public education, I witnessed so many people organizing for collective kindness and social solidarity.

Thank you to my reviewers and editors at Routledge Press, J. Michael Ryan and Helen Pritt. A big thanks goes to Vijay Shah for being the best developmental editor. What would I do without the magic of Jessica Canas-Castaneda and Luis Fonseca, two people I trust more than others? Thank you

Jewel Quilaton for always being so cool and chill. New colleagues I befriended in the past year include staff like Thais Boucherau, and all the many new faculty in Global and International Studies at the University of California, Irvine. Too many to name! My awesome chair Eve Darian-Smith has written too many letters for me and her support for me is unwavering. Colleagues that I truly value in the inter-disciplines include Paul Amar, forever my lovely guardian angel, and Bishnupriya Ghosh, who is literally everyone's favorite go-to person for a sound mind. Martin Manalansan is like the great uncle that never stops caring for us younger folks. Kalindi Vora is someone I would love to be more like, thoughtful and caring. Christina Schwenkel teaches me to keep going, and she remains a leader in the field I admire.

Krystal-Gayle O'Neill is my mutant buddy, using her superpowers to read and save the world. Thu-Huong Nguyen-Vo has always been there for me through thick and thin; I am grateful for her affection and enduring support. Li Zhang is simply too wonderful for words, and I am grateful for her friendship, as well as for Gustavo Oliveira, who does not lack for words. I want to thank mentors, family members, and old close friends for keeping me sane during the hard times. A hearty welcome goes to new folks who I met or got closer to in this pandemic journey: Jonathan Alexander, Annie McClanahan, Irene Vega, Sharon Block, and Joanna Perez. Amelle "Mel" Beauvil is my spirit twin; we need to leave this planet together.

Political change-makers and cultural tastemakers taught us all a great number of things needed to survive a catastrophe like COVID-19. These individuals were world-builders exhibiting markers of success: passion, patience, and persistence. My students carried on the torch of learning, despite the struggles of working from home or from abroad. New students I welcomed to my collective mentoring fold include Trinh Dang, Katherine Funes, Demetrius Tien, Gunn Phikrohkit, and Mary Zheng. I commend the continued success of my awesome mentees D. Alex Pina, Edward Kenneth Lazaro Nadurata, and Gvantsa Gasviani.

Stevie Ruiz is my biggest supporter, critic, and interrogator, making me a better happier person and not a grumpy one. Yousuf Al-Bulushi is not only my comrade, but he fixes my house too! He and Chelsea Schields make me want to live in academic suburbia forever. Nguyen Le has never left my side during this long journey, and I owe a lifetime of thanks to him. Thanks to the crew of Nam-Phong Le, Terry Tran, Jay Tran, Marvin Trinh, and Alex Chien.

My family had to deal with all sorts of problems like a total energy blackout for days in Texas in the freezing winter. These failing electric grids, just like COVID-19, are the by-product of bad leadership and climate-adverse political regimes. My brother and sisters are, however, the best ever group of people to find joy and humor in this world. Thank you to My Bui, Co Ha, Lena Chen, Luan Bui, Kim Bui, Christine Tran, and Lisa Bui for being the best family ever. The pandemic was one problem on top of their many woes. Besides being grateful to those workers who could not stay home, I would like to honor all those who moved on from their physical form, due to COVID-19 or not.

Lastly, I would like to thank readers and future generations of scholars, students, artists, teachers, and activists for continuing the work of social justice. This book is dedicated to those who survived and dealt with the pandemic in the best way they could. Our cultural wealth of knowledge and "viral" worlding are precious things which cannot be taken away. To endure is to live, and to live is to fight for better days. In the event of another pandemic, our global bond will lead to greater things. Renewal and revolution are things born of great reflection as well as relations.

INTRODUCTION

Quagmire, Quarantine, Query

In 2003, I felt a burst of excitement preparing for my first trip overseas. It vowed to be an unforgettable moment for this first-generation college student participating in a study abroad program. For my host site, I selected Hong Kong, lured by a childhood of watching Bruce Lee movies and martial arts flicks. In the middle of my preparation, jolting news about a malaise called severe acute respiratory syndrome (SARS) hit the semiautonomous island. With big troubles looming, my university routed me to the next best option for international education: Singapore. A split-second recalibration in plans made clear the immediacy and expanse of a modern-day pandemic.

Secure as Singapore was, this former-British-colony-turned-entrepot could not escape the new virus. Upon landing in the safety of Singapore, my mind raced with worry, overflowing with thoughts about where the threat was going next. One query revolved around the "War on Terror" and invasion of Iraq by the United States. If countries too busy fighting surrendered to a disease, failing to subdue burgeoning pandemic orders of magnitude, to whose detriment could it be? Though I spent some time learning about world cultures in Singapore, I did not need to travel so far, groping and finding my way "out there" to experience the world. Its virulent manifestations came rushing to me, bringing forth a "global sense of place."[1]

A collision of disparate events put into perspective the knotted strands of planetary life. If someone had told me as a young adult that I would return to work at my alma mater only to contend with another hovering pandemic—which strikingly resembled one that I had faced years before—I would not have believed them. Tendentious ingrained beliefs are suspended in all-consuming moments that can act as a wake-up call. Approaching a terminal global crisis requires plenty of intense learning as well as deep

DOI: 10.4324/9781032694535-1

soul-searching to find the correct path forward. Turning inward to discover the inner workings of pandemic existence, everyday people explored the new viral meanings of life. A movement for mutual aid societies grew, asking afresh what tangible strategies enabled us to not only survive but thrive on this earth—one changing faster than humans can sometimes adapt.

Pandemics invite behavioral plasticity and "personal reeducation."[2] Students began streaming into my campus in Irvine, California wearing face masks, which is so ubiquitous throughout Asia. Quite suddenly, my close friends and I developed "brain fog" and dry coughs with deep chest pains that lasted for weeks. These ailments presented not the classic symptoms of the common cold. A tight congested feeling in my airways felt like it had sharp particles nestled deep inside; I laid in bed fearing that I would choke to death in sleep. My strange persisting symptoms matched those of a British woman who at first thought all this media hype about a novel virus was overblown. Upon falling victim to the phantom menace, the 23-year-old woman said it was "like having glass in your lungs."[3] The sick had been withheld from early testing (since health officials encouraged only the very sick to become tested) due to a shortfall in kits, reserving it for the needy and elderly.

Hedging their bets against an unknown risk, my university ordered a shutdown of all on-campus operations. An unnerving mood came over me hearing about students needing to pack all their belongings and leave. Not knowing when they could come back to campus, everyone was on permanent leave until further notice. As someone who once experienced housing insecurity, I empathized with people with nowhere to go, amid an ordeal over which they had no control. Displacement due to an ascendant pandemic bestowed new meaning to my upcoming undergrad seminar on refugees and stateless people—now moved online to avoid group infection.

Listening to news of countries shutting down borders and shuttling travelers awakened inner pangs of emotion in me as a child of refugees through a shared collective responsibility. I felt attached to newly linked "communities of fate."[4] Though we humans were all on the same metaphoric boat, who would be cast overboard first? A decade-old movie like *Contagion* (2011) gave some clues with its fictional story about a fast-advancing virus that takes shape in southeastern China and spreads to the entire world. Carrying bat and pig genes, the virus whips around the air and spreads through human contact. The total collapse of global societies seemed assured as hospitals and governments were pushed to their limits. Medical staff, itinerant workers, and the poor became the first to be sacrificed. A movie that many, including myself, once dismissed as a vehicle for Hollywood celebrities now hit painfully close to home with a real-life contagion on the loose.

Viral World: Global Relations during the COVID-19 Pandemic confronts a global health crisis and its unshakable lessons for a turbocharged human planet. It attends to shocking revelations about the spread of the novel coronavirus in a world running at full speed, knocking that world off balance. That world kept on spinning though, as a viral one. While attentive to policies related to COVID-19, this book also fixates on spontaneous events, human stories, and media narratives that cropped up during this heady time. The book gathers scattered "viral" conversations from news sources as well as social media. As the novel coronavirus made its lethal trek across the planet, it poked holes in permeable social structures, the loose sinews of which no quick fix could patch. If coronavirus was another "bug" in faulty world systems, then how do we debug it? In transferring what had been previously unknown to the observable, COVID-19 sliced open societies riveted by decades of intensified class stratification, political corruption, and ecological dilapidation. Its perforations afforded an opportunity to consider the growing pains that accompanied fighting a fast-moving disease. The clock was ticking for a solution, and everyone shuddered to think about the great and incalculable loss of life as we tunneled through the pandemic's passages.

While a new disease was upending the entire world, the lifeworlds and social worlds of minoritized groups were being transformed or exposed in new "novel" ways, such as a spike in hate crimes against Asians and Asian Americans. COVID-19 brought about what I call a viral world, emanating from a common viral threat as well as the different forms of "viralized" thinking and politics that exploded across the planet from it. The book frames the unprecedent crisis in terms of "viral worlding," a process which I define as the heightening sense of global connectivity under pandemic conditions, as well as the desire for change in preexisting relationships.

The third coronavirus pandemic resulted in major shifts in world institutions, infrastructures, attitudes, ethics, identity, and well-being. World-making projects emerged in all forms, scaling across national and regional distinctions, hence the book seeks to capture them. It is known that the pandemic amplified and accelerated global inequality for the super-exploited. I juxtapose the international rise in the policing of subaltern people with demands for social justice and global democracy.

This introductory chapter opens with a personal anecdote of my study abroad experience as a starting point to think about the COVID-19 pandemic. I observe the makings of a global pandemic and how COVID-19 marks a "viral moment" looping back to old histories and quagmires. Connecting my journey back then as a student to my life now as a professor of global and international studies, I recognize new queries, but also the failure of not learning from the past with the premise that medical quarantines are the perfect analogue to political quarantines. To fight against that quarantining of worlds, one must embark on a quest to protect, save, and build other worlds.

Quagmire

Hong Kong returned to hands of the People's Republic of China in 1997 after a century under British rule. This handover came with the promise of relative autonomy for 50 years, a promise that Beijing was eager to override. Hong Kongers did not need to deal with any more problems, much less a nascent epidemic that could throw the port city into chaos. By the tail end of 2002, Hong Kong's government proposed an anti-subversion law, sparking mass protests over civil liberties. Any social gathering activity could fall foul of the restrictive law. The government's cautions over an "atypical pneumonia" struck the Asian financial center like a tsunami. Crashing onto shores of "Asia's world city," the quixotic illness exacerbated a political quagmire.

From its launching pad in China's southern Guangdong province, the malignant-named SARS metastasized into a pandemic—the first of many in the twenty-first century. In the final analysis, the formidable disease blanketed over two dozen countries. With its last gasp, SARS infected over 8,000 and robbed 800 lives. During a nerve-racking time, I watched two island territories caught up in divergent circumstances. The person who brought the ailment to Singapore, and those patients with whom she came into close contact, had been quickly put into isolation. This decision stemmed the momentum of a dreadful disease. Quick actions whittled infection down to a little over 200 people, whereas the number of people stricken in Hong Kong skewed close to 2,000. Singapore's "nanny state" bore a reputation for cleanliness and strict adherence to rules. It harbored no compunction in forcing people into quarantine, albeit under the strict eye of a "benevolent dictatorship." Experiencing protests for free speech around this time, the city-state suppressed "disorderly behavior" on grounds of protecting "law and order." That hardnosed efficiency appeared in a task force, where local agencies coordinated scaled-up screenings across private clinics and regularly updated the public. Believing it was in the clear, Singapore roared with sterling confidence in its victory. The Lion City laid waiting for the next big event, which came soon enough. SARS proved to be no fluke or anomaly, as a new bigger viral threat was in the offing.

Meanwhile, Hong Kong juggled a ballooning health scare amid wrestling with an overbearing Beijing. It was ill-equipped to defuse a ticking time bomb. In due time, the SARS outbreak reached epidemic proportions, owing to a paucity of information and interjection measures. The Department of Health asked contacts to respond to queries, but few answered. Hong Kong stood endangered with no specialized infectious disease hospital or isolation center.[5] Chinese-owned businesses, like grocery stores in Canada, faced boycotts and vandalism, spelling out the racial terms of a disease that carried the winds of hate that sailed along with it.

But just as fast as it came into the world, SARS flickered away, soon relegated to relative obscurity as global attention was diverted to the U.S. invasion of Iraq—under false pretenses of searching for weapons of mass destruction. Initiating hostilities for an unjust war a mere three days before confirming its first cases of SARS, the superpower took little notice of the irony in rummaging for hidden enemies when one was at its doorstep. Political fallout from the strange respiratory illness called SARS forced the hand of the Chinese Communist Party, which always closely guarded its secrets. The one-party regime begrudgingly shared details with the international community, facing disparagement for suppressing information. Communist officials prided themselves on their rather slow-going measured response. The worst was over, it seemed for now.

Fast forward two decades later, I am a college professor employed at my former undergraduate institution. The déjà vu of coming back to work as an employee at the former haunt rekindled old memories from my youth. But other holdovers of the SARS past came to the surface. In my second year as a faculty member, another pneumonia-like illness dominates the headlines much like the one I dealt with before. Teaching global and international studies at the University of California Irvine, I encountered a more diverse student body than as a student. There was now a large population of international students, mostly from mainland China, whose visa woes worsened from a U.S.-China trade war. Almost like clockwork, the Chinese government rammed through a new national security law to evacuate Hong Kong of its basic sovereignty, a loss of autonomy reminiscent of 2002. Mass protests erupted again in the city, despite instructions to stay home with a fast-approaching new virus. With history as my guide, I charted the course to this blockbuster sequel to SARS.

Nothing was ever serendipitous in this cliff hanger. It was all about the global synchronicity of localized events. The arc of time swung back hard, even if the results looked different. An overprepared Singapore experienced a big surge in infection cases among its growing numbers of foreign-born workers. Babies were now born with antibodies against this more resilient virus. Hong Kong wiggled out of total lockdown as people recalled the memory of SARS. The semiautonomous region obtained a handle on this new pandemic, but the bigger problem this time was the Communist Party attempting to seize control of the island's civil authority while people were falling sick.

The same happened with the COVID-19 pandemic, with a turn back to politicking, despite all the perils of a brand-new pandemic. This disease was so bad that some observers drew on the painful touchstone memory of acquired immunodeficiency syndrome (AIDS) decades earlier to make sense of it all. From a parallax view, historians knew what would happen when out-of-touch governments heartlessly abandoned the sick and unaccounted-for. Nothing could compare to the terror of the early outbreak of AIDS, and yet this new pandemic foretold untold suffering in a similar fashion, with most vulnerable dying needlessly, bringing the same kind of pain.

Taking the long view of community protection, the usable past of AIDS activism taught a whole new generation how to take care of one another and use "frail bodies, always endangered bodies, sometimes even dead bodies— to fight."[6] Organizers braced for another big fight, regrouping and leaning on one another against unfeeling leaders who refuse to care for their own citizens.

Query

Pandemic relations captured authoritarian dreams of domination by world powers and bad actors wishing to exploit pain for gain. It equally tapped into collective visions and entreaties for popular sovereignty by common people. As new contagion hot spots began to dot the map, what newly imagined worlds were made from the mind-bending force and frictions of COVID-19? What becomes of a "newly discovered" disease able to slip "in and through cracks between states and borders" to effect systemic and social mutations?[7] What is the world-*building* impact of this primordia and how do we build a better world or worlds from it? What are the colliding viral forms of desire, knowledge, and hope ushered in by a pandemic? How did it affect global relations to make them "go viral" with information and memes buzzing around as fast as the virus itself?

To link viral and worlding, I draw on thoughts of scholars like philosopher Judith Butler who considered the worldliness or worldly dimensions of the pandemic in *What World Is This?* In the book, she asks what is "the sense of the world given by the virus?"[8] I respond to this question by tracking the pandemic and its impact on the world through a finite sense of time.

COVID-19 offered refractive mirrors through which we all differently perceive the world, helping humans discern the relationship between the world-at-large and the one perceiving or knowing that presence. It moved us from cogitating over the question of what in the world is this (thing called COVID-19) to what is the world doing to save itself and also "what kinds of worlds are needed to address ecological crises"?[9] In *Viral World*, I track the specific vectors of struggle found in the imaginative process of "worlding" or the art of being global for governments, political actors, and diverse groups. Here, I study geopolitics, social movements, and cultural critiques as worlding (and unworlding).

Worlding as a concept has been taken up of late to explain the complex dimensions of living in an ever-changing global terrain. The term was first popularized a century ago to capture how humans perceive and move through the world. The term denotes the constant interplay between subject and object, the existential meaning of being-in-the-world and being *thrown into the world.*[10] The term's recent resurgence speaks to the ways that old frameworks for conceiving the world are being reconstituted over and over. The worlding of the global arises from network associations of people making worlds together.[11] As a global assemblage of viral thoughts and actions, the COVID-19 phenomenon blurs the perceptual lines between First and Third World, core and periphery, east and west, the Global north and Global South.

It is known that the COVID-19 pandemic was a global phenomenon since it blitzed across multiple regions and territories. That fact had grown clearer as the scale of infection progressed, but this book asks how did COVID-19 reveal viral forms of *worlding*, an ethical and engrossed investment in the concerns of the present world, especially for the most marginalized in society. How did this world(ing) crisis subsequently affect global relations?

My sense of global relations departs from international relations concerned usually with government-to-government interactions. In a viral world with biological and political contagions, I consider a range of relationships: civil society-state tensions, intercultural exchange, moral publics and media counter-publics, human-environment interactions, historical memory, and futures. COVID-19 did more than change our relations and relationships (connection, bonds, associations), it changed our relationality, the state or conditions of being relational and connected to others. Parsing through the reconfigurations of viral relations, being, and communication, I decipher jumbled conflicting messages within COVID-infected networks, some of which appeared malfunctioning and falling apart at the seams. Studying the escalators of the pandemic through viral worlding helps appraise a major "world-class" threat that bore many faces.

States of disorientation are awakened by a pandemic and its viral relations. Their metabolism is derived from living in global times characterized by an "unprecedented pathology" within our social immune system.[12] The "sign-value" of COVID-19 radiated in all directions, and as it gathered pace, people were either drawn into humanitarian decision-making or fell back into the orbit of fear. How did new experiences clump within old circuits of money and power? How extensive was our detachment from the lives of others? How did COVID-19 make pervasive the feeling of globalness?

As COVID-19 ripped through the flow of time, it ignited new pathways for "viral justice."[13] Under a fast time frame, we can trace long smoldering public indignation with social problems and official abuses, which persisted in the form of "pandemic inequality." Sociologist J. Michael Ryan posits that the pandemic required ideological solutions that underscore *global connection.*[14] He discusses the pandemic as a "blessing" to neoliberal, neoconservative, and nationalist ideologies that constructed an Other to promote inequality.[15] Yet, I recognize that resistant ideologies from the Other also came to the fore to challenge those restrictive global forces.

Viral World indicates that the novel coronavirus opened the doors to grasping "viral worlding" or worlding by viral means. Recognizing the "virus of ideology," I suggest racism, sexism, ageism, speciesism, ableism, internationalism, evangelicalism, cosmopolitanism, capitalism, environmentalism, socialism, feminism, and abolitionism were brought into a tighter ever closer orbit by the pathogen's ingress.[16] In these viral moments within the body politic, I juxtapose the rise in authoritarianism, nationalism, and policing (closing of worlds) with demands for democracy, freedom of mobility, and political solidarity (opening of worlds).

This new gravitational pull allowed those thought paradigms to be revamped, allowing world-making and world-building to go viral. A health crisis catalyzed by a novel coronavirus made even more "viral" our beliefs and actions—all of which disseminated like a plague. The pandemic's timescale amplified and sped up technocultural knowledge production. COVID-19 brought a "whole person" and "whole world" lens to everything.

Focusing on broad transformations in global society, many COVID-19 books were written to grasp a disease that has irrevocably altered global relations. They include *Pandemics, Politics, and Society* by Gerard Delanty; *COVID-19: The Great Reset* by Klaus Schwab and Thierry Malleret; and *Aftershocks: Pandemic Politics and the End of the Old International Order* by Colin Kahl and Thomas Wright.[17] These studies speak to an array of political topics from policymaking to religious theology to cosmopolitanism. They all agree that the pandemic will transform global culture and society. In *Pandemic Education and Viral Politics*, the editors combine viral biology and viral politics to build a "viral theory" of power/knowledge.[18] They refer to the power by the immuno-states directed toward governing and controlling populations, but one simultaneously built on the virality of chaos and social disorder. Building on these scholars, *Viral World* sheds light on how existential pandemic concerns are understood by global subjects in the making and unmaking of a crisis. What "worlds" are made when people are experiencing the pandemic differently? How did this world-altering event change all of us, exploding and reinforcing existing global divides? Thinking of COVID-19 as a singular problem conceals the specific material legacies of colonial exploitation and capitalist exclusion that have ended worlds for queer people, racialized ethnicities, migrants, women, the poor, and nations in the Global South.

Viral World recognizes virality in terms of worlding and the global treatment of social Others as pollutants. Insofar as the novel coronavirus can come from any human, or animal, or earthly source, this political virus "became viral" in more ways than one. Through a three-year span of consistent writing and meticulous updating and broad thinking that gives it robustness and heft, *Viral World* is distinct from other rush-to-print books or theme-specific books.[19] With many illuminating examples and case studies, this expansive global project demonstrates the viral ways less powerful nations are treated and how Indigenous/Black/people of color (BIPOC), workers, women, the poor, refugees, queer trans folks, prisoners, religious minorities, and animals are again rendered under a state of emergency. Construed as dangerous viruses that need to be contained, these social figures fall within intersectional or international lines of control.

Yet, I document the "viral" messages of resistance by collectives to oppressive rulership under the guise of pandemic protection. Focusing on the pandemic as an inflection point, my critical examination draws on the power of COVID-19 to activate viral meanings and actors across all levels of social life.

Quest

My book engages pandemic viral consciousness, asking whose worlds are affected by the pandemic and what world(s) do we truly want to live in. One concern is how virality became part of globality. As the globalized world became more viral, I embarked on a quest to study the virality of meaning-making that proliferated among individuals, groups, communities, and countries.

The pandemic's time warp laid out an unclear inventory to search for viral origins and antidotes. Its monumentality can be found in the multiplicity of "viral" media or socio-physical situations that bled into one another. Here, we can refer to a quote from the Greek philosopher Heraclitus, known for his doctrine of universal flux, which underscores that everything is in constant change: "If you do not expect the unexpected you will not find it, for it is not to be reached by search or trail."[20] Moving through the pandemic train as an *expected* journey—an epic odyssey to be painfully undertaken—ventures toward knowing our self-inflicted calamities. Disentangling pandemic-changed lives sets in motion a deft exploration of all things tangentially related. Marking time between the novel coronavirus' outbreak in March 2020 and ending in May 2023 when the World Health Organization (WHO) officially declared the end of this global health emergency, the book sets out to graph a disease which killed 7 million people and broke all world records.

Viral World builds on the observation that this unprecedented global health crisis was more than a worlding-crushing event; it was a leveling opportunity for rebuilding the world and "re-worlding" global society. Against the world ordering power of capitalism, militarism, racism, sexism, and imperialism stands the heightened sense of pandemic consciousness that travelled haphazardly alongside a mercurial disease. My work is primarily inspired by global media scholar Bishnupriya Ghosh's work in *The Virus Touch*, where she notes the epidemic intensity of COVID-19 effected a "worlding of things." Epidemic media enabled state and nonstate actors to collaboratively "make worlds," an interactive process in which "the world is always emergent."[21] Practitioners accommodate "worlds within worlds," a transformative thinking and feeling that moves beyond universal reason.

Sometimes these viral worlding projects follow particular ideologies like eco-socialism, anti-racism, pan-African Blackness, transnational feminism, prison abolitionism, queer radicalism, and Indigenous internationalism. While Ghosh focuses on the viral media cultures that add fuel to the fire of a mercurial infectious disease, I focus on a broad range of political projects that tarry with our "viral emergence" as global actors.

This book emphasizes social worlds torn apart and bonded together by the pandemic. So many things were happening at the same time, but I track all that was happening *with* the pandemic as much as what was made possible *by* it. The use of alliteration in title chapter sections (i.e., Pandemic, Planet, Promise) indicates the looping disjointed sense of time and everyday people trying to be *everything, everywhere, all at once.*[22] With pandemic-induced trauma, life went on repeat. Temporal disintegration and the lost sense of self came with a "once-in-a-lifetime" event.[23] Structural issues of ecocide, human rights, sexism, and unemployment all came roaring back.

With *Viral World*, I tell only one slice of the global COVID-19 saga. These critical insights occur through key themes and terms that emerged in the froth and swirl of the pandemic: (1) "foreign virus," (2) flattening the curve, (3) physical distancing, (4) frontline labor, and (5) coronapocalypse. This grand play does not follow events in unilinear way as the pandemic never spread in orderly fashion. Even as it took center stage, COVID-19 never managed to steal attention from other crucial, local, or regional issues.

A study of a global-scale problem and its multifaceted issues must cull from "various perspectives at multiple levels and across spatial and temporal dimensions."[24] Insofar as the mutating agent jumps scale and different strands of life, we too must assiduously follow this rambunctious disease, globe-hopping across frames of reference. This new "viral turn" in planetary consciousness insists on holism in turbulent times. The pandemic's endurance and our own stamina as pandemic survivors give us more than a few lessons about the rate by which humans and others were moving through a viral world.

Notes

1 Massey, Doreen, *Space, Place and Gender* (Hoboken, NJ: John Wiley & Sons, 2013).
2 Long T. Bui, "The Debts of Memory: Historical Amnesia and Refugee Knowledge in *The Reeducation of Cherry Truong," Journal of Asian American Studies* 18, no. 1 (2015): 73–97.
3 Mia Jankowicz, "A 39-Year-Old Coronavirus Patient Who Could Hardly Breathe Posted a Video from the ICU to Warn People Who Think It Won't Happen to

Them," *Business Insider*, March 20, 2020, www.businessinsider.com/coronavi
rus-woman-hospital-warns-people-who-doubt-will-affect-them-2020-3

4 John S. Ahlquist and Margaret Levi, *In the Interest of Others: Organizations and Social Activism* (Princeton, NJ: Princeton University Press, 2013).

5 Lee Shiu Hung, "The SARS Epidemic in Hong Kong: What Lessons Have We Learned?" *Journal of the Royal Society of Medicine*, 96, no. 8 (August 2003): 374–378.

6 Masha Gessen, "What Lessons Does the AIDS Crisis Offer for the Coronavirus Pandemic?" *The New Yorker*, April 8, 2020, www.newyorker.com/news/our-col umnists/what-lessons-does-the-aids-crisis-offer-for-the-coronavirus-pandemic

7 Arjun Appadurai, "Disjuncture and Difference in the Global Cultural Economy," *Theory, Culture & Society* 7, no. 2–3 (1990): 295–310, 306.

8 Judith Butler, *What World Is This?* (New York: Columbia University Press, 2022).

9 Common Worlds Research Collective, "Worlding," *Common Worlds Research Collective*, July 16, 2022, www.commonworlds.net/organizing-concepts/worlding

10 Martin Heidegger, *Being and Time* (Albany, NY: Suny Press, 2010).

11 This contemporary gesture moves beyond a worlding of the world that Spivak came up with in her worlding conceptualization after Heidegger. Gayatri Chakravorty Spivak, "Three Women's Texts and a Critique of Imperialism," *Critical Inquiry* 12, no. 1 (1985): 243–261.

12 Quoted in Mike Gane and Michael Gane, *Jean Baudrillard: In Radical Uncertainty* (London: Pluto Press, 2000), 29.

13 Ruha Benjamin, *Viral Justice: How We Grow the World We Want* (Princeton, NJ: Princeton University Press, 2022).

14 Ryan, J. Michael. "The SARS-CoV-2 Virus and the COVID-19 Pandemic," *COVID-19: Volume II: Social Consequences and Cultural Adaptations* (London: Routledge, 2020).

15 Ryan, J. Michael, ed., "The Blessings of COVID-19 for Neoliberalism, Nationalism, and Neoconservative Ideologies," in *COVID-19: Volume II: Social Consequences and Cultural Adaptations* (London: Routledge, 2020), 80–93.

16 The virus of ideology term I got from Slavoj Žižek, *Pandemic!: COVID-19 Shakes the World* (Hoboken, NJ: John Wiley & Sons, 2020).

17 Colin Kahl and Thomas Wright, *Aftershocks: Pandemic Politics and the End of the Old International Order* (New York: St. Martin's Press, 2021); Delanty, Gerard, ed., *Pandemics, Politics, and Society: Critical Perspectives on the COVID-19 Crisis* (Berlin: Walter de Gruyter GmbH & Co KG, 2021); Klaus Schwab and Thierry Malleret, *COVID-19: The Great Reset* (Geneva: Forum Publishing, 2020).

18 Michael A. Peters and Tina Besley, *Pandemic Education and Viral Politics* (London: Routledge, 2020).

19 One exception is the fantastic collection of essays in Maya Mirchandani, Shoba Suri, and Laetitia Bruce Warjri, eds., *The Viral World* (New Delhi: ORF and Global Policy Journal, 2020). The book has contributions from a diverse set of thinkers and policymakers. My book is almost like a bookend to this volume three years later in the study of the viral world.

20 Roger Von Oech, *Expect the Unexpected (or You Won't Find It): A Creativity Tool Based on the Ancient Wisdom of Heraclitus* (Oakland: Berrett-Koehler Publishers, 2002), viii.

21 Bishnupriya Ghosh, *The Virus Touch: Theorizing Epidemic Media* (Durham, NC: Duke University Press, 2023), 10.

22 This is an obvious allusion to the 2022 Oscar Best Picture winning film. The story is about a woman who tries to take care of her family, deal with finances, while pondering her life across a multiverse spoke to our fragmented senses and fears of fate.

23 E. Alison Holman, Nickolas M. Jones, Dana Rose Garfin, and Roxane Cohen Silver, "Distortions in Time Perception during Collective Trauma: Insights from a National Longitudinal Study during the COVID-19 Pandemic," *Psychological Trauma: Theory, Research, Practice, and Policy* (2022), https://doi.org/10.1037/tra0001326

24 Eve Darian-Smith and Philip C. McCarty, *The Global Turn: Theories, Research Designs, and Methods for Global Studies* (Berkeley: University of California Press, 2017), 226.

1

GLOBAL CRISIS

Anthropocene, Animal, Antibody

It burst onto the scene like something from a post-apocalyptic movie—except that this terror was very real. What began as an epidemic in the city of Wuhan in China's Hubei province zipped across air, land, and sea at breakneck speed to contaminate close to 200 countries. Scheduled meetings at factories, schools, airports, libraries, restaurants, gyms, clubs, bars, concerts, sporting events, banks, theme parks, and all manner of human congregation were shelved. Restaurants, theaters, and hospitality businesses temporarily shut their doors or closed in perpetuity. School graduations, birthday anniversaries, weddings, and funerals were put on hold. Governments closed their borders to visitors, inadvertently stranding some of their own citizens abroad. Public shaming and new restrictive laws sought censor against people going out for parties. New criminal codes that limited public outings clamped down on refugees moving to safe harbor. A father from India presumed he caught the nasty bug and hung himself from a tree to protect his family.[1]

The main culprit to blame for this spike in fear was COVID-19, a baleful virus of unknown origin with eerie resemblance to the enigmatic SARS that struck Asia almost two decades earlier. Those victims succumbing to this new sickness reported flu-like symptoms that run the gamut: difficult breathing, chills, fever, muscle body aches, shivers, digestive issues, and chest pains from inflammation. The glassy lungs of COVID-infected survivors under chest X-ray radiographs looked honeycomb with perforations. This disease presented a hitherto unknown human pathogen, against which no one had inherent defense. There was no prior medical knowledge about the ailment and no vaccine was readily available. A barrage of inquests riddled the public's mind: Where did this virus come from? How exactly do we catch it? What precautions or actions need to be taken? More than a blip in time, the pitched

DOI: 10.4324/9781032694535-2

battle against the virus would effectuate tectonic shifts in how humans live, work, learn, and love in the twenty-first century. With SARS as a front-runner, COVID-19 bore the imprimatur of something to be long remembered for many lifetimes. SARS was the dress rehearsal for this blowout.

COVID-19 illuminated seismic shifts in globality and how processes are global. By 2020, it was becoming less common to say the world was globalizing or undergoing globalization. Coronavirus proved it was already global, even if everything we knew was being rearranged under a *de-globalization* movement. Like a time capsule, COVID-19 takes a snapshot of history to capture and carry messages forward into the future, asking us how to think globally as well as how to reimagine the world differently.

Pandemics along with other global crises like climate mutation, famine, nonsensical wars all offer a great learning curve for earthlings who can no longer afford to be detached beings. Social control and a feeling of helplessness relinquish over to viral knowledge, posits theorist Bruno Latour, which "can become global just by going from one mouth to another… If you spread from one mouth to another, you can viralize the world very fast. That knowledge can re-empower us."[2]

In a more-than-human world stained by the hand of SARS-CoV-2, it is easy to repeat the classic line from poet John Donne that "no man is an island." Even if some felt though they were stuck in their social islands, others were found on actual islands in a viral stream of consciousness.[3] Philosopher Michel Montaigne delivered a warning shot to the world in his essay "Of Cannibals" that would resonate centuries later with "coron-colonialism." Overconsumption, environmental destruction, and social exploitation, he anticipated, would lead to ultimate disaster: "I clearly see that this is an extraordinary disturbance, for if it had always gone at this rate, or was to do so in the future, the face of the world would be turned topsy-turvy."[4]

The freefall from the novel coronavirus turned the world upside down. But wily humans will do what they have always done as world-shapers and meaning-makers. With the impetus of such a "world destroyer" like COVID-19, the project of re-worlding takes even greater viral form than it did before. With so many future worries, COVID-19 forcefully turned humans into worldlings, devoted to the interests of the world. But as revealed with the pandemic, there are "worlds within worlds," and these viral worlds are intimately connected to each other. As more people became infected, they learned to scale down their feelings to the personal through "micro-learning" and to "scale-up their ability to recognize the patterns of the social world."[5]

While humans were experiencing a viral form of in/worlding, SARS-CoV-2 floated in and out of posh business offices and decrepit refugee camps, took flight in industrial shipping containers, and crawled across letters written by loved ones sent in the mail. Pandemic geographies give countenance to viral information-sharing as well as shared illness. A public education in pandemic matters imparted private teachable moment about the interlaced world(s) we live and die in, big and small.[6]

The grand proscenium of COVID-19 turned into a viral moment for worlding. After the economy shut down, busy lives quieted to a hum and the human-driven planet found a hiccup with "corona-time."[7] Stoppage acted as a propellant for time travel, conjuring the yet-to-be or solutions not-yet-known. Not unlike other deadly diseases, COVID-19 cast a magnifying glass over global affairs, while exposing structural flaws and mental pitfalls. It revamped the state–society dynamic in our interlocking worlds to effectuate a new global consciousness and (viral) connectivity. Humans can always develop preventive medicines and prophylaxes for up-and-coming diseases, but how do we find a cure for the successive violence and decimation washing over the planet? Like many earth-shattering events, one could claim there was a time before and after COVID-19. And yet, like so many events of huge magnitude, this global crisis was a long time in the making. The politics of the Anthropocene, animals, and antibodies offer background to this pandemic and its viral world.

The chapter presents "viral worlding" as a concept to interrogate the global entanglements in which we find ourselves in these viral times. Focusing on issues of the Anthropocene as well as speciesist arguments that often blame human problems on animals, it recognizes that the solution or antibody to a viral threat is predicated on addressing the social rationales of human oppression. One concern involves the way major pharmaceutical giant Pfizer had previously lost a class action suit for secretly experimenting on Nigerian children. This case disturbs how we treat these COVID-vaccine manufacturers as potential saviors or problem solvers, especially for the Global South. This chapter reappraises the normative categories and popular modes of knowledge by which we view the planet and its living things. Considering the outbreak in relation to the racist and ageist concept of "herd immunity," it captures the early moments when COVID-19 became a global issue, tracking key events and establishing the setting for the powerful emergence of a full-blown pandemic.

Anthropocene

Biologists and geologists are calling our present epoch the Anthropocene. This neologism puts a name to the ill-gotten global impact of fossil capitalism and carboniferous human activity. Anthropocene follows the end of the Holocene and the period of climate stability that began almost 12,000 years ago with retreat of the glacial period and taking off with the Industrial Revolution. The concept takes a critical approach to the grand march of modernity, civilization, and globalization by focusing on anthropogenic disasters. Proponents of the term are not lulled into a false sense of human invincibility, activating global awareness toward our errant ways. Under the stranglehold of a "new" historical agent like COVID-19, predictions about the end of human meddling became more routine and pronounced with fragile transformations "effected by virus vectors carrying a new developmental code."[8]

COVID-19 brought huge commotion but also newfound cognitive powers for reshaping the Anthropocene. Gender studies professor Jane Caputi deems the Anthropocene a male-driven concept to describe the rape of Mother Earth and her treatment as an inert thing. For Caputi, there are various fates for the earth, one of which might realize the feminine powers of the earth: "Chaos, the Grandmother of all that is, now comes among us … she is the source of all order and that she is infinitely generative."[9] The befuddling pandemic compelled humans to re-world and scuttle total mastery, order, and wholeness in favor of partiality and human "error."[10] Stories of endless mistakes—like what we notice with an undulating pandemic—stand poised to capture a human-centric world in all its flaws.

Not all human beings are equally complicit or suffer the same in the Anthropocene, as it is poor communities of color that buffeted the extractive harm of petrochemical and mining industries. With Indigenous, Black, and Brown people for so long facing down undue harms, *ongoing* colonialisms "have been ending worlds for as long as they have been in existence."[11] But if time is circular, scribe Amrah Salomón waxes poetically, "then our future is within our hands now, uncolonized, unending, a seed pregnant with possibility…. for the regeneration of land and life."[12] In marking the Anthropocene as a set of compulsions, it offers foresight into planetary pluralism. By rejiggering meaning systems and resetting the course of life, the pandemic's suspended animation allowed for reimagining the world-as-we-know-it.

How this revision works out depends on what groups are being most impacted. On January 20—the same day as the United States and South Korea reported their first COVID-19 cases, and China's National Health Commission confirmed that a novel coronavirus can be transmitted between humans—the U.N. Human Rights Committee ruled favorably in a landmark case involving a Kiribati national seeking refuge in New Zealand. State legal obligations potentially accorded free movement to so-called climate refugees, reinterpreting the process as "migration with dignity."[13] Without demurring to countries perched at a cushier remove, the I-Kiribati underlined their urgent situation. Islanders did not experience macroscale environmental changes as "everyone else"; they have been busy building up protective barriers of their own worlds against environment threats long before COVID-19.

Indicators of mortal danger like COVID-19 are the fluctuating "vital signs" of an existential threat. In January 2020, as news of the novel coronavirus was breaking, researchers from 153 nations representing the World Alliance of Scientist warned about climate change on the 40th anniversary of the first world climate conference in Geneva. Taking the pulse of the planet, they demanded the deceleration of population growth, forest despoliation, excessive meat eating, and plastic consumption. They sketched out a clear map for reparative justice via planetary and human diversity.

Underscoring how risk societies function or interact with teetering ecosystems-at-risk, the science collective enunciated "unequivocally that Planet Earth is facing a climate emergency ... to secure a sustainable future, we must change how we live ... on planet Earth, our only home."[14] Members indicated salutary developments: climate emergency declarations, schoolchildren going on strike for the planet, successful ecocide lawsuits, and grassroots citizen-science movements. The pandemic made it nearly impossible to fulfill a promise by rich countries to make recompense for the loss and damage of climate change by paying $100 billion upon the 50th anniversary of the first Earth Day.

The political tide was turning even as sea levels were rising. COVID-19 called on all denizens of the biosphere to heed the call for respecting the planet's health. Edging toward a "circular economy" and slow growth based on renewables, time was running out or rather it had run out. As more arctic ice sheets melt and permafrost diminish, this year-to-year change uncovers long-gestating microbes lying dormant in the icy cryosphere. Once uncovered, primeval organisms like a virus become "novel" for modern humans. Humans did not fare marvelously to date, as 2019 was the second-hottest year ever on record (in the hottest decade up to that point).[15] Death Valley hit boiling temperatures in the cooker year of 2020, when greenhouse emissions reached their highest point in the hottest year ever recorded thus far.[16] The interminable "longest year ever" under the bog of COVID-19 earned the most named tropical storms in the Atlantic.

In a time when feverish heat waves can kill without warning, planet Earth required a "social autopsy."[17] Throughout the year, uncontrollable brushfires raged on, and Australians gaped at the sight of charred koalas and singed kangaroos. Veldfires burned in Central Africa and Siberia experienced record fires, as did California.[18] Ineffable weather patterns trended upward with no end in sight. Given the indolence and idiocy of petulant leaders unable to differentiate between inclement weather patterns and climate change, it fell to citizens to stop the carnage. But despite these wise voices, there were missed opportunities for tapering off carbon emissions.

Global infrastructures were on life support the moment COVID-19 arrived. Weaning off oil dependency and increasing carbon capture/storage does not mean much without good maintenance of existing household utilities, food production, and transportation. Despite an estimated 37% of the cumulative world population being holed up at home to avoid infection, there emerged reports of reports and photographs of a clear atmosphere in many urban areas. Yet, there registered only a slight dip in carbon dioxide emissions with a 5.8% in overall drop, according to the International Energy Agency. To reach zero CO_2 in absolute terms, there had to be large-scale behavior change, especially in the Global North—other methods for traveling, eating, heating, and cooking that did not rely too much on natural gas, oil, and coal. Global energy systems, mainly reliant on mass electrification and nonrenewable resources, were now at their breaking point.

COVID-19 made it much harder to reach carbon "Net Zero." It was no longer feasible to even say climate *change* and more apt to say this was our "climate reality."[19] Embracing these all-too-real anxieties, global youth responded with calls to action. Facing apathy from international power brokers, firebrands like Greta Thunberg, Vanessa Nakate, Varshini Prakash, Jamie Margolin came with prescient messages about a warming planet, despite a near-total scientific consensus on the matter. Concerned citizens of the world pushed the message to anyone willing to listen and change tack. LGBTQ+ disability activists like Vanessa Raditz and Patty Berne viewed the Anthropocene as an invitation to others to enter the hidden lives of the multiply marginalized: "In the moments when we're in pain … and we feel defeated by the sheer scope of everything that's wrong in the world, we don't have to give up on life or on humanity … Welcome to our world."[20] Despite pandemic weariness, hope for a just world and world-building could still go viral.

Sometimes, that world-building extended beyond planet Earth. In tandem to the U.S. Space Force being established in 2020 as a new independent branch of the armed forces, privatized manipulation of resources was precondition for the expropriation of biomes within the cosmos. President Donald Trump signed an executive order to commercially mine outer space for mineral resources, saying that "the United States does not view space as a global commons."[21]

With colonization of the moon and Mars a near possibility, commercial ambitions for "space capitalism" matched Iran's Revolutionary Guard Corps launch of its first military satellite into space through ballistic missile. Planet Earth was not made uninhabitable by a "colonizing" disease, but rather by the disease of military surveillance finance capitalism.[22] Security regimes and capitalist markets were in no way prepared for an ensuing pandemic.[23] The protean character of COVID-19 and other opportunistic diseases shrank borders even if it enlarged nationalist defenses against emerging threats.

Hendra in Australia. Nipah in Malaysia. Lass fever in Nigeria. West Nile Virus in Uganda. Langya virus in China. Like COVID-19, these lesser-known diseases made global transits after persisting in dormant local form. Their influx lights up the runaway costs of environmental degradation. Malaria and yellow fever reemerge when pristine forests are disturbed or razed for residential sprawl and urban agglomeration. Other disease take off when rich marine life and coral reefs are steadily wiped out by "dead zones" made from industrial runoff and over-tourism. Massive fish die-offs and beached sea animals with plastic in their guts were becoming common. Eroded biodiversity meant less organic sources to beat back diseases that spring up from sea trawling and other human-induced destruction are gone. Something wicked like COVID-19 comes to make matters worse.

Swine flu (officially H1N1) was the last pandemic declared by the World Health Organization (WHO before COVID-19. In 2009, 70 countries reported mounting cases of the novel influenza A as its multispecies "viral clouds" radiated to 1/4 of the human sphere.[24] The pandemic was declared over a year later, and H1N1 became part of the regular seasonal flu. COVID-19 bears more severity and infects twice as much as H1N1 (1.5); its case fatality and hospitalization rates are much higher. The lack of studies on novel coronaviruses kept the detrimental properties of COVID-19 under public concealment. People still wondered how this serial killer stayed one step ahead of us, when it was hiding in plain sight.

The insidious end for the globalized world was creeping near unless humans curbed their excesses. Swelling peri-urban settlements with incomparable loss of wild habitat fostered the perfect storm for new pathogenic encounters and sparked co-pathogenic forces. Astute commentators warned that COVID-19 could put a final stake in the sense of human invincibility, laying to rest any doubt the man-made world is waning. There was no turning back now, once we go past the tipping point.

For reasons not always clear, most of the world's governments wasted precious time by promising fast changes to public policies. They either neglected them or backtracked on assurances to do so. In the month before the discovery of COVID-19, Trump's administration notified withdrawal from the 2015 Paris climate agreement, a pledge signed by 200 countries to ameliorate greenhouse gas emissions. Not privy to addressing the global crisis, aggressive capitalists and their outworn rules faced an illusory endgame.

The United States strayed far from the global environmental norm, though it was pivotal in shaping the language that holds high-income nations accountable for paying for costs associated with decarbonization. Claiming the Paris Accord shortchanged U.S. sovereignty and economic "competitiveness," Trump's decision put the global pact in peril.[25] Refusing to let profit take precedence, states and cities independently committed to the accords and stewardship of the planet over and against Trump's administration. Presaging a (White masculine Christian) world turned to ashes, Sinophobes from Trump's camp associated COVID-19 infectiousness and Chinese "dirtiness." However, China's mode of production, which was cause for the disease, exploited a monopolized, vertically integrated system "perfected here in America and then exported to every corner of the world," one that "prioritizes concentration of wealth and maximum profitability for a gilded elite, while offloading the death and destruction it causes to everyone else."[26]

Breaking from his predecessor's green polices, President Trump gutted the independent watchdog Environmental Protect Agency (EPA), putting at its helm a denier of climate change with close ties to the fossil-fuel industry. After choosing as his secretary of state the CEO of oil company ExxonMobil, Trump steamrolled federal limits on mercury emission as well as carbon. Monitoring standards slackened off during the *terra incognita* of the pandemic. Before that, the businessman-cum-president had put up federally protected public lands for leasing to special interests, letting exploitation remain unchecked and enriching the pockets of mining companies. The economic ravages wrought by corporations downgraded public infrastructures long before the pandemic ate into them. They made a husk of state welfare programs, which were starting to show their age. Putting a brake to frenzied human activity, COVID-19 exposed political landmines, and countries like the United States were caught off guard upon the debut of the novel coronavirus.

The pandemics' ripple effect launched a watershed "viral" moment, pushing for overhauls in the existing global order. Without a straight path forward, government corona-counterstrategies operated in fits and starts. There were lapses in judgment by countries devoted to neoliberal austerity, but the structural adjustments afterward were indeed world changing. The pandemic's upending was so brashly felt that it came to be known as the Great Reshuffling, Great Unsettling, or Great Reset.[27]

Instead of committing to lasting change, short-term snap decision-making came with last-ditch efforts to save the global economy. There happened a redoubling of public sanitation standards, but a beguiling disease waits for no one, much less slow-to-act government functionaries who could not deal with the economics of a pandemic. Once enough people woke to the death grip of COVID-19, last-minute emergency lockdown measures stalled the throttle of industrial production profoundly. China's polluted skies turned clear for an extended amount of time due to a massive drop in nitrogen dioxide.[28] It would take such an unrivaled event to shock the system and bring it to a near-standstill. Commerce found its humming locomotive ground to a screeching halt, and many parts of the world went silent. In the final analysis, humans tried to outplay COVID-19, but the virus played its own game.

Lockdown gave pause to consider the meaning of laboring, living, and loving in a viral world. Students learned to take "Zoom" classes online, while folks given time and opportunity to seclude at home mulled over life–work balance. Others became unexpected caregivers to sick loved ones. Some welcomed the home isolation as a change of pace, a reprieve from everyday stress of work, a sort of "stay-cation," even as downtime churned up real concerns about civics, food security, transportation, health, and housing. Diagnosing "cave syndrome" that verged on chronic illness, psychologists believed COVID-19 "threatens to bring a wave of Hikikomori to America," invoking the maladaptive behavior of homebound persons who suffer from social withdrawal in Japan.[29] The homebound found themselves in a lived-in downstate in which "our homes became our *worlds*."[30]

Those worlds came crashing down like dominos with the viral impact of COVID-19. Sequestering for the masses occurred as medical professionals and service workers put themselves at risk to carry on "essential operations": taking care of vulnerable populations like the elderly who died at the highest rates. Blithe commentators called this pandemic's way of "culling" the superannuated and "thinning the herd." Some were more specific like a cold-hearted California planning commissioner who lost his job after posting on Facebook that the aged and the houseless are a drain on society. Ridding ourselves of these "defiled" social burdens, as he put it, would ensure a Darwinian ranking that sorts out who should be left-for-dead meeting a "natural course in nature."[31]

Drawing on eugenics and the pseudoscience of "population control," financial advisors in London vowed to ensure "herd immunity, protect the economy, and if that means some pensioners die, too bad."[32] This cost–benefit analysis chimed with a Brazilian government aide in the Finance Ministry who was unabashed in his rhapsodizing of senicide: "It's good that deaths are concentrated among the old. That will improve our economic performance as it will reduce our pension deficit."[33] Government stooges claimed that there must be a selective sacrifice of a few to save the rest. These viral messages of organic worldly renewal rang false with a desire of eliminating the dregs of humanity. Less glum environmentalists hoped this would muzzle climate change deniers and make them care for the planet. Meanwhile, "ecofascists" held fast to a deep sighting of *all* human beings as parasitic organisms. We are the virus, they argue, causing cancer on earth with COVID-19 as the cure for an invasive parasitic species.[34] In the echo chamber of human nihilism, keyboard warriors typed away on their computers, contending that Mother Nature was fed up and she was now "fighting back" with new human diseases.

Once the COVID-19 pandemic began in China, one thing that came to mind for many was from whence in nature did this malevolent come from. If it did not originate from within "us," then what is responsible? Was it another animal?

Animal

Video of what appears to be a Chinese woman eating bat soup caused a stir on social media and defined COVID-19's outbreak visual narrative. Filmed for a travel show three years before the pandemic, an Internet celebrity tasted the winged creature in the Micronesian island country of Palau, not in China. Viewers amid the SARS-CoV-2 scare balked at the inanities and barbarism of those strange Chinese who consumed weird things and exotic delicacies.[35] Pulled out of its original frame of reference, the image garnered heavy rotation in global mediascapes, marshalling abhorrent comments from rankled online users who wanted another reason to bash the animalistic, savage Chinese. Little separated race, species, and nature in new taxonomies of power and knowledge.[36]

Other animal-related videos cropped up. Unverified screen captures showed sea wolves reoccupying the beaches of Ecuador, desert goats and boars roaming the parks of Israel, penguins roaming the streets of South Africa, swans swimming in the canals of Italy, and "electric" dolphins lighting up the beaches of the United States (an effect of bioluminescence by dinoflagellate plankton). A viral video from Thailand supplied a visual panorama of "rival gangs" of monkeys laying siege to a city, whose residents stayed indoors to avoid the tenacious novel coronavirus. The brawling mobs looked like a scene from *Planet of the Apes*. Such sightings are meant to elicit shock and awe in "the birth of the post-Anthropocene epoch" where feral deer, bobcats, and parrots recolonize the planet "in the name of wildlife."[37] The primates have been regularly fed by tourists, and upon spotting no humans around decided to roam freely in a new *terrapolis*. They were not trespassing on human territory but claiming what was rightfully theirs: wide open spaces.[38]

Though "wild" creatures were seen as "replacing" humans through COVID-19, the fact remains that humankind's earthly dominion knows no bounds with ongoing species extinctions. Pinning global mayhem on other animals shirks human responsibility and due diligence to other species. The human-animal-nature relationship opens neural pathways, says anthropologist Ruth Goldstein, who believes we must cross-pollinate ideas across the species divide. The union fertilizes visions that reach toward collaborative survival for all creatures.[39] Feminist scientist Donna Haraway advocates for an interspecies conversation based on "viral response-ability" and "multispecies worlding" where "animals everywhere are full partners in worlding." Both animality and humanity co-constitute the viral world.[40]

Rare as they are, zoonotic leaps bring new viruses from "them" (animals) to "us" (humans) in ways that suggest we are still animals. This viral re-worlding gives weight to the premise that humans, too, are animals, and thinking in anthropocentric terms only reinforces speciesism, the belief in "natural" hierarchies and human exceptionalism. In the political ecology of things, human and nonhuman viral worlds are tangled within an assemblage of life. We humans must recognize our "viral becoming," moving beyond a mechanistic politics of disease toward a biocultural worlding or "oneness" with animals and environments, which are full of deadly viruses instead of ignoring or destroying them.[41]

Interspecies exchange moves beyond animal welfare and modifying eating habits. It entails initiating a sea change in intensive relations with nonhuman animal brethren as commodified food or captive slaves. With Thailand's tourist industry pounded by the country's soft lockdown, millions of elephants in Chiang Mai were relieved of "duties." Many walked miles back to their homelands in Mae Chaem to be tended to by the Karen people who have historically taken care of them. Tellingly, that just-in-time meat production ruled by corporate oligarchies could not "replenish" their supply of meat, forcing restaurants and grocery stores to adopt vegetarian options. Planetary change that opposes self-devouring behavior and stratospheric economic growth asks no less than multispecies relations with our animal kin, finding common cause with "interspeciated familiars."[42] What awfulness proceeds from killing rare endangered species for human pleasure or consumption? In the surround of Earth's profusion, humans are nothing less than animals and *metabolic* beings.

COVID-19's pathogenicity depended on social context. In the Gregorian calendar year of 2020, close to eight billion people occupied Earth, sharing this decreasingly habitable blue planet with countless other organisms. Our undisputable presence as the most dominant species could be felt all over the planet, touching various aspects of life through solid waste, noxious fumes, forever chemicals, and radioactive waste. Most pollution originates from state-supported corporations, vulturous cronies, global elites, and gilded classes with high-net worth living beyond their means. This pilfering of our bounty occurs as the world's poor are extruded from the public commons, crammed into inhospitable quarters, eking out life within unsanitary conditions.

A novel coronavirus takes advantage of the voluminous amount of new host bodies, adapting to fertile environs in which humans dwell in close proximity to other species. If not stopped, the novel coronavirus could metamorphosize into something worse. No doubt, it can interact or fuse with another coronaviral strain to be unruly. There were at least eight similar strains of SARS-CoV-2, but fortuitously they took genetic flight haltingly instead of finding "immune escape," when a strain hides its presence from antibodies after exposure to other versions of the virus. When zoo animals and house pets tested positive for COVID-19, it relayed the message that humans could now infect other species. Hybridization, reassortment, or swapping of genetic material give rise to other viral events and diseases.

A planet-in-peril engenders the ripe conditions for submicroscopic entities to co-evolve with humans. Monocultural farming and agribusiness push resource-extraction past known capacities that induce viral evolution. Three-quarters of agricultural land on earth gets cleared for livestock or soya, increasing immense environmental pressures harmful in the long run. Periodic inoculation of industrially farmed chickens (harboring the H5N1 influenza A) will be certain to cultivate the next superbug, one with complete resistance to antibiotics.[43] *Escherichia coli* scares are now regularly expected from contaminated crops, while the flesh-eating methicillin-resistant *Staphylococcus aureus* (MRSA) has overtaken hospitals. The "novel" coronavirus' arrival hints at global crises that are not novel at all. Marketized demand for wild animals was too wedded to heavily processed "Western" diets with its mainstay as meat and other foodstuffs or food products. These staples are fueled by nonlocally sourced, consolidated global food systems.

These social exigencies are part of the indeterminacies of the Age of Coronavirus. Coronaviruses are named for the crown-like protein spikes around their cellular membrane that resemble the sun's fiery corona layer. Short for coronavirus disease 2019, COVID-19 is the name of the disease and respiratory illness caused by the specific coronavirus, SARS-CoV-2. In popular parlance, they are used interchangeably. COVID-19 is one of a suite of zoonotic diseases that can jump across the species barrier (70% of infectious human diseases are of zoonotic origin). The pacing measure of zoonotic diseases signals the fact that humans never exist too far apart from "other" animals. "We," broadly speaking, are *coeval* reservoirs of disease, and our shared risk from any coronavirus becomes evident when discussing fellow mammalian inhabitants that can live almost everywhere and go anywhere.

Bats carry coronaviruses harmlessly within their bodies, but so do many other animals. These creatures of the night became identified as a prime culprit by scientists for COVID-19's emergence. The bat's resilient immune system and unique physiology protect them from pathogens, but coronaviruses reside in their intestines and are found in feces, which is cultivated as guano, a prized fertilizer by farmers. In a time when ever higher numbers of people dwell in megacities, colonies of bats come into close contact with crowds of humanity (Wuhan with its 11 million residents appeared to form the perfect incubator in the most populous country on earth). A Chinese team of scientists yoked the novel coronavirus to a bat-borne coronavirus.[44] Ebola, Nipah, Marburg, and SARS are deadly human diseases with genetic material tagged to horseshoe bats. Many scientists speculate that the novel coronavirus of 2019 may have derived from the "wet markets" like the Huanan Seafood Wholesale Market in Wuhan, which trade in all sorts of fauna. A buyer with a taste for freshly slaughtered animals can request on the spot the killing of rats, peacocks, beavers, foxes, turtles, crocodiles, wolf cubs, and, of course, bats. The blood from animal carcasses mixed freely with human bodily fluids and secretion in a viral soup of sorts.[45]

Part of the Chinese government's promotion of market-oriented breeding and e-commerce of wild animals, wet markets reflect the path-dependent processes of global consumerism and domestic efforts to ease rural poverty. These agricultural bazaars cropped up after the mass famines of Mao's

Great Leap Forward, a condensation point when the starving had been forced to eat anything they could find and when an estimated 40 million people perished.[46] Such collectivization policies are extreme, but they caution against ecological abuse and torture of animals, and what transpires when economic concerns are put before anything else. A third of the earliest cases of COVID-19 in Wuhan involved people who never visited wet markets, and so epidemiological tracing faces a roadblock if patients were infected already from somewhere else without knowing. Was COVID-19 then human-made or animal sourced?

Insofar as China was the geographic source of past flu episodes (1957 Asian flu, 1968 Hong Kong flu, and the 1997 Avian flu), virus hunters guessed the country would be "ground zero for a future pandemic."[47] Scientists conjectured COVID-19 originated in some wild animal (Beijing scientists thought snakes at first). It then moved into intermediate hosts before infecting humans.[48] In 2017, virologists from Wuhan processed the genetic building blocks for SARS in masked palm civets and horseshoe bats. COVID-19 contained many novel features, chief among them are the spiked receptor proteins that coat its shell. These proteins allow it to latch onto cell surface proteins, baiting and hijacking host cells. They differ somewhat in humans and bats, so no one knows for sure how and when it made the jump, and if the novel coronavirus came through the civet, tree shrew, or ferret.[49] From the outset, the search for animal origins was pure conjecture.

After COVID-19, China permanently pulled the plug for all wildlife trade, even though the merciless kill-off of animals goes unabated. Banning the trade runs the risk of forcing underground vendors unable to ply their trade, making tracing sources of disease harder; and yet doing nothing is far more treacherous path. The Chinese government reversed the wildlife ban but reinstated it when a woman in Guangdong caught SARS after contact with some living creature. Civets were punished instead of humans. As David Quammen describes in his book, *Spillover: Animal Infections and the Next Human Pandemic*,

> More than a thousand captive civets were suffocated, burned, boiled, electrocuted, and drowned. It was like a medieval pogrom against satanic cats. This campaign of extermination seemed to settle the matter and made people more comfortable … [except] civets aren't the reservoir of SARS.[50]

In the guesswork about the novel coronavirus' provenance, pangolins gained greater purchase as the "world's most trafficked mammal."[51] Just like elephant tusks, tiger claws, and rhino horns—pangolin scales are prized by buyers for their scaly keratin, the same material as human fingernails. As an ingredient in "traditional" folk medicine, it is thought that their scales have "healing properties" to treat sexual dysfunction, cancer, menstrual problems, poor lactation, skin diseases, and arthritis.

Despite a global ban on trade of pangolin in 2017, the animal is captured in Southeast Asia and in western Africa as a food source for poor people or for the middle class who consider them a luxury item.[52] China already banned the sale and trade of pangolin with up to a decade of prison time for offenders, but regulation remains vexing for a trade that stretches all the way to Gabon, where the meat is prized more than scales. The pandemic begat rumors that the ant-eating mammal—whose only intrinsic defense against predators is rolling up in a ball—might be a primary source for the disease.[53] Memes celebrated SARS-CoV-2 as the "pangolin's revenge" against humanity.[54] That viral recombination happened, if not in the pangolin, then in some animal, but which one? Was it a raccoon dog? An international team of scientists cited the possible origins of SARS-CoV-2 to this species, after analyzing gene sequences from genetic database (some Chinese researchers, however, said samples were bereft of animal DNA).

Leaving aside the wild goose chase for COVID's natural origins, science journalist Sonia Shah observes that the animal most responsible may have been known all along—humans: "In the end, there is no mystery about the animal source of pandemics. It's not some spiky scaled pangolin or furry flying bat … The true animal source is us."[55] *The Guardian* writer John Vidal notes how

> it is actually humanity's destruction of biodiversity that creates the conditions for new viruses and diseases such as COVID-19 … a new discipline, planetary health, is emerging that focuses on the increasingly visible connections between the wellbeing of humans, other living things and entire ecosystems.[56]

Until then, no peaceful coexistence of humankind with nonhuman animals and microbial creatures can exist, which means more viral pandemics unless we change course.

Something eventually comes along to hurry along that process. Then came the game changer: COVID-19. Theorist Mel Chen posits that we are near the horizon of intimacy with molecular particles. A deadly virus is an accelerant of transspecies relations or "animacies," says Chen, in which "myths of immunity are challenged, and sometimes dismantled."[57] A drop-off in natural barriers spells a recipe for disaster but also new viral relations between humans and nonhuman beings.

COVID-19 marked the most powerful entry into the coronavirus canon. From genetic analysis done on SARS1, scientific experts came to some consensus that cross-species transmission occurred through "amplifier hosts" like the civet cat. Cross-contamination of DNA material often happens through handling or eating flesh. China's crackdown on Wuhan's market after SARS made a small dent in an illicit trade that baits humans and their pets into close contact with "exotic" animals from every imaginable hot spot. Doing most harm when it first crosses over, mutant viruses flourish in this global mixing. Zoonotic "spillover effects" can be hard to gauge, and SARS caused some considerable damage before mysteriously dissipating and slinking off into history. Unlike SARS, COVID-19 adapt well to human genes, making it an utterly "humanized" coronavirus.[58]

COVID-19 moved with wild abandon and singular force in a world out of whack. Upon first impression, it was just one global pandemic. It soon became clear that we were dealing with multiple pandemics or different versions of the pandemic with so many variants. As a product of blighted times, the rapidity of COVID's translocation kept pace with the dizzying speed and faster tempo of modern trade. Whereas globalization made countries "interdependent, not just economically but also biologically," COVID-19 took advantage of the closing distance between people, places, and objects.[59] It narrowed the gap between humans and natural environments, which could be recently noted by the uptick of Lyme disease or Lassa fever.

If the Spanish flu pandemic in the twentieth century hitchhiked onto military cargo freight and colonial shipping routes, the novel coronavirus hopped around on ridesharing cars, nonstop long-haul air flights, and round-the-clock multi-destination cruise ships. It thrived in the gaps of globalization's spinning wheels, a miniscule particle able to breach our failing immune systems as well as human systems buckling under the crush of capitalism. The first step in the fight against the novel virus was to find a proper antibody.

Antibody

As one of variable number of zoonotic diseases that can move from species to species until it comes to pass in *Homo sapiens*, SARS-COV-2 comes from a large family of viruses named CoV (*Coronaviradae*). With the novel coronavirus grinding down the immune system, one can experience a range of unpleasant symptoms, ranging from mild to severe. They include fatigue and hot temperature upon touching the back or chest. A crude mortality ratio of around 3% means it is deadlier than the seasonal flu, which claims more lives with a mortality of 1% (SARS has 10%). As vaccines rushed to trials, the ever-changing coronavirus tore into overlooked populations.

There remained the abiding presence of the disease in "silence spreaders," especially children who were not yet effective transmitters of 2019-nCoV. There was the lingering question: if SARS-CoV-2 could be airborne (not acknowledged by the WHO until July 2020) and if asymptomatic people posed a potential threat. This conjecture fired up dustups among international bodies, public health officials and scientists, and local governments. Specialists kept disagreeing or changing their minds on wearing masks. Adaptive human thinking and brain circuitry suffered under constant shuffling back and forth among the "experts."

With "circuits of doubt" beginning to entrench in public discussions, medical scientists sought to find linkages between human structures and "natural" causes of disease.[60] Like SARS and MERS, coronaviruses are a viral family endemic to mammals and birds often in benign form. Genetically related to Sars-CoV (almost 80%) and MERS-CoV (50%), SARS part II, as some people called it, was exceptional.[61] While some virus-hunting scientists began feverishly combing the world for the animal origins of COVID-19, others spent much time on developing emergency-use vaccines in the lab. This critical lifeline jerked back into enemy territory and *realpolitik*, when Russia became the first country to roll out a national vaccine called Sputnik V ("V" for victory) in homage to the world's first satellite that inaugurated the space race. In the vaccine arms race, the Cold War threat of worldwide destruction found its rebirth in coronavirus. The Pentagon ordered all military outposts to stop public reporting of its COVID-19 cases, the goal being viral nonproliferation kept under military secrecy. Government cover-up does little to dampen a free viral agent.

Antigens are foreign substances that cause disease, and their enemy is the antibody, disease-fighting cells or molecules churned out organically by the body's own immune system that it recognizes as an invader. The relationship between antigens and antibodies remains tenuous though, since one's immune system can attack itself. Overreacting to a disease not seen before, the body's immune system unleashes a cytokine storm that causes inflammation which can kill the healthy alveoli lining of the lungs.

This reaction fills the lower respiratory tract with fluid, pus, and dead cells—a burning odd sensation that some stress feels akin to drowning. Unlike the immune memory that comes from infection by chickenpox, which induces the production of antibodies for the rest of our lives, we can get reinfected by COVID-19, since its greater virulence is 100 times more lethal than chickenpox. Cross-reacting with comorbidities, COVID-19 brings irreversible harm to kidneys or heart or the neural system, while remaining for days in semen and feces. It contributes to scar tissue and diminished lung capacity due to pulmonary fibrosis. Impaired oxygen flow may require a ventilator, which was in short supply, and there were reports that even using those ventilators could sicken us. Vitamin D deficiency (not scientifically proven) and living near polluted areas seemed to affect severity. Others lost their sense of taste and smell.

Looking like an alien death star battleship from outer space, the microscopic coronavirus can damage immune cells like lymphocytes while seizing control of the healthy host cells that it enters. In a secret attack, it sends off genetic instructions to trick the host into plugging with the enzymes found on the cell membrane to replicate, reassemble, and repackage the RNA enzymes of the trespasser through transduction and reverse transcription. Our own cells become a virus-making factory to make imperfect copies of the invader. SARS-CoV-2 is a special type of virus, able to proofread its own copying, correcting its own mistakes. Once it takes over, a phalanx of new coronaviruses floods air sacs, and the penetrating diffusion of infection leads to neurological problems, liver toxicity, and heart failure in organs. Humans can muster antibodies to snuff out the new infection, but not all can do so, which is the major fear. With a 3% mortality rate based on early data from China, COVID-19 and its related complications impose more severity than the swine flu or second H1N1 pandemic, which originated throughout North America but was blamed on Mexico. That disease hit a billion people worldwide with a mortality rate of 0.02%.[62]

As the third coronavirus known to have crossed over into humans, SARS-CoV-2 falls into special company with the likes of SARS and MERS. Unlike those diseases, COVID's distinct behavior and unusual features threw a curveball to scientists and their maverick solutions.[63] As a second-generation SARS, the novel coronavirus gave East Asian countries a lead in finding a cure, allowing them to come out ahead, but others did not possess any headway. Even more frustrating was the fact that COVID-19 symptoms were showing up in people with no travel history.

Strangely, young children did not initially become febrile from SARS-CoV-2 in the same rates as adults. Some were of the belief that perhaps their receptor cells are not susceptible to the novel coronavirus' ferocity, while others were of the mind that the disease was nature's way for clearing out the old world for a new younger generation. Adults soon wised up to the fact that children came to suffer too from COVID-19, exhibiting symptoms of Kawasaki disease. Black children bore most of the brunt of multisystem inflammatory syndrome (MIS-C). It soon dawned on everyone that the novel coronavirus spared none. Further, it aimed its poisonous arrows toward the most vulnerable like the medically unprotected, who could not easily build up their immunity walls. With no clear definite leads on a vaccine, the scramble for a cure proved more urgent than ever. Both vaccines and therapeutics were necessary. While science and scientists have always moved at their own pace, responding more quickly to emergencies, the COVID-19 pandemic made science and vaccine production go fast and move now at lightning speed.

Coordinated cross-national teams of scientists began to decode protein snippets of SARS-CoV-2. On alert for strain mutation or "antigenetic shift," scientists worked round the clock to unearth promising medical balms. Modern medicine answered the call, but so did traditional medicine. Thailand's health ministry approved the use of herbal plant extracts to treat early stages of COVID-19 as a pilot program amid a viral flare-up in a country experiencing a suicide epidemic.[64]

Before the word pandemic became commonly uttered, it was more common to hear about epidemics: the obesity epidemic, the loneliness epidemic, the gun violence epidemic, the drug epidemic. The term epidemic had been used by activists to describe the hundreds of women raped, abducted, and killed in Mexico. Johnson & Johnson, a big COVID-19 vaccine maker, settled a landmark class action suit; courts cleared the way for the largest U.S. drug distributors and drugmaker to pay for the costs of the opioid epidemic. Syndemic epidemics molded the pandemic as an accumulation of extant problems. It does not so much introduce anything new but reinforces what has been happening for a while.

Offering a new form of "biological citizenship" reliant on old therapeutic regimes, the pandemic was the signal event for refurbishing political authority.[65] COVID-19 inspired deep thinking about the crosscurrents of statecraft.[66] In *The Origins of COVID-19*, political ecologist Li Zhang scrutinizes the ways the People's Republic of China (PRC) faced a squall of blame for something larger than itself. China watchers accused the PRC of ruining the world, when blame should have been laid at the feet of global capital's profit motive infused with scientific management. This paradigm does not center collective survival but is focused on the utility-maximization and economization of life itself.

Searching for that shared moment of collective survival is a theme echoed by Native American studies scholar Alicia Carroll, "We researchers did not yet know what we were looking for. We found it only through the process of searching together … Finding is a form of remembering."[67] The cure to COVID-19 needed to be procured sifting through currents of memory to remember how we made this colonized viral world.

This task remains a tall order, as we still want easy solutions. With biotech companies in league with governments and philanthropic groups, prospective drugs and antiviral therapies came from all over. But the recent memory of what those companies had done had been forgotten in the pandemic craze. One British medical study suggested fermented antioxidizing kimchi as reason for low fatalities in South Korea, as did sauerkraut cabbage in Germany. Researchers in Canada took at face value the drug remdesivir—used for treating hepatitis C as effective in treating SARS, MERS, and COVID-19.[68]

Mumbai hoped to administer this "miracle cure" in Dhavravi and Worli, the largest most crowded slums in the country. This active experimentation on the downtrodden poses ethical dilemmas that worsen a vulgarized climate of mistrust and inertia. A fear that sensitive information from circulating peer-review studies on new diseases like COVID-19 can be used by terrorists affects scientific exchange; what can be known drifts away from an institutional context to acquire a kaleidoscope of meaning that can be described as viral.[69]

After falsifying studies pulled and retracted from *Science*, a chronic fatigue expert rebranding herself as an anti-vaccine expert put out a documentary titled "Plandemic," putting responsibility on American Big Pharma. Despite being pulled down by YouTube and Facebook, it amassed millions of views. An unvetted poisonous court of public opinion was the petri dish to breed contagious lies.

Groping for facts about coronavirus turned into a full-time job for professional scientists, particularly so when public officials start dispensation of lies or deception. Without any levying charges of wrongdoing, the main agency responsible for funding biomedical research abruptly cancelled EcoHealth Alliance's six-year multimillion dollar grant for a project called Predict.[70] The termination of funding by National Institutes of Health (NIH) came a few days after President Trump said he would zero out this research proposal called "Understanding the risk of bat coronavirus emergence." Despite collaborating with the Wuhan Institute of Virology and other institutes in Shanghai and Singapore, the entity—the only one in the United States—that had been studying bat coronaviruses for a decade found their work under heavy scrutiny. A damning 2023 report later revealed that the NIH did not properly track federal funds to conduct gain-of-function research, which alters and boosts viruses to study their evolution. Despite this lack of scrutiny, the director of the organization says, "Once we've overcome COVID-19, what about COVID-20? What about COVID-21? Who is going to go out and find those?"[71]

Someone that is no stranger to government incompetence is David Ho. The prominent AIDS researcher had witnessed the horror of state inaction during the early 1980's outbreak of HIV. He and other scientists still found a way to create a protease inhibitor that broke down the life cycle of the immunocompromising virus. Dr. Ho started to work on a COVID-19 solution immediately after requesting blood samples from two convalescent patients in Hong Kong. Ho might have seen faster progress had it not been for funders losing interest in his SARS research after the immediate panic subsided. Ho's lab developed antibodies that he and his team wished to treat SARS, but the $20 million needed to continue this research had come to naught.[72] Had more money been found, Ho would be one step closer to treating the novel coronavirus. Beyond the economic backers not caring, the doctor held the belief that the lack of licensed testing in the United States was "an outright failure in leadership."[73] A quick polymerase chain reaction (PCR) test to look for antibody presence—offering quick turnaround results in minutes, similar to HIV home testing—had been available in Europe, South Korea, and China, but they were not approved by the U.S. Food and Drug Administration.

Such are the context-specific events surrounding a dispiriting pandemic that appears shapeless. As a force to be reckoned with, its blows left a lasting impact, never with a single solution in sight. Pandemic social circumstances were driven by competing instincts to "protect the public" and a propensity to grant indemnity to selfish individuals and corporate finks. If nations ceded ground to COVID-19, it would be largely their own doing.

Left to their own devices, humans could let the disease run free. By letting their guard down and not exercising self-restraint, this relaxed public attitude gave scientists little time to find an antibody to COVID-19 before it mutates. Dithering on "physical distancing" can cause rough spots for disease prevention, especially for the immunocompromised, and those patients with underlying medical conditions like heart disease, renal failure, diabetes, or cancer. Even without any prior medical issues, individuals could die suddenly by not hewing to recommendations to stay put. A wait-and-see approach drained much energy from the plan to trace, track, and isolate a virus that was constantly shape shifting.

Early correlations of regular seasonal bouts of flu with COVID-19 led many astray, losing critical weeks and months through missteps and a lack of coordination. China took six weeks before it told other countries about the novel coronavirus. This lax attitude culminated in a groundswell of high fatalities in the equally lax Trump America, where anti-vaxxers got to know what a "vaccine-free" world looked like. Immunologist Roberto Tinoco called for ending the "Trump virus" with the virality of democratic participation: "Tenemos que curar el virus. Trompudo con la vacuna que es nuestro voto!" [we have the cure for the virus. "Trump" it with the vaccine of our vote].[74] In others, the vote was the vaccine.

New global developments like COVID-19 could not sway certain enthroned leaders with their stalwart views and ineffectual authority. Though condemned by the WHO, the concept of "herd immunity" was promulgated by the heads of the United Kingdom and the Netherlands. They claimed that the virus should run its course, and people should just become sick; survivors could amass greater COVID-19 resilience. Dutch Prime Minister Mark Rutte averred,

> As we wait for a vaccine or medicine, we can slow down the virus spreading and at the same time build up herd immunity in a controlled manner … The reality is also that in the coming period a large part of the population will be infected with the virus.[75]

Epidemiologists from Johns Hopkins University warned that nearly half a million US-ians would need to die before reaching herd immunity, defined as reaching at least 60–70% up to a 90% saturation point within an aggregate population. Talking heads like Rush Limbaugh said California already obtained herd immunity, but scientists stated unequivocally that collective immunity "will not be achieved at a population level in 2020, barring a public health catastrophe."[76]

If COVID-19 hit hard even the most prepared, then catastrophe struck the least suspecting. The British government took a lax "pragmatic" approach to the WHO's recommendation to "test, test, test" by singing the unflappable slogan "keep calm and carry on." Prime Minister Boris Johnson himself landed in intensive care for COVID-19. Johnson pitched the idea that Britons should allow the viral nomad to plow through the population. The WHO opposed the call for "herd immunity," which immunologists refer to when groups are not inoculated. The Executive Director of Health Emergencies explained,

> Humans are not herds ... We need to be really careful when we use terms ... because it can lead to a very brutal arithmetic which does not put people, and life, and suffering at the center of that equation.[77]

Herding the nation around his cult of personality, Johnson sought to exploit the pandemic situation to his advantage. COVID-19 was one transient grifter, he claimed, that we tolerate, a thief of lives sneaking in the night like the infamous Jack the Ripper. When the conservative leader referred to his assailant as an "unexpected invisible mugger," this symbol was a fitting allusion to his tough-on-crime promises to expand prison sentences. Johnson stepped down and resigned, after revelations of ethics violations and rule-breaking, when he was fined for attending a party during lockdown.

Pandemic readiness asks what actors can speak and what normative claims they can make for others.[78] Two prominent doctors in France made overtures to experimenting on Africans on live television. They proposed a new coronavirus vaccine should be tested first in Africa, since it lacks medical infrastructure. One of them made an analogy to Africans and prostitutes used in AIDS studies as human aggregates that "don't protect themselves."[79] Some proposals toyed with the racist and historic treatment of Africa as a living laboratory. This colonial mentality explained vaccine hesitancy in Ghana, the first Africa country to receive COVID-19 treatments. President Nana Akufo-Addo publicly endorsed the medicines and decreased worries that they alter DNA, cause infertility, and implant a tracking device in the body:

> Fellow Ghanaians, I know there are still some who continue to express doubts about the vaccine, others have expressed reservations about its efficacy, with some taking sides with conspiracy theorists who believe the vaccine has been created to wipe out the African race. This is far from the truth.[80]

The plant *Artemisia annua*, a sweet wormwood of the daisy family, came to attention of the president of Madagascar, who took it as a cure for COVID-19. Despite calls for more evidence by its national scientists, 20 other African countries cast their lot with Madagascar. The president questioned the patronizing attitudes toward African innovation: "If it was a European country that had actually discovered this remedy, would there be so much doubt?"[81]

Beyond the influence of Europe, political theorist Paul Amar infers that quarantine brought *insurgent intimacies* between Africa and China "fused into a global cultural megaproject with the PRC presenting itself as a leader in responding to the COVID-19 pandemic in the Global South."[82] At a time the PRC has officially branded as its "Rejuvenation Era" in stepping out into the world, China sought to create the viral world made in its image—a worlding from the Global South.

Pandemic politics cut through a wide swath of modern life. In one sense, it helped cast aside some of the petty trifles and usual tribulations of statecraft. However, the novel coronavirus broke open social pressure cookers already coming to a head at its arrival. India and South Africa asked the WHO to waive coronavirus-vaccine patent protections to jump-start manufacturing worldwide and speed up economic recovery. Pharmaceutical companies balked, insisting that vaccines are too complex and expensive to hastily scale up and bring to market. Yawning clouds of doubt hung around the more than 150 vaccines in development, amid the possibility of corporate capture of government resources.

Heading into the rocky months of a long winter, the United States, Great Britain, Canada, Germany, and other countries saw their biggest surge. No collective relief was yet possible or in sight. In the high-water mark month of December 2020, the world received stunning announcements about viable vaccines with 90–95% effectiveness. We could breathe a sigh of relief again. Rare cases of unusual blood clots that killed people could not delay vaccine development. But then consumers eyed the jaw-dropping price tag for these new drugs.

The people of Brazil paid a steep price in human lives. As their country hit a million cases of infections by June 2021, protests engulfed the streets over political corruption. Nongovernmental organizations criticized President Jair Bolsonaro and his desperado associates guilty for producing a toxic environment in government, which made it near impossible to find meaningful solutions to the pandemic. Brazilians were incensed over officials secretly making deals to buy the vaccine Covaxin from India, instead of lower-priced Pfizer products from the United States. Despite the Parliamentary Commission of Inquiry dropping this bombshell, the vaccine corruption scandal stoked rumors of genocide as overpriced medicines (for emergency use) became a sign of the *coronatimes*. For the casual observer, it was hard to deny the global stockpiling and misdistribution of vaccines.

Vaccine populations were sorted out along price points and wealth. Bilateral deals between pharmaceuticals Pfizer and Moderna and rich WHO member states Canada, the United States, the United Kingdom, and Chile secured vaccines for those recipients who could afford them. Providing that the poor did obtain anything, they received Cuban or Russian homegrown vaccines. Cheaper "alternatives" came in the form of CoronaVac from Chinese companies (Sinovac/Sinopharm) and drugs developed in India (Covidshield/Covaxin). Striving for protection against *vaccine nationalism*, the WHO began working with Pfizer to distribute its vaccines to lower-income countries like South Africa, which had paid 2.5 times more for the Oxford-made AstraZeneca vaccines than EU members. The WHO worked with Global Alliance for Vaccines and Immunization (Gavi) and COVID-19 Vaccines Global Access (COVAX), a worldwide initiative for equitable access to vaccines.

Technoscience gave no easy remedy for global societies built on unequal power structures. A deeper respect for science reached a crescendo with the pandemic, but the answer to the racist manifestations of the novel coronavirus was not "non-racist" science, but one centered on diversity and attracting more scientists of color. As science studies professor Anthony Hatch posits, "When you're dealing with an institutional structure like global science, one of its core features is that it has been a racial structure."[83] Even if enough vaccines were manufactured for everyone on the planet, how would it put into the hands of those people who needed them most like communities of color?

How does a global rollout not go to waste when half of all medical vaccines are thrown away every year? With big cracks in the global supply chain, pharmaceuticals operate from the fantasy that certain lives matter more than others and death should be averted for a privileged few. With the quick "miracle" of a COVID-19 vaccine, we discovered again that some lives were deemed worth more than others. Desired new medicines as a product of capitalist dreamwork are "felt projections built into the world that tended to erase their own conditions of creation."[84] Who are worthy to be saved and who are consigned to "sacrifice zones" overseen by biotech companies?

Flushed with billions in government aid, U.S. drug giants like Moderna and Pfizer obtained fast approval of COVID-19 vaccines based on emergency use. Their much-touted frontrunners were not true vaccines (vetted after years of trials) but were considered safe due to their noninfectious nature as they did not integrate with DNA. A lack of trust around new drugs mirrored the distrust around those that made them. No stranger to controversy, Pfizer hoped to make a profit after a year of losses. During its early heyday, the U.S. megacompany bore much scrutiny for paying little-to-no income taxes, while earning billions through offshoring profits and receiving government refunds.

Moderna, another U.S.-government subsidized vaccine maker, refused to stop its vaccine sequencing but did not enforce its intellectual property. This small window of opportunity gave the United Nations license to ask a South African start-up to decipher Moderna's recipe, sharing it with manufacturers around the world. Pressured to help but locked up by orders from the Global North, Moderna finally agreed to sell over 100 million shots to the African Union, a deal brokered by U.S. President Joe Biden.

Pfizer followed suit with promises to build vaccine factories in Africa and saving lives. One matter that becomes conveniently forgotten is how the pharmaceutical giant stood accused of medical experimentation on poor children in West African countries. In 2001, 30 families sued Pfizer in a federal court in New York, alleging that Pfizer carried out medical experiments on poor foreign children without consent.[85] The plaintiffs charged sick children were given the experimental oral antibiotic called Trovan during clinical trials. Pfizer did not inform families that it issued a low-dosed control drug, when a real better antibiotic was available.[86] Three years before COVID-19, Nigeria's government released its official report that Pfizer had experimented on its children during a severe meningitis epidemic in 1996. Pfizer denied the charges but paid out the families whose children died or were disabled. Such transgressions do not augur positive thoughts for Pfizer's development of experimental COVID-19 trial drugs on a global scale.

Drug giant Merck, which had knowingly put out drugs that harmed users in the past, entered the virus-busting game in earnest. As elite countries set about to monopolize the business, India's homemade MRNA vaccine Gennova compressed years of late-stage human trials into weeks, so it could be shipped out to a billion citizens. The Serum Institute, the world's largest manufacturer of vaccines, promised to export medicine to other countries that paid for them, but needed to redirect supplies to its domestic base in India, due to poor rationalizing and planning by the Indian government. With different stories being told of who was to blame for vaccine shortage, those supplies were never enough, explained the company, due to lack of raw materials from the United States and price caps by the government.

Not too dissimilar to the response toward HIV/AIDS, countries in the Global South elected to find cheaper vaccine alternatives. Questions circled around who would receive the treatments first, if any at all. Would poor nations and people need to pay for the dereliction of duties by rich countries who hoard medicines for themselves? Would vaccines come in the form of loans or be free? As predicted, wealthier nations gobbled up shares of vaccines using property rights. After a billion doses had been distributed by the start of summer of 2021, it was discovered that 87% of vaccines had been administered in rich countries with only 0.2% of doses dispensed in low-income ones. Even highly polarized nations like Israel and the United States managed to vaccinate half of their populations. COVID-19 proof of vaccination records soon proved to be a badge of honor, and lacking this credential proved shameful while blocking access to public places. Due to extensive refusal among Americans, vaccines went unused when they could have been used abroad. The narrow band of vaccinated nations did not seem to transect the worlds of others. We were living in a viral world without universal vaccines.

A pandemic invites painstaking conversations and reconciliation of opposing viewpoints. This convergence is where the deadly symptoms of our viral worlds are actualized, their entanglements discernible in politicized moments where a coronavirus appears as something foreign to humanity.

Notes

1 Srinivasa Rao Apparasu, "Fearing He Had Contracted Coronavirus, Man Locks Family, Kills Himself: No Coronavirus Case Has Been Reported in Andhra Pradesh and Telangana," *Hindustan Times*, February 12, 2020, www.hindustanti mes.com/india-news/man-suffering-from-cold-and-fever-commits-suicide-in-and hra-pradesh-feared-he-had-contracted-coronavirus-says-family/story-nECI2mh rvB5FiX2vHruFcK.html

2 Jonathan Watts, "Bruno Latour: 'This Is a Global Catastrophe That Has Come from Within," *The Guardian*, June 6, 2020, www.theguardian.com/world/2020/ jun/06/bruno-latour-coronavirus-gaia-hypothesis-climate-crisis

3 Mamyrah Dougé-Prosper, "An Island in the Chain: The Geopolitical Fallout of the U.S. Wars on Drugs and Terror Reveal How the United States Continues to Exploit Haiti as a Tool for Guarding Global Power," *NACLA Report on the Americas* 53, no.1 (2021): 32–38.

4 Michel De Montaigne, *Complete Essays* (Stanford, CA: Stanford University Press), 1965, 151.

5 Darren Byler, *Terror Capitalism: Uyghur Dispossession and Masculinity in a Chinese City* (Durham, NC: Duke University Press, 2021), 37.

6 Michael A. Peters and Tina Besley, *Pandemic Education and Viral Politics* (London: Routledge, 2020).

7 Purnima Mankekar and Akhil Gupta, "Future Tense: Capital, Labor, and Technology in a Service Industry: The 2017 Lewis Henry Morgan Lecture," *Journal of Ethnographic Theory* 7, no. 3 (2017): 67–87.

8 Donna Haraway, *Simians, Cyborgs and Women: The Reinvention of Nature* (New York: Routledge, 1991), 179.

9 Jane Caputi, *Gossips, Gorgons and Crones: The Fates of the Earth* (Santa Fe, NM: Bear & Company, 1993), xx.

10 There exists a plethora of Anthropocenes: Pyrocene, Capitalocene, Plantationocene, Neologismcene, Black Anthropocene, Asian Anthropocene, and Feminist Anthropocene. See, for example, Richard Grusin, ed., *Anthropocene Feminism* (Minneapolis: University of Minnesota Press, 2017); Elizabeth Chatterjee, "The Asian Anthropocene: Electricity and Fossil Developmentalism," *The Journal of Asian Studies* 79, no. 1 (2020): 3–24.

11 Kathryn Yusoff, *A Billion Black Anthropocenes or None* (Minneapolis: University of Minnesota Press, 2018).

12 Amrah Salomón, "Decolonizing the Disaster: Defending Land and Life during Covid-19," *Political Theology*, October 24, 2020, https://politicaltheology.com/ decolonizing-the-disaster-defending-land-life-during-covid-19/

13 Arielle Duhaime-Ross, "The Tiny Nation of Kiribati Will Soon Be Underwater— Here's the Plan to Save Its People," *Vice*, September 22, 2016, www.vice.com/ en_us/article/a39m7k/doomed-by-climate-change-kiribati-wants-migration-with-dignity

14 William J. Ripple, Christopher Wolf, Thomas M. Newsome, Phoebe Barnard, and William R. Moomaw, "World Scientists' Warning of a Climate Emergency," *BioScience* 70, no. 1 (2020): 8–12.

15 Lijing Cheng, John Abraham, Jiang Zhu, Kevin E. Trenberth, John Fasullo, Tim Boyer, Ricardo Locarnini et al., "Record-Setting Ocean Warmth Continued in 2019," *Advances in Atmospheric Sciences* 37 (2020): 137–142.

16 2019 was also their coldest year due to a "Polar Vortex" and northern winds breaking off from the Arctic Circle.

17 Eric Klinenberg, *Heat Wave: A Social Autopsy of Disaster in Chicago* (Chicago, IL: University of Chicago Press, 2015).

18 Xiaodan Zhou et al., "Excess of COVID-19 Cases and Deaths due to Fine Particulate Matter Exposure during the 2020 Wildfires in the United States," *Science Advances* 7, no. 33 (2021): 1–11.

19 Kyla Schuller, "Losing Paradise," *The Rumpus*, June 2, 2020, https://therumpus. net/ 2020/06/ losingparadise/

20 Patty Berne and Vanessa Raditz, "To Survive Climate Catastrophe, Look to Queer and Disabled Folk," *Yes! Magazine*, July 31, 2019, www.yesmagazine.org/opin ion/2019/07/31/climate-change-queer-disabled-organizers/

21 Jeff Foust, "White House Looks for International Support for Space Resource Rights," *Space News*, April 6, 2020, https://spacenews.com/

22 Paul Amar, "Military Capitalism: In Egypt and Brazil, the Foundations of a Terrifying New 'Para-Populism' Are Taking Shape at the Intersection of International Finance, Mega-Construction, and Military Rule," *NACLA Report on the Americas* 50, no. 1 (2018): 82–89.

23 This explains why COVID-19 infections first gyrated in the busiest global markets and metropoles of Western Europe, North America, and Northeast Asia.

24 Celia Lowe, "Viral Clouds: Becoming H5N1 in Indonesia," *Cultural Anthropology* 25, no. 4 (2010): 625–649.

25 Rebecca Hersher, "U.S. Formally Begins to Leave the Paris Climate Agreement," *National Public Radio*, November 4, 2019, www.npr.org/2019/11/04/773474 657/u-s-formally-begins-to-leave-the-paris-climate-agreement

26 Phil Hearse and Neil Faulkner, "The Coming Social Collapse," *Mutiny*, April 3, 2020, www.timetomutiny.org/post/the-coming-social-collapse

27 Manfred Steger and Paul James, "Disjunctive Globalization in the Era of the Great Unsettling," *Theory, Culture & Society* 37, no. 7–8 (2020): 187–203.

28 This despite the rollback of China's Environmental Impact Assessment Law in 2019.

29 Carol W. Berman and Xi Chen, "COVID Threatens to Bring a Wave of Hikikomori to America," *Scientific American*, January 19, 2022, www.scientificamerican. com/article/covid-threatens-to-bring-a-wave-of-hikikomori-to-america/

30 Rachel Uda, "Beyond Brain Fog: What the Pandemic Has Done to Our Memory," *Katie Couric Media*, July 29, 2022, https://katiecouric.com/covid-19/covid-pande mic-memory-loss/

31 Peter Wade, "California Official Ousted after Saying Herd Immunity Killing Elderly and Homeless Would Fix 'Burden on Society,'" *Rolling Stone*, May 3,

2020, www.yahoo.com/entertainment/calif-official-ousted-saying-herd-000143 108.html

32 Lisa Tilley, "Saying the Quiet Part Out Loud: Eugenics and the 'Aging Population' in Conservative Pandemic Governance," *Discover Society*, April 6, 2020, https:// discoversociety.org/2020/04/06/saying-the-quiet-part-out-loud-eugenics-and-the-aging-population-in-conservative-pandemic-governance/

33 Brendan Cole, "Brazil Government Aide Says COVID-19's Toll on Elderly Will Reduce Pension Deficit as Country's Outbreak Escalates," *Newsweek*, May 27, 2020, www.newsweek.com/brazil-government-aide-says-covid-19s-toll-elderly-will-reduce-pension-deficit-countrys-1506830

34 Sierra Garcia, " 'We're the Virus': The Pandemic Is Bringing Out Environmentalism's Dark Side," *Grist*, March 30, 2020, https://grist.org/climate/were-the-virus-the-pandemic-is-bringing-out-environmentalisms-dark-side/

35 Mei Zhan, "Civet Cats, Fried Grasshoppers, and David Beckham's Pajamas: Unruly Bodies after SARS," *American Anthropologist* 107, no. 1 (2005): 31–42.

36 Claire Jean Kim, *Dangerous Crossings* (Cambridge: Cambridge University Press, 2015).

37 Héctor Tobar, "Letter from Los Angeles: On a Generational Uprising," *Literary Hub*, June 5, 2020, https://lithub.com/letter-from-los-angeles-on-a-generational-uprising/

38 Los Angeles laid ground to what many called the world's largest wildlife crossing in 2022.

39 Ruth Goldstein, "Ayahuasca and Arabidopsis: The Philosopher Plant and the Scientist's Specimen," *Ethnos* 86, no. 2 (2021): 245–272.

40 Haraway has been criticized by some for her "eugenist" take on human population control and facile conflation of animals with people of color as racially marked. Donna Haraway, *When Species Meet* (Minneapolis: University of Minnesota Press, 2013), 301.

41 Nadine Voelkner, "Viral Becomings: From Mechanical Viruses to Viral (Dis) Entanglements in Preventing Global Disease," *Global Studies Quarterly* 2, no. 3 (2022): 1–12.

42 Julie Livingston, *Self-Devouring Growth: A Planetary Parable as Told from Southern Africa* (Durham, NC: Duke University Press, 2019).

43 Ellen K. Silbergeld, *Chickenizing Farms and Food: How Industrial Meat Production Endangers Workers, Animals, and Consumers* (Baltimore, MD: Johns Hopkins University Press, 2016); Rob Wallace, *Big Farms Make Big Flu: Dispatches on Influenza, Agribusiness, and the Nature of Science* (New York: New York University Press, 2016).

44 Ren, Li-Li et al., "Identification of a Novel Coronavirus Causing Severe Pneumonia in Human: A Descriptive Study," *Chinese Medical Journal* 133, no. 9: 1015–1024.

45 Melinda Liu, "Infected with 2019 Novel Coronavirus in Wuhan, China," *The Lancet* 395, no, 10223 (2020): 497–506.

46 China's preeminent leader propagated communist pseudoscience through the "Four Pests" campaign that called for wanton extermination of crop-eating sparrows alongside flies, rats, and mosquitoes. The near extinction of sparrows gave way to swarms of vermin like locusts due to ecological imbalances, and that is when China did a volte-face to import a quarter million of them from the Soviet Union.

47 Melinda Liu, "Is China Ground Zero for a Future Pandemic?" *Smithsonian Magazine*, November 2017, www.smithsonianmag.com/science-nature/china-ground-zero-future-pandemic-180965213/

48 Megan Molteni, "Snakes?! The Slippery Truth of a Flawed Wuhan Virus Theory," *Wired*, January 23, 2020, www.wired.com/story/wuhan-coronavirus-snake-flu-theory/

49 David Cyranoski, "Bat Cave Solves Mystery of Deadly SARS Virus—and Suggests New Outbreak Could Occur," *Nature*, December 2017, www.nature.com/articles/d41586-017-07766-9

50 David Quammen, *Spillover: Animal Infections and the Next Human Pandemic* (New York: W.W. Norton & Company, 2012): 37.

51 Genomic comparisons of COVID-19 and the coronavirus in pangolin found high concordance (90–99%) but less so for bats (77%).

52 Sales of pangolin came down during the pandemic in Gabon and other African nations after hearing news of the novel coronavirus in China.

53 A social media source cited data from unpublished research from scientists in Guangzhou found that 99% of viruses found in the pangolin resemble the novel coronavirus cycling through the planet.

54 Alexandre Hassanin, "Coronavirus Could Be a 'Chimera' of Two Different Viruses, Genome Analysis Suggests," *Science Alert*, March 24, 2020, www.sciencealert.com/genome-analysis-of-the-coronavirus-suggests-two-viruses-may-have-combined

55 Sonia Shah, "Think Exotic Animals Are to Blame for the Coronavirus? Think Again," *The Nation*, February 18, 2020, www.thenation.com/article/environment/coronavirus-habitat-loss/

56 "'Tip of the Iceberg': Is Our Destruction of Nature Responsible for COVID-19?" *The Guardian*, March 18, 2020, www.theguardian.com/environment/2020/Mar/18/Tip-Of-The-Iceberg-Is-Our-Destruction-Of-Nature-Responsible-For-Covid-19-Aoe

57 Mel Y. Chen, *Animacies: Biopolitics, Racial Mattering, and Queer Affect* (Durham, NC: Duke University Press, 2012), 8.

58 Trina J. Wood, "Can Pets Contract Coronavirus from Humans or Vice Versa?" *UC Davis Veterinary*, February 6, 2020, www.vetmed.ucdavis.edu/news/can-pets-contract-coronavirus-humans-or-vice-versa

59 Maru Mormina and Ifeanyi M. Nsofor, "What Developing Countries Can Teach Rich Countries about How to Respond to a Pandemic," *Quartz Africa*, October 19, 2020, https://qz.com/africa/ 1919785/what-africa-and-asia-teach-rich-countries-on-handling-a-pandemic

60 Sherine Hamdy, *Our Bodies Belong to God: Organ Transplants, Islam, and the Struggle for Human Dignity in Egypt* (Berkeley: University of California Press, 2012): 13.

61 Jeong-Min Kim, et al. "Identification of Coronavirus Isolated from a Patient in Korea with COVID-19," *Osong Public Health and Research Perspectives* 11, no. 1 (2020): 3.

62 Kimberly Hickok, "How Does the COVID-19 Pandemic Compare to the Last Pandemic?" *Live Science*, March 19, 2020, www.livescience.com/covid-19-pandemic-vs-swine-flu.html

63 With almost half of deaths stemming from cardiovascular complications according to a *Lancet* journal paper, COVID-19 came into focus less as a purely respiratory disease and more a vascular blood circulation disease that attacks endothelial cells.

64 Athira Nortajuddin, "Suicide: Thailand's Epidemic in a Pandemic," *The ASEAN Post*, March 18, 2021, https://theaseanpost.com/article/suicide-thailands-epide mic-pandemic

65 Vinh-Kim Nguyen, *The Republic of Therapy: Triage and Sovereignty in West Africa's Time of AIDS* (Durham, NC: Duke University Press, 2010).

66 Li Zhang, *The Origins of Covid-19: China and Global Capitalism* (Stanford, CA: Stanford University Press, 2021).

67 Alicia Carroll, "Autobiographical Indiscipline: Queering American Indian Life Narratives," PhD diss., University of California, Riverside, 2014, 112.

68 These drugs meant for Ebola may also counter coronaviruses. Despite the patchy record of hydroxychloroquine in warding off malaria, this drug (commonly used for arthritis) had not undergone clinical trials for COVID-19. University of Alberta Faculty of Medicine and Dentistry, "Drug Meant for Ebola May Also Work against Coronaviruses," *Science Daily*, February 27, 2020, www.scienceda ily.com/ releases/2020/02/200227122123.htm

69 Carlo Caduff, "The Semiotics of Security: Infectious Disease Research and the Biopolitics of Informational Bodies in the United States," *Cultural Anthropology* 27, no. 2 (May 2012): 333–357.

70 This provoked 77 Nobel laureate scientists to put out an open letter opposing this dangerous precedent.

71 Kim Hjelmgaard, " 'What about COVID-20?' U.S. Cuts Funding to Group Studying Bat Coronaviruses in China," *USA Today*, May 9, 2020, www.usatoday. com/story/news/world /2020/05/09/coronavirus-us-cuts-funding-group-studying-bat-viruses-china/3088205001/

72 Robert Langreth and Susan Berfield, "Famed AIDS Researcher Is Racing to Find a Coronavirus Treatment," *Bloomberg*, March 20, 2020, www.bloomberg.com/ news/features/2020-03-19/this-famous-aids-researcher-wants-to-find-a-coronavi rus-cure

73 Lori Dajose, "The Tip of the Iceberg: Virologist David Ho (BS '74) Speaks about COVID-19," *Caltech*, March 20, 2020, www.caltech.edu/about/news/tip-iceberg-virologist-david-ho-bs-74-speaks-about-covid-19

74 Robert Tinoco, Facebook post, August 19, 2020, www.facebook.com/roberto.tin oco.92

75 Vice, "The Netherlands Is Letting People Get Sick to Beat Coronavirus," March 23, 2020, VICE, www.youtube.com/watch?v=ozmh40wwAGc&feature=youtu.be

76 David Dowdy and Gypsyamber D'Souza, "Early Herd Immunity against COVID-19: A Dangerous Misconception," *Johns Hopkins Research University & Medicine, Coronavirus Resource Center*, May 8, 2020, https://coronavirus.jhu. edu/from-our-experts/early-herd-immunity-against-covid-19-a-dangerous-miscon ception

77 Hilary Brueck, "The WHO Made a Thinly Veiled Dig at Sweden's Loose Coronavirus Lockdown, Saying 'Humans Are Not Herds' and Old People Are Not Disposable," *Business Insider*, May 11, 2020, www.businessinsider.com/ herd-immunity-few-people-have-had-the-coronavirus-who-2020-5

78 Antoine de Bengy Puyvallee and Sonja Kittelsen, " 'Disease Knows No Borders': Pandemics and the Politics of Global Health Security," in *Pandemics, Publics, and Politics: Staging Responses to Public Health Crises*, ed. Kristen Bjørkdahl & Benedicte Carlsen (New York: Palgrave MacMillan, 2019): 59–73.

79 Julian Kossoff, "2 Top French Doctors Said on Live TV That Coronavirus Vaccines Should be Tested on Poor Africans, Leaving Viewers Horrified," *Business Insider*, April 3, 2020, www.businessinsider.com/coronavirus-vaccines-france-doctors-say-test-poor-africans-outrage-2020-4

80 "Taking COVID-19 Vaccine Will Not Alter Your DNA, Ghana President Says, *Reuters*, February 28, 2021, www.reuters.com/article/uk-health-coronavirus-ghana-president/taking-covid-19-vaccine-will-not-alter-your-dna-ghana-presid ent-says-idUSKCN2AT1L3

81 Afua Hirsch, "Why Are Africa's Coronavirus Successes Being Overlooked?" *Microsoft News*, May 21, 2020, www.msn.com/en-ie/news/coronavirus/why-are-africas-coronavirus-successes-being-overlooked/ar-BB14pbLy

82 Paul Amar, "Insurgent African Intimacies in Pandemic Times: Deimperial Queer Logics of China's New Global Family in Wolf Warrior 2," *Feminist Studies* 47, no. 2 (2021): 427.

83 The Time to Dismantle the Racial Structures That Pervade Global Science Is Now, Devin Williams on June 23, 2021, www.scientificamerican.com/article/the-time-to-dismantle-the-racial-structures-that-pervade-global-science-is-now/

84 Michelle Murphy, *The Economization of Life* (Durham, NC: Duke University Press, 2017), 53.

85 Kovac, Carl. "Nigerians to Sue US Drug Company over Meningitis Treatment," *BMJ* 323.7313 (2001): 592.

86 They cited a settled whistleblower lawsuit filed by a former Pfizer medical director, who had claimed that his former company sacked him after he warned its study methods were improper.

2

THE FOREIGN VIRUS

Panic, Propaganda, Prison

On New Year's Eve of 2020, China notified the World Health Organization (WHO) about an unknown virus with SARS-like symptoms. Three months later, the supranational body declared COVID-19 a pandemic. Whenever a new disease takes global precedence, questions dominate over its geographic and biological originations and ultimately how to contain it. The big question of "who" brought a disease from "where" often sidesteps the question of what "it" is. This panicked thinking about disease becomes reposed as how do "we" protect against "them." As the pandemic inched closer to a full-scale disaster, public officials acclimated populations to lockdowns and quarantines to deflect worries of being infected. Those public interventions devolved into panic, politics, and imprisonment.

The pandemic hit several publics, which did not always find common ground in the viral world. As science writer Pat Morrison observes, an infectious disease "makes a mockery of all the ways that human beings like to divide themselves up, by class, by wealth, by color, by religion, because everybody is vulnerable."[1] An all-encompassing pandemic, able to wrap itself around our busy, hurried schedules, fixes attention on stasis and the "time (waiting) that structures people's lives, leaving them in limbo or giving them hope."[2] It might crumble some of the walls people erect to socially separate ourselves from others. Woven into the fabric of a new *corona-collectivity*, we might still hold some cognitive dissonance or disconnect with this fictive kinship. New vocabularies needed invention to flesh out this novel time: *pandemic brain, corona-somnia, vaccine passport, vaccine dictatorship, pandemic polarization, quaran-tinis, frontline fatigue,* and *vaccine apartheid.*

Pandemics and extremist reactions commonly go together, but their symbiosis can be quite revealing. As science journalist Laurie Garrett

DOI: 10.4324/9781032694535-3

expounds, collective panic seldom occurs or matches the gravity of a situation. The public's responses to new disease are often peculiar or unpredictable. In the "total war society," where disease prevention follows the logic of preemptive first-strike wars, it seemed "now the scientists couldn't shoot straight. They were pointing their guns, it seemed, incorrectly."[3] With a new global enemy, the question of "whose world is this?" turned out to be "whose war is this"?

At the turn of what some observers call the Coronavirus Century, the United States subsumed pandemic preparedness to military preparedness. It becomes evident that biosafety stands out as a gap in national security. This counterterrorist attitude of "toughing it out" could not deal with a slippery virus that left societies breathless. In 2018, Donald Trump's biodefense preparedness adviser firmly warned that a flu pandemic was the number one security threat to the country, one that "cannot be stopped at the border," and the United States was ill-prepared.[4] Bypassing a "pandemic playbook" briefed to Trump by the National Security Council (NSC), the White House dismantled the NSC's office of health security—an elite team of health experts disbanded numerous times by previous administrations.

Though he was the first U.S. president to order a pandemic preparedness plan, George W. Bush eliminated the office after winning election only to bring it back during the 2001 anthrax terror, which occurred a week after the 9/11 attacks. Outlining contingency plans for biosecurity federal agencies, the Pandemic and All-Hazard Preparedness law in 2006 sprang up under the War on Terror, the military doctrine of defense was concerned with bioterrorist counterproliferation and medical countermeasures.[5] President Barack Obama abolished the pandemic office and then brought the office back after Republicans thrashed him for his lagging response to the Ebola virus crisis. Instead of activating a rational "public sphere" based on enlightening interchange of ideas, a global pandemic like COVID-19 did not convince some that health was a public good necessary to protect. National security advisor John Bolton dissolved the Global Health Security team as part of across-the-board cuts and programs axed.[6]

With a brain-racking pandemic in tow, bedlam reigned but there was a method to the madness. *Gendarmes* in Peru and South Africa shot back at starving citizens and locked them up for flouting lockdown policies—a predictable response from regimes that had recently descended into political instability. As the South American country hit the hardest by COVID-19 after Brazil, Peru saw a standoff between a crooked president and bad legislators in 2020. SARS-CoV-2 pervaded the country as it dived headlong into a constitutional crisis, after the fall from grace and jailing of the country's main conservative leader, Keiko Fujimori, for corruption. This crisis-prone time sat atop "ethnocide by inaction" in the state's refusal to shield Indigenous tribes from COVID-19 in the Peruvian Amazon.[7] With the president impeached, the vice president took over only to step down after serving short of a week, rattled by mass protests over corruption, the economy, and the pandemic.

When South Africa declared a national state of disaster in response to COVID-19 (and protests for the end of corruption), it felt like a logical progression of events there. In its 2019 general election, the African National Congress (ANC) held onto power despite an economic slump, fending off the left-wing Economic Freedom Fighters (EFF) party, which courted the vote of poor Black youths in the closest electoral face-off since the end of apartheid. This retention of power remained despite the assassination of high-profile ANC leaders Sindiso Magaqa, one of many whistleblowers slain for exposing the party's racketeering. Both Peru and South Africa opened the spigot of COVID-19 funding, instituting the most generous stimulus packages in the name of protecting the nation. Economic shock absorbers could not compensate for the death spiral of "thug states" that will do anything to destroy their enemies, foreign and domestic.[8]

This chapter starts with the perception of the COVID-19 as a "foreign disease." It probes social exclusion or censoring laws, based on the perception that the novel coronavirus originates from elsewhere. The so-called "China flu" or "Wuhan virus" activated intense national responses over the import of ventilators, quarantine masking, and closing the border to refugees or immigrants. Through the themes of panic, propaganda, and prison—this chapter scrutinizes key incidents produced at the outbreak that gave rise to pandemic politics. It stresses concern about the increasing surveillance in countries like China, which suppressed political freedom and protest as strongly as it did infection. It pairs this example with the pileup of disaster in the United States, the epicenter of the early pandemic. The chapter distills the popular racialized assumptions made about Asian bodies and touches upon China-bashing at a pain point when countries like Israel, Uganda, and Hungary unleashed xenophobic policies and took an aggressive stance toward a "public menace," human and microbiological. The result is a move toward mass incarceration of people to control a disease during a time of great panic.

Panic

COVID-19 time-stamps the year of discovery for a new coronavirus, asking future historians and generations to uncover the circumstances which allowed a trial-by-fire pandemic to spiral out of hand. As new infectious diseases fan out, their names capture raw combustible emotions. COVID-19 was called the "Wuhan virus" in the international media before it found an official name from the WHO. Mindful of grave mishaps made in retrospect, the international body took extra precaution to name the disease under new scientific guidelines set in 2015, which avoided stigma for "a geographical location, an animal, an individual or group of people."[9] Ascribing stigma prevents infected people from coming forward, thwarting strenuous mitigation efforts. This new etiquette of naming diseases responds to a history of labelling disease like the Hong Kong or Spanish flu, Crimean–Congo hemorrhagic fever, Middle East respiratory syndrome coronavirus, and Ebola viruses (Zaire ebolavirus, Sudan ebolavirus, Reston ebolavirus). A new preference was to leave out names of specific places, so COVID-19 was special for doing so. While a country or region was not named, panic invariably followed the virus in a viral world where certain places and people are already stigmatized.

Within the high-stakes game of cat-and-mouse with the novel coronavirus, mealy mouthed leaders and media ringleaders played loose with facts. It is not hard to understand why mass panic blasted off. The power of "infectious fear" oozed out to become a viral worlding for the paranoid who saw the threat of disease from traditionally marginalized groups.[10] Played out as a dramatic *coronanovela*, one also dressed up in the theatrical language of war, the COVID-19 pandemic managed to rip off the social band-aid to reveal deep emotional "woundscapes." Feminist scholar Jennifer Terry indicates that panic is a logical human response to threat. However, the free run of fear is political: "In the face of imminent and emergent pathogens, all bodies are conceived as potentially threatened or threatening … war is waged on, through, and with microscopic pathogens. Panic is a marketing tool."[11] As a marketing tool for war, prison time and panic mode set in a viral world when little is known or foresworn. All bodies might be threatening, but some are deemed more so.

Countries began evacuating their nationals out of China. African nations like Senegal and Uganda thought their international students were better off in China in case they need to be looked after, despite recommendation by the Africa Centers for Disease Control and Prevention (CDC) to bring all students back home. A fair number of African countries had not yet stopped travel from China in the stormy months of the outbreak. The first African to test positive for the novel coronavirus was a Cameroonian student studying in China, whose status was found out by dismayed family members from an online post. South Sudan received its first four cases, all brought by U.N. workers, and when one staffer fled the country to avoid quarantine.

No continent was spared the hand of COVID-19. This behemoth bore all the markings of something long-lasting, memorable, and far enduring than SARS. The latter seemed more like a flash in the pan compared to its younger cousin. As the first pandemic wrought by a coronavirus, SARS burbled out from China in 2002–2004, around the same time the People's Republic of China joined the World Trade Organization, with China ramping up to become the world's manufacturing hub. The number of infected business merchants, overseas students, and tourists had not yet flared to the levels during COVID-19.

The first SARS-CoV-2 cases for Italy, Thailand, Japan, the United States, Singapore, Vietnam, and so many other countries were pinned to travelers from Wuhan, China. The hunt for the original index patient in Wuhan proved elusive, even though the first confirmed COVID-19-related death came from an older man who had visited the seafood markets. China could not exactly point to who brought the virus to marketplace, and how it escaped to splash down on other shores, suggesting perhaps it came from outside the country.

With a hungry coronavirus making landfall and aching to infect an ever-climbing number of people, a slew of measures came to pass. This procedure included closing all wildlife markets and mass human quarantining, an action commended in a report from a WHO-China joint mission: "In the face of a previously unknown virus, China has rolled out perhaps the most ambitious, agile, and aggressive disease containment effort in history."[12] China's valiant attempts could not stop COVID-19 from fomenting into a full-blown pandemic. The international community fumed at China's overdue action, blaming the secrecy of the Communist Party as a springboard for COVID-19 to snake its way to the rest of the planet.

Deep ambivalences over the novel coronavirus were bound up with a lack of public trust in shambolic governments. Governing bodies plotted an uneasy response, letting both disinformation and disease get out of hand. Believers of conspiracy theory thought 5G technology in cellular networks was a way for SARS-CoV-2 to be spread by global elites to the masses. Aggressive steps to limit social gatherings lit the fuse for pranks that were not too far from reality. A random text phone message was sent around to individuals where the progenitor claimed a friend high up in military ranks, who overheard the U.S. president was going to order martial law. A viral meme from India shared by thousands took things further. It claimed Russia's leader Vladimir Putin released lions on the street to keep people in their houses (the doctored photo was taken from a movie set in South Africa). Such malarkey draws on the credulity of people to become easily duped. The director of the WHO chimed in: "We're not just fighting an epidemic; we're fighting an infodemic. Fake news spreads faster and more easily than this virus, and is just as dangerous."[13]

Pandemic panic is part of a constant state of emergency in which mass demonstrations and extremist violence are more and more frequent.[14] Russia's imperialist overtures in the country of Georgia put national borders at risk way before the novel coronavirus. When the former banned flights from Georgia in 2019 in retaliation for anti-Russian protests there, travel bans based on vindictive political reasons had already been regular before the pandemic's shake-up. Rather than be concerned with slaying the dragon of COVID-19, Russian kleptocrats turned guns on their own people in a revolting showcase of state thuggery. Protests across 100 cities in Russia itself tested the resolve of Putin, whose personalist regime and "power vertical" made little distinction between disease and dissension. In the throes of a biopolitical crisis, striking parallels between the Iron Curtain and a pandemic-directed curtain of secrecy could hardly be clearer.

Jockeying for power appears benighted amid a rolling pandemic, and yet that is exactly what happened. As China returned to some semblance of normalcy after control measures and the United States became the viral epicenter, a Chinese news anchor said that all humans need to follow the grand scheme of a shared global community, a noble ambit waylaid by social fissures and the whims and fancies of politicians: "When I saw Governor Cuomo of New York begging the federal government to step in to get ventilators, I thought, wow, what a difference different systems can make."[15] A nervous Singaporean public health official commented on the raucous American coronavirus soap opera: "I am deeply concerned about the U.S.... . It's become politicized, making it difficult for the average citizen to know who to trust or what to believe."[16] Singapore's Minister of National Development added a comment with the addition of other European countries:

> We are watching America quite closely ... the number rising there as well ... It's not just about the numbers, but the fact that these countries have abandoned any attempt at containing the spread of the virus. They have said so, especially the United Kingdom and Switzerland.[17]

Singapore was one of the first countries to leap into action, monitoring temperatures of any traveler from Wuhan and mandating masks. Persons sick with flu or pneumonia were tested for free, employers could not subtract sick days from employee quarantine, and the government footed the hospital bill, roping in international travelers who were grounded for a compulsory two weeks. On social media, one foreigner documented her stay at luxury hotels replete with room service and ocean views. Videos online captured the gratitude of elated foreign workers confined to dormitories; this footage though plays into the gloss of state beneficence as migrants were given health check-ups and daily food packages loaded with vitamins. Singapore is not a socialist welfare state by any means, but a pro-capitalist autocracy (Singapore's high court upheld colonial-era laws criminalizing same-sex relations at the height of the pandemic to reinforce gay people as the enemy Other). It is unrealistic to export the Singapore success story to the United States, a much bigger country with 100 times the population of the Asian city-state. Despite achieving the lowest mortality rate of any country, Singapore's shiny patina as a safe country belied troubles at home.

The island bolstered its national branding, protecting its nationals while eliding the "canned human lives [that] are packed and accounted purely as a labor force."[18] But in mid-April 2020, the country experienced a turnabout in its prior standing as the gold standard for trouncing COVID-19. An outbreak tripled the numbers, toward a daily intake of 1,000 new case counts with no more than a dozen Singapore nationals. Most new cases emerged from imported workers from India and Bangladesh who prop up Singapore's economy, many forced to sleep with 10 to 20 other people to a cramped, poorly ventilated rooms. Comprising one-fourth of the country's residents, these migrants initially escaped Singapore's regulatory oversight, which disavowed their existence in early pandemic reports. Transient Workers Count Too, a migrant labor advocacy group, impugned Singapore's entire economic model, asserting that it reaps

> the benefits of the cheap labor of the Third World in order to create our so-called First World economy … The only problem is a virus comes along that does not respect this apartheid-type of segregation, and then you have an explosion.[19]

Singapore's ruling party, the People's Action Party (PAP) squashes any show of dissent and represses anyone reporting bad news. Predictably, disease prevention became awash in the morass of a "post-truth" viral world.

Australia's federalist system of power sharing with states supposedly hindered the prime minister (a climate change denier) from directly ordering school closures. Federalism and "state rights" discourses in the United States brought about regional disparities under a worn-down democratic political system.[20] But as the monarchal kingdoms of Saudi Arabia and the United Arab Emirates boarded up their schools without haste, Jordan's king dissolved parliament and the government banned people from even walking outside and driving, closing all grocery stores in one of the harshest lockdowns in the world. He broadcasted his message for unity and peace on state media but shut down social media to thwart "dissidents."[21]

COVID-19 tracking fed into the surveillance state and platform capitalism.[22] Governments gave chase to infected persons by keying into the common practice of tracking consumer behavior. A girl from Hong Kong had to wear a quarantine tracking bracelet and was followed, taped, and shamed online after going to a restaurant. Similar to Israel, Singapore internally tracked its nationals and returnees, forcing them to share their phones' location data every day per quarantine directives (the state utilized Bluetooth signals sent between phone users to keep track of their contacts).[23] Politicos argued that countries where people report on their neighbors accede to rules and authority unlike in "large Western countries where people might chafe at the harnessing of CCTV cameras or immigration records for the health of the nation."[24] East European countries like Poland required citizens to prove they are prostrating to the yoke of authorities by using a selfie monitoring app.

No less impressive were Rwanda, Colombia, Chile, and Senegal, countries able to handle COVID-19 well but differently through their state surveillance technologies.

In Latin America, the political pendulum swung hard in both directions. In Chile, the quirky tantrums of the conservative billionaire president bowed to public pressure to change the country's martial-law constitution made under dictator Augusto Pinochet. This new charter would be drafted by the people rather than legislators in response to social unrest over increasing inequality and metro tax hikes in 2019. People leaned in on feminist eco-socialist ideas to cajole the government, demanding more education and rights for Indigenous people. Two short years later, voters rejected the "left leaning" constitutional draft for going too far in legalizing abortion, adopting universal health care, and protecting the environment. COVID-19 demanded wholesale changes to all these things, but some felt change came too fast.

When France's President Emmanuel Macron declared "we are at war" with COVID-19, the leader up for reelection overleveraged his own political ambitions. Skeptics of the "Asian way" of handling the pandemic such as Macron postulated that communist countries like China consistently lie and underreport their numbers (Vietnam and North Korea often claimed no COVID-19-related deaths). Naysayers suggested that it would be naïve to believe closed-off authoritarian regimes. For their intents and purposes, *all* countries undercount due to tests with false positives and inability to test the entire population.

A posted article by an unknown diplomat on China's French embassy website caused an international row. It claimed French nursing homes were leaving people to die (a day after France raised death tolls by including nursing homes), and falsely reported that Taiwan had called the head of the WHO a "negro." After French senators derided embassy tweets that cast the country in a bad light, the Chinese ambassador was called to task by the foreign minister to quiet the negative buzz.

In top-secret classified reports, the U.S. intelligence community concluded that China, alongside other countries like Egypt and Indonesia, fakes their infection numbers, painting an incomplete picture by covering up their veracity. The Department of Homeland Security traced how Chinese state-owned companies were swooping up and hoarding medical supplies right before admitting about the novel coronavirus—a clear violation of the 2005 International Health Regulations, which China signed. In mid-April 2020, Wuhan city admitted that its death toll was 50% higher than it had reported due to a lack of data updating by hospitals and state officials. The Chinese government admitted to issuing orders in January to dispose coronavirus samples at unauthorized labs, but many viewed this disposal as a cover-up, though it coincided with guidelines at the time for labs to avoid any media information about the furtive virus.

A sound shellacking from dissatisfied Chinese citizens brought down the heap of naked lies told by the powers that be. Accustomed to communist publicity stunts and posturing from party chiefs, Wuhaners heckled a vice-premier when she came to visit their city. In videos shared online, residents shut in by China's zero-COVID-19 policy seethed with anger, yelling profusely from their windows, "Fake! Fake! It's all fake! Everything is Fake." At first, China refused to admit fault for its bungling of the pandemic. Mistakes were made, but some hardy lessons were imbibed from the SARS crash course and pandemics decades earlier. China took a much shorter time to take ownership of its errors with COVID-19 but kept a tight lid on information about the novel coronavirus weeks before sharing with the WHO. Doctor Ai Fen, the director of emergency care at Wuhan Central Hospital had been blacklisted from speaking out and discouraged from mandating masks, since the hospital's head said this warning will only cause "panic" and harm social "stability."[25]

Communist party apparatchiks punished any local reporter who talked about COVID-19. It reprimanded the Wuhan-based ophthalmologist, Doctor Wenliang Li, for sounding alarm about the new disease to his colleagues on a WeChat chatroom.[26] Local police forced him to write a "self-criticism" after summoning him in the middle of the night. The whistle-blower's death from COVID-19 transformed the 34-year-old into an icon of resistance for people fed up with government overreach. China's normally stringent censors let this story of good and evil play out in public, given the viral media response to his death. Expressing a torrent of grief for Li and vitriol against the Chinese Communist Party (CCP), grieving mourners still wrote to the deceased doctor and posted confessionals on his social media page.

Days after Li's death, the central government dispatched an investigative team to Wuhan. It found local authorities acted "inadequately," not in agreement with "proper law enforcement procedures" to deal with this "rumor" spreader, though the group never recommended what punishment need to be meted instead.[27] Two officers were disciplined, and Li's family received an apology from the government, which included dropping Li's official reprimand posthumously. In 2004, China had set up a national almost fail-safe mechanism for reporting disease after SARS—the Contagious Disease National Direct Reporting System. But the onerous fear of rattling Beijing's nerves led local authorities to silence those dissidents who did not toe the line. A world of secrecy and suppression led to the next great pandemic.

Throughout January 2020, the Wuhan Municipal Health Commission disseminated statements that there is no living proof of human-to-human transmission of the new illness, despite personal anecdotes to the contrary by medical workers. This injunction was repeated by the WHO, which declared a pandemic months later; by then, millions had contracted the virus. "I regret that back then I didn't keep screaming out at the top of my voice," said a doctor at Wuhan Central Hospital, "I've often thought to myself what would have happened if I could wind back time."[28]

China's top brass kept everything shrouded in secrecy, policing media dispatches that could leak information about the country's COVID-19 woes, especially about its hasty lockdown of Wuhan. To protect its tarnished reputation and conduct damage control, China faulted the United States for starting the pandemic. Military officials and policymakers pinned the human carnage unleased by the shapeshifting novel coronavirus to the Central Intelligence Agency and the U.S. military. Even though Twitter is banned in the country, China's Foreign Ministry spokesperson tweeted that the U.S. CDC

> was caught on the spot. When did patient zero begin in United States? How many people are infected? What are the names of the hospitals? It might be U.S. Army who brought the epidemic to Wuhan. Be transparent! Make public your data![29]

Zhao had based the tweet on discredited articles from the CCP-approved tabloids like *Global Times* and the *People's Daily* that claimed a Japanese TV show (offering no link) found COVID-19 originated in the United States with help from Taiwan. The message claimed it did not come from mainland China, and perhaps the country was introduced to the virus via the 2019 World Military Games in Wuhan, when China first hosted this event. The tweet assisted in doubling the number of followers for the ministry. China's ambassador to South Africa concurred with the tweet, "Although the epidemic first broke out in China, it did not necessarily mean that the virus is originated from China, let alone 'made in China.' "[30]

A video called "Once Upon a Virus" was uploaded to the Twitter accounts of the Chinese embassy in France and the *China Daily*. Made of toy Lego figures wearing face masks, the illustrated figures bear the symbols of the United States and China: one side has terra-cotta warriors and flanked by medical workers and and the other had a lone Statue of Liberty hooked to IV fluid. The two interlocutors go back and forth with the former telling Americans to "wear masks" and that "it's time for lockdown" to which the latter responds with "human rights violations" and "you lied to us."

Manufactured hoaxes abounded. One held the position that China tampered with a microparasite to make COVID-19.[31] *The Washington Times* quoted an unknown military source that the virus started in a lab supported by China's military bioweapons program. Just as SARS-CoV-2 variants took on a life of their own, defying active resistance, so too did conspiracy theories that overwhelmed new research on the novel coronavirus. The U.S. government pulled funding for a nonprofit that for years sent a team to China to study and monitor the location of bats, raising suspicions that COVID-19 leaked from Wuhan Institute of Virology, which repudiated this claim. Italian far-right personages Matteo Salvini and Giorgina Meloni claimed it was manufactured in a Chinese lab to unleash upon humankind. Scientific organizations and the WHO put out statements to confirm COVID-19 is not man-made.[32]

Fabrications about germ warfare may not seem far-fetched if we brood over the long sordid history of secret government experimentation on citizens. Whether it is in the United States or China, governments turned residential areas into public laboratories and sites of military target practice.[33] Before wide speculation emerged about COVID-19 as a biological weapon, many conjectured such a threat would come from labs close to Wuhan that were priming to acquire biological agents abroad. The year 2020 saw federal investigations into university and national microbiology labs in the United States and Canada based on these hunches.[34] Australia's dictate for an independent probe into the origins of COVID-19 prompted a warning from the ambassador of China. The Chinese newspaper *Global Times* mocked Australia as "this giant kangaroo that serves as a dog" of the United States.[35]

Viral wounding as worlding exacerbated a global incitement toward mass violence. 2019 was already the deadliest year of gun violence in the United States. *The Atlantic* proclaimed a "mass-shooting epidemic is contagious" and "spreading like a disease."[36] In 2022, a Swastika-wearing gunman killed and wounded dozens of students in central Russia, while a former policeman murdered 36 people, mostly children at a youth center. Even in low-crime Japan, former prime minister Abe Shinzo was assassinated by a lone-wolf gunman. Canada experienced tragedy when a shooter gunned down people in Nova Scotia with weapons smuggled from the United States.[37] After the biggest mass shooting in that country's history, Canada immediately announced plans for immediate ban on all assault-style weapons. In 2021, Mexico's government brought a lawsuit against ten U.S. gun manufacturers and suppliers for illegally selling their military-grade weapons to drug cartels.

State orders to "hunker down," "lockdown," and "shelter in place" mirror instructions stamped into the minds of school children gearing up for active shooter drills. Even though many institutions closed, mass shooting violence in the United States crested overall in 2020—the largest increase in history. For the next few years, gun violence became the leading cause of death for U.S. children, surpassing car accidents. Parents needed to sign "death waivers" for their children forced to return to school where the novel coronavirus and other serial killers waited.

Go-for-broke efforts to drive down COVID-19 deaths looked farcical, given little-to-no government action on civilian deaths by military-grade weapons. Ban attempts were met with gun rallies and neo-Nazi threats. This reaction happened when Democrats tried to wring out a gun control law to no avail, forcing the governor of Virginia to declare another state of emergency. A security guard was shot to death after simply asking a woman to wear a mask before entering the store to shop. Rather than appreciate his effort to save her life, she and her male accomplices ended his.

Beneath the coverage of pandemic prevention, sovereignties engaged in building viral deathworlds, where viralized populations are made disposable. The logic of bodily sacrifice and redistribution of social risk forms another form of necropolitics, since COVID-19 democratized the state's "power to kill" to the point where "now we all have the power to kill."[38] There is no guarantee that humans will be here forever, and life will continue without us, say philosopher Achille Mbembe. A glorified humanity might be on its last legs, given the toxic political atmosphere.

Above all, the Cameroonian-South African scholar emphasizes, creative humans manage to remain in "permanent generation, re-creation, and resignification of life [which] flows in the face of the forces of capture, extraction, and desiccation." Public panic enhances life-restricting powers, but this viral politics and practice will rewire our balance of relations in the face of pandemic propaganda.

Propaganda

Saluting their merits on top of blaming others, governments ended up fueling propaganda without any panacea. By March 2020, the "Chinese virus" became the "American virus" when the United States reported cases than any other country, and COVID-19 was now a principal cause of death (two months later the disease became the leading cause of death in the world).[39] Trump set social media abuzz after jokingly calling the virus "the China virus" and blithely ribbed the public about the "Kung flu." The former reality television star engaged in dog whistle politics (Facebook removed his cheeky reelection ads using Nazi symbols).[40] Earlier, Trump had labelled COVID-19 "the foreign virus" and the "China plague."[41] A *Washington Post* reporter took a photograph of his written speech, noting the word "Corona" had been crossed out and replaced with "Chinese."[42] Coded racial doublespeak characterized Trump's political ascendancy, alongside the certitude that "the market" will cure all social ills. Pitching a pathogen of amorphous origin as "foreign" redounded more animosity at foreign places and people. This all panned out as Trump invoked the Korean-War era Defense Production Act (DPA) to remit automobile manufacturers to make medical supplies.

Cold War 3.0 indoctrination was now in overdrive. Born in the era of McCarthyism and red scare hysteria, Trump sought total victory over an imperceptible foe that resembled the communist enemies with which he grew up. In defending his use of labels, the truth-bending president sowed further discord, suggesting Asian Americans agreed with him on calling

COVID-19 the "China virus" without any evidence. Subterfuge downplayed the pandemic's reach, while the president gave the constant runaround in terms of facts. A *pandemic of propaganda* magnified a viral culture of fear, where countless rumors saturated the media's "coronascapes" with whirling "scamdemic" theories.

Inundated by a steady stream of bad news, fretful citizens burrowed at home. People needed clarity of direction and a new tack as well as moral guidance and emotional soothing. But rather than receive succor, they heard inaccurate information from unsavory fickle leaders. Though not one to speak softly, Trump himself was quite evasive during the worst public health crisis in a century. He waived the usual rituals of mourning for the dead, bypassing homilies to victims and ceremonies befitting of somber occasions, celebrating a premature win against the novel coronavirus. Unwilling to be the Comforter-in-Chief, Trump hammered instead benefits of untested long-shot treatments like hydroxychloroquine, an immunosuppressant that doctors have been discouraged from prescribing to patients. Without a doctor's prescription, Trump took the drug as a prophylaxis, claiming all the world's leaders use it. El Salvador's president admitted to taking it as well (an announcement made conveniently right after the U.S. donated ventilators to his country). In an inexplicable move, Trump sarcastically promoted injection of disinfectants to rid oneself of COVID-19, which prodded the manufacturer of Lysol to dispel rumors that cleaning agents are a not a cure-all for disease. Trump made a baseless claim that 99% of COVID-19 cases were "totally harmless" as caseloads spiraled. He later pivoted back to the United States being the best at everything, including testing, and that "one hundred and eighty-nine countries and China must be held fully accountable" for spreading the virus.[43]

When Trump asked during a public meeting, "Why don't we let this wash over the country?," his top infectious disease expert weighed in with, "Mr. President, many people would die."[44] Contradicting the president's fast-track program to spring the market back to life, the flummoxed Dr. Anthony Fauci made a swipe at his boss: "You don't make the timeline, the virus makes the timeline."[45] Upon this rebuttal, Trump doubled down on unverified claims, calling the alarms raised around COVID-19 a hoax to bludgeon him by enemies, before conceding to the pandemic's enormity. This small concession did not stop the CDC from being forced to route all hospital data through the White House, making the whole process of COVID reporting opaque.[46] After a volley of belittling insults against state governors, Trump astoundingly caved in to pressure, letting them call their own shots.

Then in an incendiary tweet, Trump riled up his epigones to "liberate" Democrat-controlled states and cities to ensure the constitutional right to bear arms. Hong Kong protesters seized on this message of liberation to beseech the Trump administration for help, forging an alliance between U.S conservatives and Chinese pro-democracy activists. Political theater and pandemics make strange bedfellows, especially when anti-quarantine protest becomes associated with anti-communism.

The blistering command from the head of state to fight the enemy of liberalism and socialism kick-started a nationwide movement of the self-proclaimed Freedom Party. Spurring on charges of state interference in people's lives, the sentiments of this "aggrieved" group twitched with racial anger. Here, White Americans felt indignant about their social circumstances, their emotions made more legitimate than non-Whites who suffer more by every metric before and during the pandemic.[47] Joined by anti-vaxxers refusing to take any shot to the arm, anti-maskers cried for an end to lockdown. They compared their ferment to the brutalized lives of African Americans under Jim Crow segregation, putting their "discrimination" on par with experiences of racialized minorities. Rallygoers, who ran afoul of masking mandates, went so far as calling it a muzzle, not dissimilar to the mouthpiece worn by enslaved people. Dubbed "coronavirus crusaders," these fabulists compared enforced quarantine to Nazism and faulted Jews for the COVID-19 plague. A scrum of Baptist pastors launched a lawsuit against stay-home order, equating their domiciled status to detained Japanese Americans put into concentration camps during World War II.

The usual politics of distancing from social outsiders came back with a twist. Using a little-known law, Trump by executive order stopped all visas for foreign worker and international students on account of the novel coronavirus, a pincer on immigration that put the number of newcomers at historic lows. Pockets of Trump supporters accosted healthcare workers, blocking them from entering their workplaces, testifying to the ways underequipped medical professionals were on multitudinous frontlines—one against far-right populism and another against coronavirus/science denialism. Refusals to accept the pandemic's horrifying reality led to the squandering of millions of government dollars poured into "Rona 4 Real" and "This is Real" campaigns. Public service announcements repeated ad nauseum this simple truth: COVID-19 exists. Working from their own sense of the "viral real," many COVID-19 deniers were willing to die than to admit that.

Before COVID-19 found stature as public enemy number one, the nemesis of humanity had been already marked in the cultural Other. The spectral density of coronavirus as a foreign threat gained traction in efforts to target "bioterrorists," what Venezuela's government called emigrants returning from abroad. Via an encrypted messaging app called Telegram, neo-Nazis in the United States targeted law enforcement officers and communities of color for diabolical plots, which included obtaining spray bottles with COVID-19-infected saliva and putting them on door handles and elevator buttons.[48] In a precipitous move, the U.S. State Department designated for the first time a White ultranationalist group as a terrorist organization, the Russian

Imperial Movement. Among a parade of terrorizing global figures, the novel coronavirus spoke to the virality of international hate networks in an age of extremes.

Lacking foolproof solutions, most governmental efforts to contain SARS-CoV-2 came to nothing. With easy answers beyond reach, they fail to nourish alternative ideas outside the prism of war, often to their own demise. This failure portends a dire future for polarized societies mired in stifling power games. Presidential partisan politics made a show of force that politicized public health, rendering inoperable effective disease prevention.[49] When the problem is the buffoonery of leaders, the so-called war against COVID-19 will not go to plan. Commentators made bizarro comparisons of the tally of COVID-related deaths in April 2020 to the death toll of 9/11 attacks by Al-Qaeda, while the U.S. Surgeon General called the pandemic "our Pearl Harbor moment." When the number hit 200,000 deaths (September 22, 2020), comparisons were made to all fatalities in combat involving conflicts since the Korean War combined. Swathed in the acerbic rhetoric of war, the market imperative geared itself toward the viral contagion of militarism. "We're in a war to contain this virus ... everybody has the same common enemy across the whole world," said the CEO of Bank of America.[50] A viral world mobilized against disease was the opening salvo of a bigger conflict.

Pandemic messaging never fails to hew close to propaganda. It is thought that the deadliest pandemic in modern history was the "Spanish flu" of 1918. The disease lifted and took off in military barracks, caught up in the crosshairs of World War I. The flu reached its apotheosis in India, where independence leader Mohandas Gandhi was sickened.[51] India's British rulers found themselves in an unflattering position, ill-positioned to address an outsized crisis that fleeced 18 million lives. The pandemic fueled an independence movement with anti-imperialists using it as an opportunity to kick out colonizers.[52] With COVID-19, India experienced mass protests with homegrown oppressors and Hindu nationalists accused of recolonizing Muslim-majority areas. Hindsight, as the saying goes is 20/20, and 2020 was a palindrome year for looking back on bygone times. Within the fog of history, COVID-19 offered a rearview mirror to times gone wrong.

Tenacious diseases in wait strike down the most confident of skeptics. The Spanish flu brought down the leader of Brazil, a cautionary tale of how a pandemic is not an improbable event that can be taken lightly. An almost similar fate befell alpha men like Jair Bolsonaro and Donald Trump, both of whom survived COVID-19 after they bucked scientific opinion and trivialized health warnings. Time and again, leaders underestimated the superpower of a tiny piece of protein and RNA. Others who came down with the novel coronavirus were not so fortunate, such as the prime minister of Eswatini who died a month after announcing his positive test result. Trained on providing armed security instead of biosecurity, political figureheads took the selfish path, calling the usual shots without a clear path of action.

Despots believed the pandemic made them beyond reproach. They thought COVID-19 gave them untrammeled liberty to make decisions carte blanche and engage in abuses of power. From Sudan to Kazakhstan to Israel, military governments reined in human rights and civil liberties in the name of "public safety." As protests in Occupied Palestinian Territories pulsated with higher frequency, the longest ruling prime minister was swept out of office.[53] Benjamin Netanyahu would return to power in 2023 with a right-wing government that swerved further to the far right.[54] Hungary used this unparalleled crisis to forfeit civil rights. It did so in the name of protecting public health. Prime Minister Viktor Orban claimed at a press conference that COVID-19 is enough reason to abolish migrant asylum, making "a certain link between coronavirus and illegal migrants" (there were no confirmed cases in Hungary at the time of his statement).[55] Similar to the strident mode in Poland, Hungary voted to allow the prime minister to rule by unconstrained decree for as long as he sees fit. With no set time limits on executive power, new elections could not be held or anything that could "interfere with the protection of the public." Calling on special "emergency powers," Orban helped push through a ban on "propagandic" portrayals of transgenderism or homosexuality in education. These extremist measures launched protests and legal proceedings from the European Commission. Hungary had invited reprimand by European Union (EU) Parliament for breaching the continent's core democratic values. An op-ed piece in the *Washington Post* did not mince words when it said: "Coronavirus Kills Its First Democracy."[56]

Political propaganda circumvented slapdash efforts to bring emergency provisions to Iran, the West Asian country rocked most by COVID-19. Iran was verging on war with the United States and its neighbors. The call to combat promised to derail all and any methods to mitigate the coming pandemic. Iran's clerics claimed the United States was "weaponizing" the pandemic to further its imposed economic sanctions and choke the country's oil revenues. Both countries had teetered on the brink of open conflict before the pandemic as the United States government dealt a blow to a nuclear energy deal and put to death an Iranian general who had been targeting U.S. embassies. When the U.S. offered the olive branch of COVID-19 humanitarian aid, Supreme leader Ayatollah Ali Khamenei called U.S. leaders terrorists, charlatans, and liars before finishing with this missive: "Several times Americans have offered to help us to fight the pandemic. That is strange because you face shortages in America."[57] Given the perpetual enmity, it came to no surprise that Khamenei accused Americans of bringing medicines to spread poison since he believed the novel coronavirus was "specifically built for Iran using the genetic data of Iranians, which they have obtained through different means."[58] A propitious moment for rapprochement between Iran and United

States once seemed possible before. Standing in-between them now was a new third party: COVID-19.

While transfixed over who hatched the novel coronavirus, the United States and China were knee deep into a querulous trade war. The rudiments of this conflict were temporarily paused with a tariff-heavy trade deal signed five days before detection of the first case. The novel coronavirus could not slow viral contagion by other means, like spying, so tech apps like Tik Tok and WeChat were banned by the United States, even if they helped millions to connect and stay entertained amid the pandemic. China was bent on revenge with its own regime of sanctions against the United States. In controlling the pandemic story, Xi Jinping government's covert action delayed full cooperation with the WHO, speedily rewriting its status from global victim to world savior. When Jinping visited Wuhan to survey the situation six weeks after its lockdown, he waxed lyrical on how "daring to fight and daring to win is the Chinese Communist Party's distinct political character, and our distinct political advantage."[59]

That unstoppable will to fight by the CCP remains circumspect when it keeps at bay courageous voices. Much noise has been made online about the publication of the *Wuhan Diary*. Composed by acclaimed writer Fang Fang, the personal treatise gave a first-person eyewitness account during the initial outbreak. By celebrating the perseverance of the Wuhan people, the diary turned book stirred the political waters. Academics were investigated for posting or tweeting on social media about it. The book's elderly writer loudly reminded Wuhan's people that they did not bear alone the consequences or ignominy of this disaster. The "conscience of Wuhan," as Fang Fang was called, reminded the people that governments should not shake their faith in people power or pass over their feelings of rage either. Her most quoted line, which became the slogan for a soul-crushing quarantine was, "a grain of ash of the era, if it falls upon the head of an individual, will become a big mountain."[60]

The uphill mount to fight disease drove forward a battle of words and chest-pounding by capricious, pugilistic leaders. But such a test of mettle requires nimbleness, dexterity, flexibility, and common decency—qualities not exhibited by hard-liners. By this measure, COVID-19 came at a bad time, making its appearance at a juncture when ultra-conservative parties and boorish leaders triumphed on the world stage. Contested national elections across countries inspired new electoral rules, wedging open the question of who counts. The canards on Facebook against posting false information or incendiary material threatened to derail elections in Uganda, whose president harshly ruled his country for almost half a century. Uganda, Myanmar, Belarus, Ethiopia, and Venezuela blocked the social media platform ahead of their elections, preventing round-the-clock news and protests from going viral.

With ethnonationalist populism on the rise, established democratic republics used the pandemic to slide into greater repression and move toward the extreme right. Turkey, Poland, India, Russia, Brazil, Poland, Zimbabwe, the Philippines, Hungary, United Kingdom, and the United States elected authoritarians. In 2022, Italy ushered in a neo-fascist government. Nationalist populism was only the tip of the spear in a viral world in which political ideologies become viral and toxic. In the face of a big world full of worries and dangers, nations closed themselves off and shut their opponents down.

Civil liberties took a huge hit from the scaleback of democratic norms. The Democracy Index indicated that the hammer of freedom had swung lower in 2019, an abysmal year for representative democracy as a whole—its lowest rating since the survey began. Democratic governance was backsliding, caught in a most worrisome free fall.[61] In 2020, the United States had been reclassed by the Democracy Index as a "flawed democracy" (China sat at the bottom of the list). Despite the power of a pandemic as a change-agent, political tyranny was not going away soon, even with the changing of the guard. Alpha Conde, Guinea's first democratically elected authoritarian president had been deposed by military forces, which dissolved the constitution, closed all borders, and ordered a national curfew. This *coup d'état* was justified in the interest of protecting the people from COVID-19.

Economist Amartya Sen finds the project of building societal "capacities" should be based not on force but on diversity, information pluralism, and public reasoning.[62] Such capacities needed to contend with the *démarche* of sociopaths drunk on power and enthralled with their own godliness. From 2020 to 2021, Malaysia elected three different prime ministers. Voters flip-flopped on who would rule the Muslim-majority country after the resignation of the country's decades-long ruler, Mahathir Mohamed. Returning to power after being ousted in a major financial corruption scandal, Mohamed's United Malays National Organization (UMNO) took advantage of COVID-19 fears. Under the presidency of Gurbanguly Berdymukhamedov, Turkmenistan banned the word "coronavirus" from public utterance and arrested anyone from using it. Reporters Without Borders took the former rapper and quack doctor to task for violating human rights in a country ranked dead last for its World Press Index.[63]

Thailand registered the biggest drop overall in the Democracy Index. A declared "state of emergency" with imposed police curfews, media restrictions seemed almost redundant in a country that had only a few years before experienced a military coup. Under a general-turned-prime minister, public faith in the grassroots-driven healthcare system kept COVID-19 infection to a minimum, but it did little to halt pro-democracy protests. With blessings of the pro-royalist military junta ruling on behalf of King Rama X in absentia, the monarch stayed with an entourage of consorts in lavish

German Bavarian hotels, while his people suffered under the rule of the novel coronavirus.

The King governed from afar and the ruling military government slammed any political opposition. In the first month of 2021, a former Thai civil servant was sentenced to 87 years in prison for criticizing the royal family under the world's toughest *lèse-majesté* or "injured sovereignty" laws. Thai citizens wondered why so few people were vaccinated, when tourism hot spots encouraged vaccinated foreign visitors to come vacation in their pandemic-hurt country. Thai people wanted more COVID-19 shots, but also more women's rights, freedom of speech, and economic protection. Like so many in the world, they received stiffer jail sentences and prison time for their just demands.

Prisons

The arduous work in combatting pandemic propaganda compels the world to move toward greater trust, versatility, dialogue, and tolerance. By this criteria, COVID-19 might have come at the worst possible time. Word of the pandemic broke when Britain's fate hung in the balance, as the United Kingdom proposed steps to leave the EU in the drawn-out debacle known as "Brexit." China's leader Xi Jinping's upswell in political clout extended his rulership indefinitely. Nixing term limits, Jinping ascended to de facto "emperor for life." Despite differing political systems and ideological orientations, constitutional democracies shared a steadfast commitment to concentrating wealth and power, as did one-party states and absolutist monarchies.

These governments exploited pandemic politics to inveigh against old "enemies of the state." Cambodia, Venezuela, Thailand, and Bangladesh detained or expelled journalists who dared to question tepid government responses to COVID-19. This censoring delimits prevention messaging. Russia banned all form of protest, and Algeria blocked demonstrations for democratic reforms. Dictatorships tailored their reparative metrics to the pandemic's tumult. In the twisted mind of megalomaniacs, sometimes we must kill the people to "save" them. If not outright killed, they could be put in prisons to die out a slow tortuous death by COVID-19.

The novel coronavirus failed to tear up the dictator's playbook and unseat self-enthroned rulers. In 2021, Putin signed a law that reset his presidential terms and allow him to remain in power. This "back to zero" move was justified on the grounds that Putin was a stabilizing force against social turbulence, COVID-related or not. Political maneuvers could not fool citizens who staged the biggest protests in a generation. The Russian president abducted opposition leaders in exile and poisoned his main rival with toxic nerve agent.[64] Thousands of Russians braved COVID-19 to fight back, but they too were thrown in jail.

In Zimbabwe, a country ruled by Robert Mugabe for nearly four decades, protestors against authoritarianism were arrested under COVID-19 protections by Mugabe's chosen successor. The leaders of Ivory Coast and Guinea likewise ran for third terms, after pushing constitutional changes to term limits and disqualifying opposing candidates. Uganda's elder statesman bent the rules, pressing parliament to rid an age limit so that he could be reelected in 2021. Media censorship mushroomed under carceral regimes ready to impose a permanent lockdown. As people went into quarantine for the first time in their lives, millions were locked up for political reasons.

Carceral states put a premium on the strategy of maximum containment and pandemic separation. As everyday folks stayed still at home, people held captive in prisons faced pressures to remain perilously in "their place." Incarcerated populations remained under strict watch, even though the novel coronavirus promised to make prison life demonstrably worse for them. Public efforts to bottle up and contain the virus fell upon those held in human cages. Despite having 4% of the entire human population, the United States contained a quarter of all COVID-19 cases on the planet. This percentage would be entirely shocking if not for the fact that this number mirrors the country's other ugly aspects such as its extreme incarceration rates, the highest in the world (and one-fifth of all the world's prisoners). Pandemic prevention in this context became swept under the aegis of mass incarceration.

While the world was under lockdown, evil government agencies were busy trying to lock up more people. Jails crowded with political resisters and activists. Hundreds of protestors who marched against quarantine received a permit by the state highway patrol to march on California's capitol, even though other groups like Black Lives Matter (BLM) had been rejected out of respect for stay-at-home orders. A member of Trump's economic council compared the riled-up upstarts to civil rights leaders, while one woman in Orange County, California held up a sign bearing the message: "Social distancing = Communism."

The scale of mass agitation in the United States Bears similarity with far-right protestors from the Vox Party in Spain, a party hostile to women and migrant rights. It gained its first parliamentary seats in 2019 to become the third largest party, rivaling the left-wing parties of the Socialist Workers and Unity We Can. Rabble-rousers descended onto the capital of Madrid, plying the prosaic language of freedom and justice in a "Caravan for Spain and Liberty," while calling home confinement a violation of their constitutional rights, something to which a government spokesperson sarcastically recast as the "right to infect."[65] Leading Vox ideologues fell ill after orchestrating a massive rally in 2020, then apologized for the gun-toting infectious public event. The rowdy yahoos then blamed authorities for not warning enough about coronavirus dangers.

Waving Confederate flags and brandishing swastika signs, anti-government groups in the United States thronged into the capitol of Michigan, attempting to kidnap the intrepid governor, who had just announced a program of free college tuition for workers called "Futures for Frontliners."[66] Early in 2021, a mob of supporters for Donald Trump stormed the federal capitol building in a spoiled coup, a spectacle repeated in Brazil after its presidential elections in 2023. As an insurrection against the formal vote for President-elect Joe Biden, this disgraceful assault on the democratic transition of power met wide opprobrium. Currying favor with White nationalists, Trump as the Republican standard-bearer stood resolute in his support for perpetrators. Through the language of false equivalence, Trump again described these putschists and fringe elements as patriots and "great people." Anti-quarantine "covidiots" were given free rein to move about carelessly.

A far-reaching virus deemed as "foreign" brings back into picture the ideological tug-of-war between liberty and death. The state's life-or-death calculations interprets this dualism as struggle as over who can be saved or killed openly, who obtains protection or waste away in prison. Manipulative polities with a strong penal code found a way to pull its "death-making" power alongside the pandemic's crushing current. In the military state of Myanmar, hundreds of protesters were killed and imprisoned for affirming a landslide election victory for the ruling National League for Democracy and its leader, Aung San Suu Kyi. After dwelling under house arrest for over a decade before, the Nobel Peace Prize winner was confined again after an army coup declared a state of emergency. Through martial law, the junta assumed control, restricting political protests while installing orders to quarantine. However, government employees stopped working, and protestors brought fire to the streets. Hundreds died by the barrel of armed troops, if not by the bowels of a virus. Too many citizens were sent away, never to be seen again.

Dictatorial governments pulled out the stops to hold people hostage in their own homes (or prisons) and forced them to follow their whims. Ruled by the same party since 1986, Uganda halted all public transport and enlisted a paramilitary outfit, the Local Defense Unit (LDU), to help the police and army enforce curfews. Under the auspices of extinguishing the flame of COVID-19, Ugandan security defense forces deployed excessive force and tactics ranging from arbitrary detainment to public flogging. Police shot construction workers in Mukono for riding motorcycle taxis and raided a shelter for houseless lesbian, gay, bisexual, and transgender youth in Wakiso, closing the space and beating the occupants for living in cramped nonphysically distant quarters, even though there was nowhere to go for many of them. Wielding intimidation and surveillance as a blunt instrument of crowd control, President Yoweri Kaguta Museveni gave this bluster to police in addressing the country: "Beating is illegal and pointless, what are you beating for? I don't have to depend on you because my cameras are everywhere ... If you are not doing your work, we shall get you."[67]

While Museveni asked landlords to not evict people, such pandemic paternalism was buried beneath another message that he publicly gave—about how the autocratic state does not need to depend upon its security forces because it is all-powerful and all-seeing. This sends a message about lack of freedom in Uganda. COVID-19 lockdown, viewed most notably in the capital of Kampala, reflected another phase of rule by a demagogue.

Iran released thousands of prisoners from the pandemic's death trap. This contrived public act of mercy did not make up for the fact that in 2019 it laid a four-decade prison term (and 148 lashes) for human rights lawyer Nasrin Sotoudeh, a proponent for ending the death penalty and for women to appear in public without the hijab. Journalists, lawyers, and activists in Iran and the world protested in the streets after the death of Mahsa Amini. The young Kurdish-Iranian woman was in custody of the morality policy for not wearing a headscarf. Weeks after her death, Iran sent drone strikes to target Kurdish groups in northern Iraq, a move that implores global watchers to connect the personal to the political. Protests are part of the "fractured locus" of a *pandemic-prison-industrial complex*, in which pandemics offer the excuse for continued attacks on freedom and mass incarceration.[68]

The pandemic cauldron of mass detention and far-right politics formed the crux for a "global burning."[69] Indonesia arrested a West Papua activist for protesting front of the presidential palace in Jakarta (sentenced in a virtual hearing due to quarantine). The Black Lives Matter movement inspired the call for the Papuan Lives Matter movement.[70] West Papuans were placed under lockdown, due to both the novel coronavirus and colonialism. Emotive banners in Indonesia declaring infectiology and the need for communal hygiene obscured the real danger to internally colonized subjects. The *pandemic worlding* of public spaces in Indonesia—through billboards, posters, and news reports—shifted human conduct in ways that not only corseted physical movement but also managed their social and emotional life within certain viral "orders of feeling."[71]

Authoritarian regimes were not going away soon, even with efforts to oust them.[72] In summer 2019, Hong Kong activist Joshua Wong ran afoul of political authorities and could not avoid jailtime for civil disobedience. Resisting Beijing's effort to supplant local academic curriculum with communist orthodoxy, Wong called into question the prison of communist (mis)education and an axed extradition proposal to bring criminals from the special administrative region to mainland China for prison sentencing. A disdainful Beijing clamped down on people as they rose up against violations of Hong Kong's unique autonomous status.

The pandemic provided cover for a new round of police terror. On April 18, 2020, Hong Kong police rounded up leaders of the pro-democracy movement for protests months earlier, including the former chairs of the Democratic Party, the Civic Party, and Labor Party. While finalizing the stipulations of Brexit and leaving the European Union, the United Kingdom offered citizenship to Hong Kongers to flee the clutches of the Communist Party.

Foot patrols in mainland China did little to muffle social unrest. Quarantine rechanneled some parts of asymmetrical warfare into new online platforms such as the Nintendo game Animal Crossing: New Horizons, a simulation game where players live on customized tropical island where they build houses and interact with anthropomorphized animals (an apt metaphor for zoonosis). The world-making game was pulled by regulators from China's e-commerce market, as did the video game called Plague Inc., in which players unleash a pathogen to disrupt the planet. On Animal Crossing, Joshua Wong shared images of Xi Jinping and the WHO's head at a funeral with the sign "Wuhan pneumonia." He also put up a screen capture on Twitter of his animated island with the banner "Free Hong Kong, Revolution Now!"[73] The CCP introduced new laws that banned online gaming to curtail freedoms and activists through unregulated online spaces. Mandatory quarantine reworks the power of world-building games and digital activism as jailed leaders were forced to operate behind the computer screen.

Beijing's office in Hong Kong accused protestors of holding up or arresting capitalism. It frowned upon a grassroots campaign to mobilize over 2,000 pro-democracy shops as an organized economic response to the absence of tourists during coronavirus travel restrictions. A CCP spokesperson claimed activists did "scorched-earth politics with politics kidnapping the economy."[74] Banned from protesting in malls, Wong on Twitter indicated that shoppers were not trampling the free market, but actually living up to its cherished axioms. Nothing, not even a pandemic on the ascendant, could slow down the police state and its capitalistic tendencies. Hong Kong rebels were called a "political virus" for promoting the "poisonous" notion that "if we burn, then you burn with us."[75] Under the gravitational pull of COVID-19, elites arrayed themselves against commoners.

Some tribunes failed miserably in the pandemic's test of courage, but others won. Hong Kong's leader, Carrie Lam, misused the language of freedom of expression—pledging six months of jail for violators of Hong Kong's zero-tolerance quarantine—while backing anti-sedition laws to ban any disrespect toward China. Warning foreign countries from interfering in local affairs, Lam put Beijing's interests above her own constituents. She promised prison time for treason, while calling the dissidents "spoiled children." The patronizing tone set the stage for more protests by infuriated residents.

In the state of California, the governor ordered a mandatory shelter-in-place. The Golden State led the national charge and other states quickly followed. Newsom, who survived a recall election, assured his constituents, "This is a not a permanent state, this is a moment in time."[76] Semi-permanence of a lockdown did not apply to prisoners. The term lockdown had been used for years in places like California with "zero tolerance" toward crime, which caused a frisson of "moral panic" and an increase in incarcerated people of color.[77] Under a two-week "soft" lockdown in California's prisons, exhausted prison nurses ran ragged with countless rules, working overtime in a dangerous environment. Over 70% of inmates at all federal prisons tested positive, while 96% of inmates did at Lompoc Federal Correctional Complex in California, the country's viral hot spot for the incarcerated population. In a Faustian bargain, California's governor gave prisoners a "choice" of putting down and extinguishing burning forests or face down COVID-19 in the hot tinderbox of prisons. In a cruel twist of fate, they could elect to die by fire or perish in the infernal pit of prison. This executive decision came in the form of a subtle death warrant, even after a push by activists to cancel prisoner involuntary servitude. By ignoring an unmitigated disaster, dishonest politicians and inept business dealers made a bad situation woefully worse.[78]

The pandemic rewrote the global rules of engagement even as it cemented some. For California's incarcerated populations, their pandemic vulnerability was not a moment punctuated by COVID-time, since their lives already presented a semipermanent arrested state of being. The media reinterpreted Governor Newsom's order of home stay as a "lockdown," even though he did not use those exact words. Lockdown is terminology common to prison work, used to describe when prisoners are restricted from moving to corral inmates within dangerous situations. It could also mean putting an individual into solitary confinement for breaking the rules. The imprisoned knew this term all too well.

Lockdown was not tenable a solution to keep prisoners isolated from the novel coronavirus. Reformers goaded the governor to release inmates, especially the elderly and sick or those prisoners there for petty crimes. Incarcerated people took a big hit from the pandemic, which is why the state released up to 8,000 prisoners. The imprisoned population faced an early death sentence from crowded quarters without physical distancing. Los Angeles County Jail, the largest jail system in the world, ended court fees and debt collection, truncating its number of arrests as to stem the staggering rate of infections.[79] Yet, many more people remained in perpetual "lockdown."

Early on with COVID-19, meager attention had been paid to incarcerated populations, but they were core to unraveling the granular strands of the pandemic (and putting it all together). While Beirut had been rocked by a blast from the accidental detonation of improperly stored ammonium nitrate at a port, which received international attention, the incarcerated people at Lebanon's two largest prisons demanded release and amnesty. A parallel situation was found in Sudan, given the lockup of protestors and a new transitional government after the ouster of President Omar al-Bashir. Social inequality is baked into trouble-ridden societies beset by problems, especially when incarceration is transformed into "bio-inequality."[80] As prison studies scholar Martha Escobar observes, criminalization is woven into the everyday life of "undesirables," hinged upon "the ordinary" incarnations of danger, disposability, and death-row. [81]

Increased media attention to prisoners amid the pandemic did not shake governments out of their old patterns. The latter staggered on, with little regard for prisoners and treating them like removable commodities or objects of moral uplift (U.S. COVID-19 stimulus packages contained educational grants for prisoners without addressing the problems of prison enclosure). The United States and Iran negotiated prisoner swaps, while the Afghan government released Taliban prisoners as part of a brokered peace deal. The U.S. carceral state never released inmates *en masse* from its surveillance, prioritizing home confinement. This order put thousands of felons with underlying health conditions in home stay, such as Trump's former campaign chairman who was convicted of bank fraud. The Emergency Community Supervision Act decreased individuals in federal custody during a national emergency relating to a communicable disease and placed them in community supervision.

Incarcerated subjects were part of a pandemic state of exception. A live-streamed video on Facebook of detainees Karim Golding and Tesfa Miller standing on a ledge with roped bedding around their necks went viral. After a prolonged wait for sanctuary, the asylum-seekers threatened to hang themselves in objection to conditions at Alabama's Etowah Detention Center. Fed up with the prison's decision to lock down but refused testing for the novel coronavirus, Miller hoped to make it out alive to visit his daughter: "We're so far removed from everything else, it's like nobody notices. Nobody even knows that we're here, and we're just hoping that we can make it out of this place alive. These are the things that keep me fighting." No one came to rescue the men, their cry for help and distress signal to the world discounted by guards, worrying themselves about catching COVID-19.

> We're the last people to get protected. If we die, so what? This is the black hole. The entire system is working to keep this facility open because this is their money. This is politics at its finest ... Burials are cheaper than deportations,

said Golding, originally from Jamaica.[82] This quote speaks to the ways the advocacy of capitalism and mass imprisonment came together. In spite of the drastic downturn of financial markets, the prison-industrial complex remained firmly intact, especially after the ousted governor of New York, Andrew Cuomo, advertised that hand sanitizer made in prisons was superior to products on the market.

For the masses of prisoners forced further into private retreat and obscurity, pandemic lockdown drove home their status as exploitable labor. China's *cordons sanitaires* for Wuhan's residents differed from the gulags erected for its ethnoreligious minorities. Millions of Uyghurs had already been placed in concentration camps (billed as vocational training centers) due to fears of Islamic terrorism. They were rerouted to factories bereft of Han workers due to COVID-19 quarantine. A nosedive for China's manufacturing base morphed the Uyghur people into a reserve army of coerced labor, responsible for cycling through raw materials for a global supply chain weakened by pandemic disruptions. Those chains were tangled up with U.S. companies like Nike, Apple, and Coca Cola. On top of reports of forced sterilization, these concentration camps served to additionally enact demographic genocide and forced indoctrination. These practices drew opprobrium from the U.N. and the U.S. Senate, the latter introducing a bill over this human rights issue. Even if SARS-CoV-2 made powerful countries kneel, it did not send the world's second biggest economy careening. The mighty dragon was slightly brought to heel by the infinitesimal virus, tapping into an exploited minority to fuel its economy.

When we talk about viral worlds, we must also work out how certain social groups and cultural ideas are rendered as dangerous viruses, needing to be kept out of the world by keeping them domiciled. A Chinese biomedical firm was given responsibility for sequencing SARS-CoV-2, building a "Xinjian gene bank" and supplying millions of COVID-19 tests to over 80 countries.[83] Information-sharing about COVID-19 looped back into vast troves of biodata on ethnic/domestic terrorists.[84] The Xi Jinping government forced Uyghur labor to keep its factories churning out products, while the Han ethnic majority stayed home. The mistreatment of Uyghurs directs attention to the detainment of persecuted ethnoreligious groups in China, a country that contains the most political prisoners, many of whom are locked up for merely expressing free speech and thought. It expulsed international reporters to tighten its hold on the media, keeping at bay any bad press about COVID-19 and concentration camps. China's lockdown flattened its epidemiological curve but did not raise the bar of hope for tortured prisoners.

Freedom is still possible through direct action and activism. But how are such things possible for communities locked outside of society and global governance? Just as COVID-19 changed everything, abolition as a global project resurged to take on the entire reality of a world under lockdown. The undoing of all that ails us, according to prison studies scholar Ofelia Cueva, is possible through abolition as "a worldmaking and world building project," one that can help you become a subject "in the world free from pain, from worry, from anxiety, from alienation."[85] Abolition as world-making offers a source of power for prisoners and their advocates. Activist-scholar Ruth Gilmore said as much: it requires that we change everything from the ground up, not just police and prisons but also schools, housing, art, and work. To build a truly "free world" and make freedom *infectious*, she advocates that we change "the ways people think about the world ... [and] what they do to endure or change the world."[86]

Insofar as humanness presents a property that one can own, the lack of it evidences how freedom is central to *pandemic personhood*, the ways that infectious individuals are moral agents with blameworthy or praiseworthy actions. Prisoners exist on the other side of the grid of humanity since "their personhood is erased and inverted, rendering them nonpersons, beings devoid of futures."[87] For people both locked in and out of "the system," the real fight is freedom from violence and want. COVID-19 lockdown as a means to "protect humanity" promised indefinite uncertain futures for those most isolated people on the planet.

As more people increasingly stayed indoors, some compared their own homes to a prison, while others were actually sent to prison for leaving their homes. Archival projects like the Prison Pandemic Project allowed prisoners to cope with quarantine and unsanitary conditions by sharing their experiences "from the inside" of prison to the outside world.[88] The wall between the public outside and private inside blurred with new lines of command. The effect of this global convergence—what I call viral worlding—shreds the idea that we all were on the same page. Without working together, people could not stay ahead of the pandemic's curve to flatten it.

Notes

1 Patt Morrison, "What the Deadly 1918 Flu Epidemic Can Teach Us about Our Coronavirus Reaction," *Gulf News*, March 15, 2020, https://gulfnews.com/opin ion/op-eds/what-the-deadly-1918-flu-epidemic-can-teach-us-about-our-coronavi rus-reaction-1.70313751

2 Danièle Bélanger and Rachel Silvey. "An Im/mobility Turn: Power Geometries of Care and Migration," *Journal of Ethnic and Migration Studies* 46, no. 16 (2020): 3423–3440.

3 Laurie Garrett, *The Coming Plague: Newly Emerging Diseases in a World Out of Balance* (New York: Macmillan, 1994): 178.

4 The adviser left the administration soon after along with scores of other purged long-time staff. A hostile atmosphere for medical experts, environmental data collection, and scientific enterprise incited global marches for science.

5 Jennifer Terry. *Attachments to War* (Durham, NC: Duke University Press, 2017) 151.

6 Deirdre Shesgreen, " 'Gross Misjudgment': Experts Say Trump's Decision to Disband Pandemic Team Hindered Coronavirus Response," *USA Today*, March 18, 2020, www.usatoday.com/story/news/world/2020/03/18/coronavirus-did-president-trumps-decision-disband-global-pandemic-office-hinder-response/506 4881002/

7 The letter represented eight leaders and nearly 2,000 communities. Maria Cervantes, "Peru Indigenous Warn of 'Ethnocide by Inaction' as Coronavirus Hits Amazon Tribes," *Reuters*, April 24, 2020, www.reuters.com/article/us-hea lth-coronavirus-peru-indigenous/peru-indigenous-warn-of-ethnocide-by-inaction-as-coronavirus-hits-amazon-tribes-idUSKCN22639A

8 Paul Amar, "Turning the Gendered Politics of the Security State Inside Out?" *International Feminist Journal of Politics* 13, no. 3 (2011): 299–328.

9 Georgina Laud, "Coronavirus Explained: Why Is It Called Coronavirus? What Does Corona Mean?" *Express*, March 20, 2020, www.express.co.uk/life-style/ health/1241302/Coronavirus-named-COVID-19-meaning-WHO-coronavirus-lat est-update

10 Samuel Roberts, *Infectious Fear: Politics, Disease, and the Health Effects of Segregation* (Chapel Hill: University of North Carolina Press, 2009).

11 Jennifer Terry, *Attachments to War: Biomedical Logics and Violence in Twenty-First-Century America* (Durham, NC: Duke University Press, 2017): 26.

12 World Health Organization. Report of the WHO-China Joint Mission on Coronavirus Disease 2019 (COVID-19), February 16–24, 2020, 16, www.who. int/docs/default-source/coronaviruse/who-china-joint-mission-on-covid-19-final-report.pdf

13 Joel Rubin, "Coronavirus Misinformation and Hoax Text Messages Are Making the Rounds. Here's How to Spot Them," *Los Angeles Times*, March 18, 2020, www.latimes.com/california/story/2020-03-18/coronavirus-martial-law-email-message-hoax

14 Ian Millhiser, "The Fake Text Message about the 'Stafford Act' and a National Quarantine, Explained: Don't Believe Everything You Read Online," *Vox*, March 16, 2020, www.vox.com/2020/3/16/21181486/stafford-act-text-mess age-hoax-coronavirus-national-quarantine-trump; Joel Rubin, "Coronavirus Misinformation and Hoax Text Messages are Making the Rounds. Here's How to Spot Them," *Los Angeles Times*, March 18, 2020, www.latimes.com/california/ story/2020-03-18/coronavirus-martial-law-email-message-hoax

15 "PBS NewsHour," full episode, *PBS NewsHour*, April 22, 2020, www.youtube. com/watch?v=h3Xli0HpdGU

16 Laignee Barron, "What We Can Learn from Singapore, Taiwan and Hong Kong about Handling Coronavirus," *Time*, March 13, 2020, https://time.com/5802 293/coronavirus-covid19-singapore-hong-kong-taiwan/

17 CNA. "COVID-19: Singapore Concerned as Some Countries Have Given up on Containment, Says Minister," March 15, 2020, www.youtube.com/watch?v= AxAuMEo5XTs&feature=youtu.be

18 Joyce C.H. Liu, "Irregular Population and the Aporia of Communities," *University of California Humanities Research Institute*, May 2019, https://uchri. org/foundry/irregular-population-and-the-aporia-of-communities-toward-a-criti que-of-internal-coloniality-in-the-age-of-neoliberal-capitalism/

19 Shashank Bengali, "From 'Gold Standard' to a Coronavirus 'Explosion': Singapore Battles New Outbreak" *Los Angeles Times*, April 14, 2020, www.latimes. com/world-nation/story/2020-04-14/coronavirus-surges-migrant-workers-in-singapore

20 Jamila Michener, *Fragmented Democracy: Medicaid, Federalism, and Unequal Politics* (Cambridge: Cambridge University Press, 2018).

21 Jane Arraf, "Jordan Keeps Coronavirus in Check with One of the World's Strictest Lockdowns," *NPR*, March 25, 2020, www.npr.org/sections/coronavirus-live updates/2020/03/25/821349297/jordan-keeps-coronavirus-in-check-with-one-of-world-s-strictest-lockdowns; Leif Weatherby, "Delete Your Account: On the Theory of Platform Capitalism," *Los Angeles Review of Books*, April 24, 2018, https://lareviewofbooks.org/article/delete-your-account-on-the-theory-of-platform-capitalism/#!*97

22 Shoshana Zuboff, *The Age of Surveillance Capitalism: The Fight for a Human Future at the New Frontier of Power* (London: Profile Books, 2019).

23 Motoko Rich, "Why Asia's New Wave of Virus Cases Should Worry the World," *New York Times*, March 31, 2020, www.nytimes.com/2020/03/31/world/asia/coronavirus-china-hong-kong-singapore-south-korea.html

24 Hannah Beech, "Tracking the Coronavirus: How Crowded Asian Cities Tackled an Epidemic," *New York Times*, March 17, 2020, www.nytimes.com/2020/03/17/world/asia/coronavirus-singapore-hong-kong-taiwan.html

25 Lily Kuo, "Coronavirus: Wuhan Doctor Speaks Out against Authorities," *The Guardian*, March 11, 2020, https://amp.theguardian.com/world/2020/mar/11/coronavirus-wuhan-doctor-ai-fen-speaks-out-against-authorities

26 Chris Buckley, "Chinese Doctor, Silenced after Warning of Outbreak, Dies from Coronavirus," *New York Times*, February 6, 2020, www.nytimes.com/2020/02/06/world/asia/chinese-doctor-Li-Wenliang-coronavirus.html

27 Amy Cheng, "Chinese Authorities Admit Improper Response to Coronavirus Whistleblower," *NPR*, March 19, 2020, www.npr.org/sections/coronavirus-live-updates/2020/03/19/818295972/chinese-authorities-admit-improper-response-to-coronavirus-whistleblower

28 Steven Lee Myers, "China Created a Fail-Safe System to Track Contagions. It Failed," March 29, 2020, www.nytimes.com/2020/03/29/world/asia/coronavirus-china.html

29 Tanner Brown, "Inside China's Campaign to Blame the U.S. for the Coronavirus Pandemic," *Marketwatch*, March 15, 2020, www.marketwatch.com/story/inside-chinas-campaign-to-blame-the-us-for-the-coronavirus-pandemic-2020-03-15

30 The original *Global Times* article was replaced with one from U.S. Centers for Disease Control and Prevention's denial of the TV Asahi report, but the *People's Daily* reprint of this article was published on conspiracy website GlobalResearch.ca, titled "China's Coronavirus: A Shocking Update. Did the Virus Originate in the US?"; Robert Boxwell, "How China's Fake News Machine Is Rewriting the History of Covid-19, Even as the Pandemic Unfolds," *Politico*, April 4, 2020, www.politico.com/news/ magazine/2020/04/04/china-fake-news-coronavirus-164652

31 Sean Iling, "'Flood the Zone with Shit': How Misinformation Overwhelmed Our Democracy," *Vox*, February 6, 2020, www.vox.com/policy-and-politics/2020/1/16/20991816/impeachment-trial-trump-bannon-misinformation

32 A *Nature* report discovered 96% identical genome structure to a bat coronavirus. An "engineered" virus would resemble previously known coronaviruses, which it did not.

33 Leonard A. Cole, *Clouds of Secrecy: The Army's Germ Warfare Tests Over Populated Areas* (Louisville, KY: Rowman & Littlefield, 1990); Jonathan D. Moreno, *Undue Risk: Secret State Experiments on Humans* (London: Routledge, 2013); Allen M. Hornblum, Judith L. Newman, and Gregory J. Dober, *Against*

Their Will: The Secret History of Medical Experimentation on Children in Cold War America (New York: Macmillan, 2013).

34 Charles "Sam" Faddis, "Bioterror: We Aren't Ready," *The Hill*, February 19, 2020, https://thehill.com/opinion/national-security/483506-bioterror-we-arent-ready

35 Samantha Maiden, "Chinese State Media Labels Australia 'the Dog of the United States,'" News.com.au, May 20, 2020, www.news.com.au/world/coronavirus/glo bal/chinese-state-media-labels-australia-the-dog-of-the-united-states/news-story/ fb1464c8a04b61e8863038c7d0dada84

36 Derek Thompson, "Mass Shootings in America are Spreading Like a Disease," *The Atlantic*, November 6, 2017, www.theatlantic.com/health/archive/2017/11/ americas-mass-shooting-epidemic-contagious/545078/

37 A mass stabbing followed involving two men who killed more than 10 people on the territory of the Cree Nation and other areas in Western Canada.

38 Achille Mbembe, Diogo Bercito, "'The Pandemic Democratizes the Power to Kill,' an Interview," *European Journal of Psychoanalysis*. Originally published in *Gauchazh* on March 31, 2020, www.journal-psychoanalysis.eu/the-pandemic-democratizes-the-power-to-kill-an-intyerview/

39 T.C. Sottek, "The Coronavirus Is Now the American Virus," *The Verge*, March 26, 2020, www.theverge.com/2020/3/26/21196267/coronavirus-usa-cases-covid-19-pandemic-china-number-positive-trump

40 Chinese American CBS reporter Weijia Jiang tweeted that a member of the Trump administration called the coronavirus "Kung-Flu" when speaking to her (a social media user came up with the term Flu Klux Klan as a witty rebuttal to this race-baiting). www.cnn.com/2020/03/18/opinions/trumps-malicious-use-of-chinese-virus-filipovic/index.html

41 CNN, "READ: Trump's Oval Office Speech on the Coronavirus Outbreak," *CNN*, March 11, 2020, www.cnn.com/2020/03/11/politics/read-trump-coronavi rus-address/index.html

42 Jessie Yeung, Helen Regan, Adam Renton, Emma Reynolds, and Fernando Alfonso III, "March 19 Coronavirus News," *CNN*, March 19, 2020, www.cnn. com/world/live-news/coronavirus-outbreak-03-19-20-intl-hnk/h_21c623966 aa148dbeed242de4e94943e

43 David Smith, "Trump Claims 99% of US Covid-19 Cases Are 'Totally Harmless' as Infections Surge," *The Guardian*, July 4, 2020, https://amp.theguardian.com/ world/2020/jul/05/trump-claims-99-of-us-covid-19-cases-are-totally-harmless-as-infections-surge

44 Mary Papenfuss, "Trump Reportedly Weighed Letting COVID-19 'Wash Over' U.S., but Was Warned of Grim Toll," *HuffPost*, April 4, 2020, www.huffpost.com/ entry/trump-free-range-covid-19-death-toll_n_5e925a48c5b6f7b1ea82dcd7

45 Justin Wise, "Fauci on Trump Coronavirus Comments: 'I Can't Jump in Front of the Microphone and Push Him Down,'" *The Hill*, March 23, 2020, https://theh ill.com/homenews/administration/488961-fauci-on-trump-coronavirus-comme nts-i-cant-jump-in-front-of-the

46 In a briefing to governors, the contrarian leader made a comment roundly rejected, one that claimed as president his "authority is total." Remarks by President Trump, Vice President Pence, and Members of the Coronavirus Task Force in Press Briefing, April 10, 2020, www.whitehouse.gov/briefings-statements/remarks-president-trump-vice-president-pence-members-coronavirus-task-force-press-briefing-24/

47 Davin L. Phoenix, *The Anger Gap: How Race Shapes Emotion in Politics* (Cambridge: Cambridge University Press: 2019).

48 Peter Wade, "Just When You Thought Things Couldn't Get Worse, Neo-Nazis Are Trying to Weaponize Coronavirus," *Rollingstone*, March 22, 2020, www.rollingstone.com/politics/politics-news/neo-nazis-are-trying-to-weaponize-the-coronavirus-971002/

49 Shana Kushner Gadarian, Sara Wallace Goodman, and Thomas B. Pepinsky, *Pandemic Politics: The Deadly Toll of Partisanship in the Age of COVID* (Princeton, NJ: Princeton University Press, 2022).

50 Fred Imbert, "Bank of America CEO Moynihan Says 'We're in a War to Contain This Virus,'" CNBC.com, March 15, 2020, www.cnbc.com/2020/03/15/bank-of-america-ceo-moynihan-says-were-in-a-war-to-contain-this-virus.html

51 Laura Spinney, *Pale Rider: The Spanish Flu of 1918 and How It Changed the World* (New York: Public Affairs, 2017).

52 Shyam A. Krishna, "How the Spanish Flu Changed the Course of Indian History," *Gulf News*, March 15, 2020, https://gulfnews.com/opinion/op-eds/how-the-spanish-flu-changed-the-course-of-indian-history-1.1584285312898

53 With the dissolving of parliament and the collapse of coalition governments, Israel held five elections in the first three years of the pandemic.

54 Israel renewed for another year the Citizenship and Entry into Israel Law, an emergency law passed in 2003 which denies the right to family life and prohibits Israeli citizens married to Palestinians from the West Bank or Gaza Strip from living with their spouse. This follows the recent nation-state of the Jewish People Law.

55 Lillo Montalto Monella and Rita Palfi, "Orban Uses Coronavirus as Excuse to Suspend Asylum Rights in Hungary," *Euronews*, March 3, 2020, www.euronews.com/2020/03/03/orban-uses-coronavirus-as-excuse-to-suspend-asylum-rights-in-hungary

56 Ishaan Tharoor, "Coronavirus Kills Its First Democracy," *Washington Post*, March 30, 2020. www.washingtonpost.com/world/2020/03/31/coronavirus-kills-its-first-democracy/

57 Parisa Hafezi, "Iran's Khamenei Rejects U.S. Help Offer, Vows to Defeat Coronavirus," *Reuters*, March 22, 2020, www.reuters.com/article/us-health-coronavirus-iran/irans-khamenei-rejects-us-help-offer-vows-to-defeat-coronavirus-idUSKBN21909Y

58 Aljazeera, "Iran Leader Refuses US Help; Cites Coronavirus Conspiracy Theory," *Aljazeera*, March 23, 2020, www.aljazeera.com/news/2020/03/iran-leader-refuses-cites-coronavirus-conspiracy-theory-200322145122752.html

59 Vivian Wang, "China-Writer-Fang-Fang-Closes-Wuhan-Coronavirus-Lockdown-Diary," *MSN*, April 8, 2020, www.msn.com/en-us/news/world/china-writer-fang-fang-closes-wuhan-coronavirus-lockdown-diary/ar-BB11JB7L; Vivian Wang, "China's Coronavirus Battle Is Waning. Its Propaganda Fight Is Not," *New York Times*, April 8, 2020, www.nytimes.com /2020/04/08/world/asia/coronavirus-china-narrative.html

60 Jane Li, "China Writer Fang Closes Wuhan Coronavirus Lockdown Diary," March 26, 2020, https://qz.com/1825896/china-writer-fang-fang-closes-wuhan-coronavirus-lockdown-diary

61 Marc Montgomery, "2020 World Democracy Index: Worrisome Decline," *RCI*, January 27, 2020, www.rcinet.ca/en/2020/01/27/2020-world-democracy-index-worrisome-decline/

62 Amartya Sen, "Human Rights and Capabilities," *Journal of Human Development* 6, no. 2 (2005): 151–166.

63 Joanna Kakissis, "Turkmenistan Has Banned Use of the Word 'Coronavirus,'" *NPR*, March 31, 2020, www.npr.org/sections/coronavirus-live-updates/2020/03/31/824611607/turkmenistan-has-banned-use-of-the-word-coronavirus

64 Aleksey Navalny was sent to a prison labor camp, a gulag "concentration camp" known for its strict handling of convicts.

65 Joseph Wilson and Alicia León, "Spain's Far-Right Holds Car Protest against Virus Lockdown," *ABC News*, May 23, 2020, https://abcnews.go.com/amp/Health/wireStory/spains-holds-car-protest-virus-lockdown-70847709

66 Andy Borowitz, "Michigan Governor Arrogantly Forcing Residents to Remain Alive," *The New Yorker*, May 1, 2020, www.newyorker.com/humor/borowitz-report/michigan-governor-arrogantly-forcing-residents-to-remain-alive

67 Daily Monitor, "Uganda's Coronavirus Cases Rise to 53," *Daily Monitor*, April 8, 2020, www.monitor.co.ug/News/National/Uganda-s-coronavirus-cases-rise-53/688334-5518396-76ms9dz/index.html

68 Maria Lugones, "Toward a Decolonial Feminism," *Hypatia* 25, no. 4 (2010): 742–759.

69 Eve Darian-Smith, *Global Burning: Rising Antidemocracy and the Climate Crisis* (Stanford, CA: Stanford University Press, 2022).

70 Street activists recalled in 2016 when a student was pinned down and jailed by police unfairly, a moment that sparked much protest. The anticolonial activist infringed upon the criminal code of conspiracy for secession, a movement that driven by how West Papuans were treated under Dutch rule.

71 Thomas Stodulka. "Emotive Banners and Billboards: Worlding Covid-19 and Orders of Feeling in Kupang, Indonesia." *European Journal of East Asian Studies* 1.aop (2022): 1–28.

72 In 2019, China's Communist Party newspaper called Hong Kong's liberal education a poisonous "disease" that invited illegal activity that needed to be slayed.

73 Chantal Da Silva, "Coronavirus in the Age of Protest: How the Pandemic Could Change the Way We Organize," *Newsweek*, April 8, 2020, www.newsweek.com/coronavirus-age-protest-how-pandemic-could-change-way-we-organize-1496701

74 Kelly Ho, "Hongkongers' Support of Pro-Democracy Shops 'Violates' the Free Market, Says Beijing," *Hong Kong Free Press*, May 4, 2020, https://hongkongfp.com/2020/05/04/hongkongers-support-of-pro-democracy-shops-violates-the-free-market-says-beijing/

75 Helen Davidson, "China Calls Hong Kong Protesters a 'Political Virus'" *The Guardian*, May 6, 2020, www.theguardian.com/world/2020/may/06/china-calls-hong-kong-protesters-a-political-virus

76 Mario Koran and Sam Levin, "All Californians Ordered to Shelter in Place as Governor Estimates More Than 25m Will Get Virus," *The Guardian*, March 19, 2020, www.theguardian.com /world/2020/mar/19/coronavirus-california-more-than-half-gavin-newsom

77 After the first case in the state was reported, Governor Newsom banned the intake of new inmates. Newsom had previously ended all private prisons and juvenile prisons.

78 Jeff Wasserstrom, "What to Do and Not to Do amidst a Crisis If You Are a Public Representative," *The Wire*, April 13, 2020, https://thewire.in/world/california-hong-kong-leaders

79 LA Times, "Editorial: Coronavirus Makes Jails and Prisons Potential Death Traps. That Puts Us All in Danger," *The Los Angeles Times*, March 18, 2020, www.latimes.com/opinion/story/2020-03-18/coronavirus-prisons-releases

80 Didier Fassin, D., "Another Politics of Life Is Possible," *Theory, Culture & Society* 26, no. 5 (2009): 44–60.

81 Martha D. Escobar, *Captivity beyond Prisons: Criminalization Experiences of Latina (Im)migrants* (Austin: University of Texas Press, 2016).

82 Ryan Devereaux, " 'Burials Are Cheaper than Deportations': Virus Unleashes Terror in a Troubled ICE Detention Center," *The Intercept*, April 12, 2020, https://theintercept.com/2020/04/12/coronavirus-ice-detention-jail-alabama/

83 Running China's national gene bank, BGI founders signed an agreement to build this bank in 2016 working with CCP and the military to create facial recognition technology.

84 Bethany Allen-Ebrahimian, "Chinese Coronavirus Test Maker Agreed to Build a Xinjiang Gene Bank," *Axios*, June 3, 2020, www.axios.com/chinese-coronavirus-test-maker-agreed-to-build-a-xinjiang-gene-bank-f82b6918-d6c5-45f9-90b8-dad3341d6a6e.html

85 Ofelia Cuevas, "400 Years of Resistance: Race, Policing, and Abolition," UC Davis Humanities Institute, July 6, 2020, www.youtube.com/watch?v=M38dX4gnyqk

86 Ruth Wilson Gilmore, *Abolition Geography: Essays Towards Liberation* (New York: Verso Books, 2022), 268.

87 Ofelia Cuevas, "Welcome to My Cell: Housing and Race in the Mirror of American Democracy," *American Quarterly* 64, no. 3 (2012): 605–624.

88 Prison Pandemic Project, University of California, Irvine, https://prisonpandemic.uci.edu/ (accessed November 11, 2023).

3

FLATTEN THE CURVE

Control, Capitalism, Community

"Do you want us all to get sick? You all are being irresponsible, idiots!" shouted the mayor of Gualdo in a viral video paraded around the world. Presiding over the mess in his city in response to COVID-19, the Italian politician was fed up with citizens flouting quarantine orders, despite national efforts to "flatten the curve." The term, taken from public health, means controlling disease through community intervention. Under the pandemic's glare, this epidemiological precept soon became incumbent upon all humans to adopt as a collective goalpost. Plastered on television and media screens as the main focus of attention, the curving visual chart displayed the steady rate of infection and risk perception pivoted against hospital overcapacity. If no speed bumps were put in place, maladjusted societies would fall behind the curve into peril.

Missing the curve marked the danger zone of patient overflow. It stood to reason that any crowding of emergency clinics induces a bottleneck effect on local infrastructure and subverts triage. Without physical distancing, our healthcare workers and systems would be put at great risk. Moving ahead of coronavirus by slowing it down, mandatory lock-ins bought some time to dodge the virus' meteoric bullet. Surmounting the curve meant eluding a medical surge that no country or community could handle alone. While low-income patients were sent to overstretched public and makeshift hospitals for COVID-related symptoms, individuals of means acquired personalized care in expensive private hospitals. Trial-and-error attempts to flatten the curve needed to deal with the rising curve of medical inflation. In slowing the course of the novel coronavirus, the question remains who—governments, capitalists, or communities—would take control?

DOI: 10.4324/9781032694535-4

The chart's apex was a moving target that changed with daily or weekly modulations based on data points and risk analytics. Zeroing in on mitigation on a community level, this fuzzy threshold needed to be reined in through policing the behavior of people. Pastors holding service were rounded up, shoppers were charged with terrorism for coughing on food produce, and suspects faced manslaughter charges for intentionally spreading coronavirus. Videos circulated of Bolivians railing against their interim government's curving efforts and its inability to provide basic needs to the poor during lockdown. Protesters in the Riberalta region held up banners exclaiming, "The government is locking us up, hunger is going to kill us!" Charges of genocide were also levelled at Ethiopia's president, who postponed elections under the pretense of controlling COVID-19.

The pandemic politics of control can easily morph into rule by the hands of power-hungry elites. Though soap presented the best defense against germs, a good number of people could not wash their hands, a problem in water-distressed U.S. communities Flint, a rustbelt city in Michigan state, where low-income people of color were poisoned with lead and other toxins by state authorities. Detroit residents found their water flow lopped off if they could not pay. This severing left dry more than 30,000 low-income people.[1] Activists protested and sued, but the practice of water-denial to the poor held sway. The local water department had long denied a link between disease outbreaks and water shutoffs—that is, until COVID-19—and now they had to adjust to a newfound reality. From refugee encampments to cities, water-stressed areas faced willful neglect.

Quality control and population control can be hard to maintain under a pandemic. Countries like the Netherlands recalled defective surgical masks shipped from China. Basing its decision on scientific evidence, the U.S. Food and Drug Administration revised its decades-long restriction on gay male blood donations after public demands to stop discrimination, as SARS-CoV-2 flitted from one body to the next and depleted limited blood supplies. While Brazil, Northern Ireland, and Portugal revoked their blanket bans on men who have sex with men (MSM), the U.S. agency shifted from a one-year ban to a three-month waiting period, after dealing with shortages of convalescent plasma.[2] Certain types of pathologized bodies remain overregulated and stigmatized, even when blood is most needed.

Companies offered corporate perks and vacation days to employees, extenuating pandemic control to worker management. "Corona therapy," according to an op-ed in the *New Republic*, fails if our bosses continue to check in on us at home to make sure we are still doing the same amount of work under seesawing circumstances. Fundamentally at odds with productivity pressures and burnout, the writer recommends that we find ways to extricate ourselves from the "America's hustle culture—the idea that every nanosecond of our lives must be commodified and pointed toward profit and self-improvement ... the obscenity of pretending that work and 'the self' are the only things that matter."[3] Companies and countries moved toward a remote work week, sometimes to stunning success and an increase in employee well-being.

Just as the situation in China and East Asia began to calm, a second round of infection struck, one much harder than the first. As soon as people let their guard down and everything was thought to be under control, the scaling back of restrictions led to a steady rise rather than a winding down of infection. As Hong Kong, Singapore, Japan, and many other places soon learned, the idiosyncratic novel coronavirus does not rest. COVID-19 writes its own rules.

A return to before times could not boost a sputtering gross domestic product. Japan's island of Hokkaido reinstated its lockdown three weeks after ending it, as infection numbers leveled off. Plans to renormalize backfired. With incessant stress on businesses, the governor eased up on quarantine restrictions. When infection numbers shot back up, this spike muted the reset button to rev up a Japanese economy. Despite smothering the novel coronavirus early on, China locked down its northeast region again after COVID-19 cases emerged, reportedly coming from Russia, despite reopening for a month with no new cases.

This chapter examines the forms of capitalism and social control that took effect under a pandemic, but one in which local communities regained control of the situation. It illustrates an early tendency to view a major public health threat as an excuse by dictators to militarize their nations and motivate people to rise up against a terrifying "common enemy." As the "war" against COVID-19 intensified, militarized governments activated their own war machines against women and LGBTQ+ people. Through a critical analysis of the pandemic's culture wars in various countries, I critique the simple belief that Asian societies coped better than Europe. With disease prevention doubling as population control, territories like Hungary, India, Malaysia, and Brazil imposed problematic responses to the crisis due to growing authoritarianism. Insofar as corporate powerbrokers and financial investors exploited the situation for profit, "corona-capitalism" shaped the direction of communal responses and social resilience. Finally addressed are the concerns of Native and Indigenous groups, particularly the hard-hit Navajo nation, and how Tribal communities fared or struggled with their own efforts to flatten the curve.

Control

"Shoot them dead," decreed the Philippines' President Rodrigo Duterte on public airwaves, "My orders are to the police and military, as well as village officials, if there is any trouble ... Do not challenge the government. You will lose."[4] Millions of residents in Luzon were under strict lockdown orders, but this measure did not stop residents from the poorest slums to protest the government over thinning COVID-19 emergency supplies. Residents in the capital Manila did not receive any food packs for weeks. Since coming to power in 2016, Duterte raised hackles and much uproar over his reign. Reports swirled around extrajudicial organized killings of innocent people as "collateral damage" in a war against suspected drug dealers. A license to kill devolved into nearly 30,000 dead mostly in the southern Muslim parts of the country. In one of the deadliest countries for Indigenous people and journalists, Duterte's choice words sent a chilling message, giving wide latitude to soldiers to shoot at will and whipping up a frenzy over restrictions on freedom of movement. Duterte's shutdown of independent television networks touched off a media blackout in the worst time to do so, which is during a pandemic. Giving marching orders to kill labor activists protesting rights violations in the Anti-Terrorism Act of 2020, Duterte told police and military to slay all communist bandits in Mindanao and "finish them off if they are alive."[5] With the War on Terror/Drugs shading into the war on coronavirus, the enemy target could be anyone.

This counterinsurgency campaign of terror corresponds with what was happening in Brazil, where police were allowed to use lethal force with impunity when meeting a perceived imminent threat. Austria limited five or more people from gathering with the threat of police dispersal. The country flattened its curve in almost a blink of the eye, a partial vindication for a country awaiting a new interim government. Such "wins" come at a human cost. Jair Bolsonaro ordered a stop to the releasing of death toll counts and the wiping of data from official Brazilian websites. Donald Trump dismissed the heads of four organizations that comprise the U.S. Agency for Global Media, dissolving their boards, an action interpreted as a grab for power and seizing control over media platforms.

Governmental pandemic responses varied considerably. What South Korea did in a week, crystallizing a national agenda for COVID-19, took months for the United States to carry out. This variation was a sober reminder of the dire need for pandemic preparedness, despite differences in country size, demographics, and geography. From an epidemiological standpoint, it may not be wise to harp on the finer points of such national comparisons when a global pandemic is in full force. What happens in one place affects other sites. For if one country fails to stamp out COVID-19, or "the inequality virus" as it is sometimes called, in their home territories, others shall suffer. The U.S. refusal to leverage ready-made kits by the World Health Organization (WHO) and develop independent kits through private–public cooperatives allowed the pandemic play out to devastating effect. Even with early knowledge of four known cases, this was enough to jangle the nerves of public health officials in South Korea's Centers for Disease Control and Prevention (CDC). Drive-through screenings at strategic contact points were rolled out to test people daily, on average 12,000 patients per day, the same number tested in the United States over the course of two weeks. Through a patchwork of measures, the government of Moon Jae-In swiftly identified over 90% of the 8,000 infected, and the number dramatically subsided.

The United States confirmed its first coronavirus case the same day as South Korea (January 20, 2020), but it faced a bigger gauntlet of problems. Foremost among them, it never met the testing demand for its citizens, thus falling behind and below expectations. This tale of two countries living under COVID-19 indicates a distinction between "a streamlined bureaucracy versus a congested one, bold versus cautious leadership, and a sense of urgency versus a reliance on protocol."[6] Instead of drafting the private sector to scale and develop tests like South Korea, U.S. health officials, much like those in Japan, relied on government-produced defective test kits (some tainted with coronavirus), dismissing readily adopting ones served up by the WHO. The CDC misled its diagnostics capabilities and restricted private labs from conducting tests. It never finessed outside partnerships; and when it ginned up a collective response to COVID-19, it was too little too late.

South Korea squandered little time and spared no effort in releasing tests, checking their effectiveness later in original sample groups. With lots of false starts, desperate countries sought to emulate South Korea, after watching people there calmly drive up to test stations to take nose swabs while sitting in their cars. After the leaders of France, Sweden, and the United States sought advice from President Moon, the Republic of Korea became the exemplar for how to aggressively root out SARS-CoV-2 through contact chasing with no time lost.

The appearance of brisk efficiency displayed by Asian countries belies political tremors on the ground and a lack of public trust. International news media exporting images of the country as one of fastidiousness flies in the face of earlier headlines like, "How South Korea's Coronavirus Outbreak got so Quickly out of Control."[7] Potential instability from COVID-19 was squashed by Korea's militarized work culture, one carved out of state-led mergers between corporate *chaebols* and the defense industry.[8] "We acted like an army," one health expert mentioned, and diagnostic tests were activated with swift governmental approval. As part of that military-like response, the government reactivated the Infectious Disease Prevention Act, originally passed during the 2015 MERS scare and a recurrent biochemical threat from North Korea.[9] In the very early stages of the pandemic, South Korea responded sluggishly and Moon, like so many world leaders, claimed the disease would simply evaporate due to hot summer weather.

After confirmation of hundreds of COVID-19 cases, Moon's administration sent out daily real-time updates of places where infected patients went and where they were going next through smartphone apps. Moon's corrective could not pacify backlash against the patrician leader's "whole of government" approach. The majority whip in the National Assembly, called it the "Moon Jae-in virus." Reeling from the recent memory of MERS, South Koreans excoriated President Jae-in for not responding early enough to an invasive disease. Without closing any borders, his administration allowed Chinese nationals to enter, even though Taiwan, North Korea, Hong Kong, and Singapore restricted them. Many viewed this concession to keep the economy running as appeasing China, South Korea's biggest trading partner. Moon's bullhorn roar of "maximum containment" in Daegu slipped after receiving serious public blowback. The party's spokesman who made the announcement even resigned. The country's disease-prevention system came up woefully short, opined the president of the Korean Medical Association (KMA), which called for an early ban on Chinese visitors, "The biggest reason for that failure is that the government ignored the very basic principle of disease control, which is blocking the source of infection."[10]

With political control masquerading as disease control, everything circled back into the "culture wars." Anti-gay lawmakers voted against the U.S. coronavirus stimulus package because it gave sick leave pay to domestic same-sex partnerships. President Trump asked the Supreme Court to invalidate parts of the government-sponsored "Obamacare" or The Affordable Care Act at a time when people needed health care the most. A close association had been birthed between universal healthcare and universal face-masking, even in European countries with a socialized medical system. The Czech government launched a video campaign of "my mask protects you, your mask protects me," differing from Trump's axiom: *your* mask protective order infringes on *my* rights.[11] The U.S. mindset of "I have rights" was at variance with the Cherokee perspective of "I have obligations" to elders, and future generations and obligations to the planet.[12] Through this collective mindset, the Cherokee nation held off hospitalization and avoided political gridlock.

Pandemic orientalism revived old ways of seeing Asia as different and foreign in their response to a health crisis. This Othering occurred amid media coverage of the United States and European countries, where the response went awry or amiss. Foreign policy expert S. Nathan Park took issue with cultural accounts of COVID-19 as only an "Asian disease." Park elucidates how anti-Asianism stalled portable global solutions, especially when Italy's health minster undersecretary verbalized the maelstrom over COVID-19 in China as a "science fiction movie that had nothing to do with us," and the *Wall Street Journal* quipped, "The lingering cultural imprint of Confucianism gives a paternalistic state a freer hand to intrude in people's lives during an emergency."[13] Always in step with government orders, Park held South Koreans as meek, docile, and willing to sacrifice for the greater good. Diffident Americans remained unbowed in finding some solace that

"Asia's solution could be its solution too." East Asian autocratic republics, he contends, responded to COVID-19 with more efficacy than Western democracies and "getting better results." The politicalized use of disease marks a refusal to take stock of failed priorities in siloed nations.

In ascertaining the pandemic's acrimonious cultural politics, a key aspect not considered is gender and sexuality. Community partners made safe havens for vulnerable elderly Black lesbians or single Filipina lesbian parents.[14] In Germany, 17 days after the first known COVID-19 case in Berlin, hundreds of people signed up for support through an ad hoc relief line for queer womxn, femmes, and nonbinary or trans people.

These grassroots efforts combatted the international rise in hate. One of the first draft laws proposed in Hungary in 2020 was a bill that sought to end legal recognition of transgender people, a change similar to the record number of laws proposed or passed in U.S. conservative states. President Trump blocked the trans community from protection against sex discrimination in healthcare. The WHO's official declaration of COVID-19 as a pandemic on March 11, 2020, only three days after the International Women's Day (March 8), did not dampen vociferous calls for gender equity and women's empowerment. As the pandemic unfurled pushing the world over the edge, feminist activists underscored the fact that the majority of countries have never chosen a female head of state, and only 6% of all nations did so at the time of COVID-19. According to U.N. Women, political exclusion of women attenuated initiatives for open communication, delegation, competence, and global cooperation—essentials for pandemic mitigation. Valorization of male authority coupled with the reductionism of women's political abilities stood averse to the power sharing needed to govern in times of crisis.

The highest echelons of political office are far removed from the unsafe living conditions faced by poor women. In Hawai'i, women were pressured into sex by their landlords in lieu of rental payments. In a state with the highest cost of living, Hawai'i's State Commission on the Status of Women proposed a feminist economic recovery plan that included special funds for sex-trafficking survivors and domestic immigrant workers, prioritizing those with special needs (50% of deaths in hospitals from people with disabilities) and age-susceptibility (eight out of ten coronavirus deaths were elderly). Calling for deep social change at top and bottom, the executive director of the commission, Khara Jabola-Carolus attributes high coronavirus mortality to men since the burden of self-care and sickcare are relegated to women. Insofar as the feminist recovery plan's strove to "build a system that is capable of delivering gender equality," Jabola-Carolus hoped that she and colleagues could provide the blueprint for other states and countries to "build your feminist army and go beyond advocates and legislators."[15] In that vein, the Aina Aloa Economic Futures Declaration proposed a plan to recreate the tourist economy based on island values of food and energy sustainability according to the love of *aina* or land. Eternal love for the land and protection of the island's inhabitants writhe under the tyranny of colonial governments purporting to speak for all people and wringing emotion from hating Others.

Despite the pandemic's transformative power to induce social change, heteropatriarchy managed to still demonize women and sexual minorities. The "right" of countries to infringe on civil/human/social rights in the name of public health found its litmus test in Malaysia. The country's top court deliberated on a trial of whipping, caning, prison, and fines for gays, who were arrested under federal and local Sharia edicts against homosexuality. Governmental recommendations to stay home to protect against the novel coronavirus seemed moot when police were raiding private residences and dragging people of their homes on suspicions of same-sex relations. With the hashtag #WomenPreventCOVID19, Malaysia's Ministry for Women, Family, and Community Development put up an infographic poster on Facebook and Instagram, advising women to not "nag" their husbands during lockdown. It urged them to dress up in office attire (avoiding home clothing) and wear makeup. The family agency abandoned its women's campaign after much public scorn, though its cavalier attitude worsened Malaysia's movement control order. Only the male "head of the household" could go out to purchase necessities, reinforcing this sense of feminine private space (controlled by men) and a male-dominated public space.[16]

Keeping COVID-19 in check is a feminist issue that dovetails with a cross-section of issues like labor. In rankings of the Organization of Economic Cooperation and Development (OECD) (the club of the wealthiest nations), South Korea held the highest gender income gap among high-income countries (37%), even more than runner-up Japan (24%). Pressures to do the uncompensated labor of parenting and childrearing delineated the lines by which women could work outside the home. When Korea experienced peak infectivity (the second highest outside China), millions of women left their homes to brave the disease to rally in global protests capped by International Women's Day. The first feminist political party, the Women's Party, launched that same day to wrest power away from the major parties, which have relegated their needs. Aimed squarely at shaking up the old-boys club and political establishment, women and their coconspirators called for antidiscrimination laws and more female representation in the National Assembly.

Such actions compose fourth-wave feminism, a global movement for wholesale change in places like India, which fails to protect women from systemic female infanticide, gender discrimination, and rape. Indian women stood at the forefront of sit-in rallies and hunger strikes against Parliament's new Citizenship Act passed in December 2019 by the ruling Hindu nationalist Bharatiya Janata Party (BJP). The new law blocked all Muslim migrant applicants from naturalization, an egregious violation of the country's secular constitution and multicultural ethos, while the National Register of Citizens required copious documents to prove citizenship, which many rural women from underresourced communities lacked. Guwahati, in the Assam region, underwent indefinite curfews and Internet shutdown in the city after protests organized by college women attempted to end detention camps for unregistered migrants.

Women led the charge against COVID-19. Working within South Korea's male-dominated government, the KCDC's head was a woman named Jung Eun-Kyeong, whose confident pandemic leadership made her one of five global "heroes" listed by the *Wall Street Journal*. These coronavirus (s)heroes held ground as career deputies who "are rarely the bold, charismatic, impulsive, self-regarding, politically calculating alphas we've elected."[17] A study found the leadership styles of women tilted toward service and ran counter to traditional male cravings for power and personal gratification.[18] During a maddening pandemic rife with "mad men" leaders, hundreds of women marched in support of three main female opposition leaders uncowed by threats of arrest after contested elections in Belarus. As Europe's longest-running dictator, alpha leader Alexander Lukashenko sent the message that the novel coronavirus could be rid through saunas and vodka. Democracy stalled with the postelection arrest of protestors against an autocrat who ruled for a quarter century and who once shown support for Adolph Hitler. Defending the idea that the firm-hand of authoritarians provides COVID-19 protection, Lukashenko found close affinity with Russia's Putin and China's Xi. To avoid torture or kidnapping, the women leaders fled to other countries, promoting their pro-democracy messages in exile.

Gendered policing in the name of purifying or protecting patriarchal society goes hand in glove. Millions dug themselves out of social isolation to protest bans on abortion. These restrictions were seen in China, Poland, and in U.S. states like Texas. While patriarchies and pandemics appear divorced from one another, they are not, when a sick society steeped in misogyny cannot avail itself of all human resources against COVID-19. A regime of surveillance becomes synthetically concretized in place of full participatory civic culture by women. In 2019, Freedom House listed South Korea's political system as robust and "free," but ranks the country as "partly free" on its Freedom on the Net list. South Korea led the way in disease prevention, going the farthest among crisis-prone countries in utilizing online devices. Remote sensing public maps worked to the effect of pinpointing the exact whereabouts of positively identified individuals, via their purchases on credit cards and private smartphone data. This kind of state surveillance interferes with individual liberties, admits the director for the Korea Disease Control and Prevention Agency, a necessary evil for sake of "public interest."[19]

As the novel coronavirus snaked through the population putting human life at risk, South Korean women fought for their lives in other ways. Suicide rates soared over 30% in early 2020, compared to the year before. Most of these deaths or injuries were related to women working in industries most harmed by the pandemic. Activists demanded a break from imposed child-rearing, marriage demands, and rape culture. They were pushed to the edge by an "epidemic of voyeurism" in which public spycams secretly filmed women.[20] For years, the annual Korea Women's March advocated for LGBTQ+ rights, immigrant rights, disability rights, the environment, and social responsibility. Women demanded a hardier democracy in 2020 rather than just a governmental deterrence of disease. Charges of graft against President Pak Geun-hye, who consorted with a corrupt Christian cult leader, toppled the country's first female president a year earlier. Her embroilment in big scandals prompted the Candlelight Movement for political reform. Street protests had dragged down several elected officials, including the justice minister, for corruption charges in a country long overshadowed by nepotism.

The panacea to a pestilence like COVID-19 lay in a comprehensive, community-based approach to care, one rooted in restorative justice. Everything suddenly matters in a global crisis with all resources tapped to block an implacable foe that threatens all of humanity. What can become lost in "flattening the curve" is the person behind the caretaking or who is most affected. Senior citizens received more public attention than usual, and the elderly extracted themselves from the rest of society to protect their health. The cutting of social relations however compounds the isolation for those elders who were potentially most vulnerable health-wise to COVID-19. Isolation from others was both beneficial and hurtful to elders.

This vulnerability is worse for Southeast Asian, Native, Pacifika, Latine, and Black people who are less prone to have hospice care. When people of color are forced to care for others, while being uncared for, it becomes clear that "racial capitalism" is a main causative agent or driver for health disparities.[21] This social gradient of health is part of "infrastructure schemes," where racialized communities are unable to shrink from the world or access the right to abode due to their placement within public spaces and facilities.[22] Anthropologist Layla Brown-Vincent observes that "poor Black and Brown people all over the world are flowing out of their homes, and into the streets determined to fight for their lives and their livelihood."[23] Indeed, they must leave their homes instead and, out of necessity, enter the harsh cruel (viral) world.

To bottle up COVID-19 and prevent it from running loose, governments trapped people inside their homes. Videos emerged of officials in Wuhan dragging people away and bolting their front door locks. These harsh actions underlined the inhumaneness of quarantine. To mitigate despondency from physical distancing, hardest-hit communities responded to the call for help. In New York, Sikhs with gloves and face masks prepared their *sewa* service of providing free vegetarian food to thousands of people. Young people reconnected with quarantined seniors via phone check-ins, special curbside meal delivery, outside window conversations, and pooled emergency funds. Mental health, ordinarily the stepchild of physical health care, achieved a raised profile when it was reiterated by healthcare professionals that physical distance did not mean emotional separation. Self-care messages, whether shared in person or over social media, proved invaluable in coping with the stress of imposed self-isolation. People conveyed encouraging words of hope, finding ways to maintain social cohesion during (and after) long-term quarantine.

Just as the pandemic spread outward, so too did the power of love. Caring for others poses a global mission of social unification that cannot be compromised. The New Age ethos of self-care can easily shade into profit schemes and monetization by those opportunists that do not want social transformation. Self-care nevertheless offers an important corollary to the rallying point of *structural* change, a much-needed reminder in prioritizing wellness since the body serves as a social battleground. In the U.S., transwoman Layleen Xtravaganza Cubilette-Polanco died while in solitary confinement, against doctor's wishes due to her epileptic seizures. Another transwoman named Diamond was fatally shot while lying inside an ambulance waiting to be treated for COVID-19.[24] Disturbing acts of murder torqued the information overload and counterfactual data about a rampaging "silent killer" virus. To demand a life that is safe and secure, especially in a pandemic, tapped into political claims for protecting transpeople and transwomen.

Such demands serve as a structure of feeling and form of "radical love." This feminist concept is exemplified by the LGBTQ+ community in response to the HIV/AIDS crisis. With an eye toward the longest-running pandemic, we can ask why certain communities remain in crisis, touching upon "where we locate the crises ... when and how we identify, name, and categorize their impacts ... who is the exception and who is the rule?"[25]

The race to find a cure for COVID-19 proved nothing short of a major challenge in terms of vaccine quality control and testing. Actual testing turned out perplexing in terms of who matters enough to be flagged for inoculation. In times of upheaval, the picture of social inequity appears more clearly, which happened when famous movie stars with "concierge doctors" and professional athletes became tested ahead of healthcare workers and the poor. Failure came from shortage of test kits, availability of dated kits too old to effectively use, and lack of a public crisis infrastructure to test people. On Facebook, the Norwegian University of Science and Technology posted a shady comment directed to the United States that "strongly recommends" all students who are "outside Norway to return home. This applies especially if you are staying in a country with poorly developed health services and/or collective infrastructure, for example the U.S.A."[26]

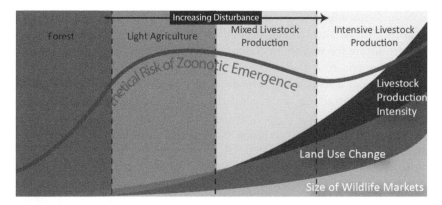

FIGURE 3.1 One health in action illustration (EcoHealth Alliance).

This slight was not without some merit. Representative Katie Porter needed to "do the math" for the CDC director, who did not know the numbers associated with cost and testing for COVID-19. This embarrassment forced his office to cover the tests regardless of insurance and ability to pay. Norway by contrast enjoys an advanced decentralized healthcare system, but with co-pays for its citizens, all insured by the government.[27] It almost seemed like some countries cared for their citizens, while others left sick people to wither away. Decisions boiled it down to schematics of free-wheeling capitalism and the bloodthirsty prioritization of wealth over health.

Flattening the curve must move beyond basic survival mode to consider how human technology can operate within Gaian theories and earth systems. A visual chart from the Eco-Health Alliance indicates how the rising threat of zoonotic threats is burned into industrial activity (see Figure 3.1). Part of the One Health movement, Eco-Health experts are part of a global consortium of people pleading for transformative changes.

With only 1% of all viruses detected so far in mammals, there is no way to ferret out the next viral killer, so geography comes in as a convenient shorthand for epidemiology. According to political ecologists, the red zoning of countries in the Global South as the next viral "hot spots" obscures the discontinuous capitalist networks across territories—funded in part by Colgate and Johnson & Johnson and other corporations—driving the levers of the pandemic.[28] Put baldly, capitalism gave birth to the novel coronavirus in the viral shape and global character it takes.

Capitalism

Despite the many unknowns of the pandemic, one thing could be certain: those capitalist robber barons who had exploited the planet would exploit this situation. Economized counterstrategies to COVID-19 unsurprisingly fell into corporate balance sheets, funding rich biotech companies rather than fully accounting for wealth inequality as a determinant of health inequality. Attempts to construe the pandemic as "temporary" mask a crumbling neoliberal order founded on false promises of endless wealth. Forced to obey market contractions as general rule, capitalist societies entered more unpredictable boom-and-bust cycles under a *capitalized* pandemic. Any faith in minimalist ad hoc response became demolished by American-style "plantation economics."[29] COVID-19 marked a turning point in global political economy, where working folks of color everywhere were left to pick up the slack of ramshackle governments who are entrusted to be the duty-bound vanguard of "the people." Ailing states with no way out of the pandemic simply fell apart.

A pandemic lifts off as a local problem before taking shape as a global phenom. Under the propulsions of capitalism, India's policies under Modi's government and the BJP gave rise to the largest strike ever. Impelled by a coalition of over 200 farmer groups, strikers demanding expansion of government aid for rural workers and those people made rootless by COVID-19. In Delhi, a quarter billion people took to the streets to protest the end of state protections over food crop production. They were upset with relaxed rules for firing workers, the running up of short-term contract employment, and depreciation of trade union activity. Work stoppages held their precedence in COVID-19 stay-home restrictions months earlier, which racked workers' lives, especially migrant laborers. Both moments merged into a "neoliberal death-spiral" that winds up as "roll-over ruination."[30]

When it comes to ruins, perhaps nothing was sadder to watch than the blast explosion at a port in Beirut in 2020, the Suez Canal's shipping crisis of 2021, or the implosion of the Sri Lankan economy in 2022. In Beirut, Lebanon's major port and capital fell into utter disrepair after a deadly sonic blast at a grain silo. Protests erupted over the corruption that contributed to this "accident." Before this welter of bad events, the World Bank had called Lebanon's economic contraction as one of the worst depressions in our lifetime. The country's currency lost more than 90% of its value in a year and half of all Lebanese fell into poverty. The "social explosion" encapsulated all the political earthquakes that left Lebanon in shambles. Shell-shocked Lebanese saw banks set on fire, a capstone to a national insurrection that began in 2019 over corruption, hunger, and poverty, which spilled into 2020. The urban "riots" needed to be repelled by military security forces in a country convulsed by austerity-driven turmoil the year before, resulting in the prime minister's resignation. African migrants trapped under the employer-controlled Kafala employment system had nowhere to go if they were fired or discharged.

On-call employees and day laborers came back to workplace hazards and conditions that they never encountered before. On Labor Day, Malaysian authorities rounded up migrant workers and raided their homes under movement-control orders. The mass arrests discouraged many migrants from becoming tested and going to work. Undocumented workers, mostly from neighboring countries, were easy scapegoats for the economic anxieties that came after (and before) the pandemic. A number of Malaysians believed migrant workers sapped state resources, though migrants kept afloat the country's factories and agricultural plantations.[31]

Beliefs that migrant worker camps could spread SARS-CoV-2 stirred up hatred in Arab Gulf states, where foreign workers make up half of the population. In Bahrain, parliamentary member Safaa Al-Hashem called for the deportation of migrants to "purify" the country from illegal workers. These workers comprised a little more than half of all nurses in the country. The call to kick out nonnationals seemed cruel, especially when they do not receive temporary pay protections like nationals. An intensive care nurse working in Bahrain said that citizens who volunteer to work with COVID-19 patients obtain compensation but "we, on the other hand, don't even get hazard pay for putting our lives at risk ... We feel that we are also not appreciated."[32] Slavery and indentured servitude became reinterpreted by the value creation of corporate stakeholders; citizens clamoring to reopen the economy (half of them on Twitter were bots one research team found) took their "civil rights" as being violated, promoting a "freedom to harm" and "freedom to infect."[33]

The rationale behind this freedom to infect and harm others contrasts with global solidarity. Despite the fact that African lives are valued differently, anthropologists Vito Laterza and Louis Philippe Römer posit,

> There is some hope though that the truly global, albeit highly uneven, dimension of this pandemic might lift the veil of false consciousness that has so far separated the North from the South, the West from "the rest." As more people in the North experience the frailty of life under the necro-biopolitics of the market, the opportunities for global solidarity will increase.[34]

Under "health dictatorships," Africans were consigned to "the freedom to die." A global "hierarchy of disposability" motivated China in 2020 to send 1,000 ventilators to New York, City, but not to all of Africa. The WHO estimates only 2,000 ventilators were sent in total for 48 African countries. There was less concern for a continent where epidemics and disease seem to happen "all the time."

Plunged into the abyss by the novel coronavirus, a financialized system of care(lessness) broke beyond repair. Venture capitalist Nick Hanauer maintains that the COVID-19 pandemic in some ways is a "uniquely American" problem. The United States is the country with biggest spending on medical care but lowest ratio of doctors and hospital beds. If the novel coronavirus was the demon seed of unbridled American capitalism, it forewarned the repercussions from the prevailing view of health care as a privilege rather than a right. Hard-wired neoliberal thinking is a starting point to explain the shortcomings of health regimes. Under Donald Trump— a multibillionaire mogul who perceives government and society working like a corporation—the United States experienced a *laissez-faire* approach to the COVID-19 tempest. The *fait accompli* of corporatist groupthink is best clarified by Trump's quote on why his pandemic team was short staffed: "I'm a businessperson. I don't like having thousands of people around when you don't need them."[35]

Coronavirus reigned supreme in redirecting the "invisible hand" of capitalism and the "big hands" of authoritarians. Driving public attention away from health and toward the market, Trump panned the media and doctors for their "anti-business" attitude. This misdirection comes on the heels after months of reports about the shortage of intensive care units(ICUs), personal protective equipment (PPE), and special lifesaving ventilators in a worst-case scenario. Purchased or philanthropic shipment of ventilators destined for other countries had been cancelled. Even though governing bodies in Canada, Germany, Cayman Islands, and Barbados legitimately procured them, medical supplies were blocked, seized, and confiscated by the United States, by executive order. One shipment of 200,000 protective masks slated for Germany went missing in Thailand. It had been reportedly intercepted, redirected by the United States, as when a shipment meant to be transported to France had been hijacked by U.S. agents in a Shanghai airport (the newspaper *Libération* reported that the Americans paid double the buying price and bribed locals). The supplier claimed the United States forced this unplanned diversion, a "modern act of piracy" according to Berlin's mayor.[36] Without much substantiated information, Germans could no longer give the benefit of the doubt to their American allies.

Renewed terms of global partnership under COVID-119 favored a "pathological insistence on shareholder values," a corporatized model of governance based on malfeasance and executive bonuses or payouts— all paid by taxpayers and generations robbed of a future.[37] Angela Merkel called the social leveling caused by the pandemic the worst disaster to hit her country since World War II, one that could tip the Europe toward the road to financial ruin. Germany did not regard the crunch in economically limited terms, rolling out a $50 billion package for the cultural sector, recognizing that artists are key to bundling the creative energy of societies to build pandemic solutions in the viral world.

In the bid for in-demand medical items, cutthroat companies and gluttonous governments found their firm footing. In September 2019, Royal Philips, a Dutch company, agreed to ship 10,000 ventilators to bulk up U.S. stockpiles but never did. It sold more expensive units for $15,000 each in the heat of coronashock. Amid instigating more rifts within international diplomatic channels, President Trump called the United States the "king of ventilators" only to goad state governors into buying their own medical supplies, but the federal government outbid them every time. Responding to one pleading governor about this prickly matter, Trump replied, "Prices are always a component of that ... maybe that's why you lost to the Feds, OK, that's probably why."[38] Maryland's governor hid COVID-19 tests bought from South Korea, directing the state's national guard to watch over them. This action was to disincentive the Trump administration from commandeering them. Responding to these impediments, Governor Gavin Newsom reiterated California was an autonomous "nation-state," enabling it to export/import freely the medical equipment that it needs, which the Feds cannot supply (the state of Missouri sued China in a federal court for lying to the world and inflicting loss and mortal suffering). Despite asking the Feds to pay for his state's unemployment benefits, Newsom's announcement seized on visions of the Golden State as the moral counterweight to Trump's "country where inequality doesn't seem to be a problem, where climate change doesn't exist, and where the greatest threat we face comes from families seeking asylum."[39]

Market volatility delivered much psychic anguish brought on by the pandemic. The New York stock market crashed on March 9, 2020, when the Dow Jones experienced its biggest decline since the Great Recession of 2008. Reporters made much of the worst quarterly finish in 135 years, but this datum points up the banality of quantifying pandemic-era profit, as though a pandemic was part of the "natural" ebb and flow of markets. Hyperinflation scares from oil in Iran to onions in India brought "greedflation." Scores of new investors fled to (and from) the erratic cryptocurrency market, which China began regulating and which El Salvador adopted as legal tender, a historic first. As China's real estate crisis rattled, major developers snowed under by unpaid debt liabilities began massive sell offs, setting off a "global contagion" for financial markets.[40]

These problems had existed way before the pandemic but were exacerbated by COVID-19. A strong domestic economy and historic low unemployment rates boosted by President Trump could not stave off the economic downdraft precipitated by the novel coronavirus. Stock values swung wildly, but they redounded, even after a momentary plummet. Renegade investors did a run on the New York stock exchange. Capital markets tumbled and rose again, even as millions of wage workers chugged away in their daily jobs, and whole industries stilled.

Shrewd financial actors went about their usual business, acting as if everything was normal even as the pandemic rewrote the rules of economic engagement. Senators cashed in on an anticipated financial crash. They banked big on market failures, while promising to voters everything was alright as the economy began tanking. Trickle-down economics collided with demands for a "bottom-up bailout" by the Women's March National to help the neediest of workers who were put into a financial tailspin.

Adhering to top-down economic policies catered to the wealthy, political elites could not wrap their heads around the lateral community relations needed to stop the person-to-person transmission of the stealthy novel coronavirus. After U.S. Congress announced a speedy market recovery in mid-2020, stocks rebounded. Yet, record numbers of people applied for temporary unemployment benefits. Meanwhile, the COVID-induced quasi-recession pushed up the year from which Social Security retirement benefits would be insolvent. As SARS-CoV-2 wound through the economy, the Dow Jones dipped only to hit an industrial all-time high average. Investors and shock troops banked on potential COVID-19 vaccines, making a financial killing.

In pandemic times, it becomes harder to fall back on a bifurcated measure of economic health based on the interests of finance, particularly when the interests by collectivized labor are subsumed to capital. Coronavirus aid packages tried to deflect the jolt to the labor/capital market. Fashioned as government largesse, it was one of the biggest wealth transfers in history. Taking advantage of an unscrupulous system of government oversight, businessowners engaged in the "great pandemic theft," which the *New York Times* called the biggest public money fraud in U.S. history.[41] Billions disappeared in this "honor system." The finance-savvy enriched themselves on market upturns precisely "because the market doesn't represent the economy; it represents the future of big business."[42]

Competing investments in capital—human and financial—found real purchase in a viral world. This dichotomy raises the intrinsic value of decoupling wealth from health, whether the goal of wealth accumulation outweighs the cost of saving lives. After only a week of lockdown, Trump announced a cratering economy would torment more people, driving up suicide attempts. Wanting to start up the market as fast as possible against advice by medical experts, the restless businessman announced the end of April 2020 as the right time to open all stores again, in only a month: a target which he had to later amend. With a slight nod to his capitalist base amid currying favor with the religious right, the president envisaged packed houses of worship as "essential" business.

After Trump's announcement, staunch conservatives and far-right provocateurs fulminated against the New Green Deal, encouraging older Americans to go back to work. Conservative Glenn Beck weighed in on the trade-off: "I'd rather die" than "kill the economy."[43] In his mixed messaging and prevarication, Trump bumped up against state governors easing restrictions. Promising that the United States will be soon open for business, his top-down prescriptions for quick economic revival boiled down to a "cure [that] is worse than the problem."[44] States hell-bent on reopening led to the deadliest day on record. President Trump appeared without a mask at many rallies attended by thousands, and one manufacturer threw out all its swabs when the president visited and perused the factory without wearing protection. When market choice is presented as the only other choice to dying, one reporter observed, "the best safeguard against the novel coronavirus is the ability to voluntarily withdraw oneself from capitalism."[45]

Eluding the clutches of capitalism is hard when its grip overlaps with that of the omnipotent coronavirus. Variants of COVID-19 first arose in major economic hubs like the United States, Japan, the United Kingdom, and China as well as the emerging major economies of Brazil, Russia, India, China, South Africa (BRICS). There is nothing unique or special about the ecological profiles of these countries that would suggest that they intrinsically give rise to new viral strains. What they commonly shared is a strong commitment to global capitalism and sometimes fearmongering, as when Brazil's minister of Foreign Affairs called COVID-19 the "communavirus." Brazil's President Jair Bolsonaro faced scrutiny with not only calling the novel coronavirus the "Chinese virus," but calling for resuming economic activities as soon as possible. This call unleashed widespread outcry from medical experts. The temperamental leader used the bully pulpit to go on profanity-laced rants. Leaked messages exposed his self-proclaimed right to control federal police. Demanding a basic income for the poor, Brazil's state governors defied the president's rush orders, hewing to WHO protocols to stay the course on the quarantine.

The "Trump of the Tropics" lashed out at them on television, describing quarantine as a "crime" and "scorched-earth policy"—a poor choice of words given massive infernos in southern Brazil the year before. Cattle ranchers and illegal loggers treaded in slash-and-burn cycles, which the pro-business president abetted by calling the fire blazes a media contrivance.[46] For the first time ever, Brazilian scientists confirmed the Amazon rain forest emitted more CO_2 than it absorbed, turning a known carbon sink into a dumpster fire.

The histrionic president cited COVID-19 as "a little flu" maintaining that death is "everybody's destiny." He reasoned that burning fears of COVID-19 were superb "hysteria" and connivance by his foes to "trick" citizens.[47] He claimed governors of hardest-hit Sao Paulo and Rio de Janeiro were destroying Brazil by shutting businesses. Multiple news sources confirmed Bolsonaro contracted COVID-19, which he refuted. Along with the heads of Nicaragua, Belarus, and Turkmenistan—Bolsonaro was one of four "strongmen" that denied COVID-19 as a major public health threat, despite the obvious warning signs.

This nonchalance by male executives contrasts with the clear thinking, no-nonsense approach of women leaders in Singapore, Trinidad and Tobago, Barbados, Finland, Denmark, Norway, and Iceland. Empathetic calm and fortitude resided in New Zealand's prime minister, who was also reliant on scientific data and direct messaging. But in a country with a 93% vaccination rate, Maori people made up almost half of Delta-related strain (though they make up 16% of Aotearoa's population). Nonetheless, we should not underestimate the power of good leadership.

It was less the case in Brazil, where President Bolsonaro dismissed his health minister to sabotage the latter's campaign for physical distancing. The president also wanted to keep open cruises, gyms, and beauty parlors. His health minister's successor resigned a month later over Bolsonaro floating chloroquine as a COVID-19 treatment. This all occurred in Brazil a few days before Trump fired his top expert on vaccines for refusing to tout untreated medicines for the president.[48] Even while his national security advisor contracted COVID-19, Bolsonaro held no appetite for playing by the rules.

His administration released a video titled "Brazil Cannot Stop" that only drew scathing public flak. The vaccine skeptic shut down public institutions that supported quarantine. When accused of deflating the power of democracy, he thundered, "I am actually the constitution." As Brazil gained the highest number of reported cases after the United States by the end of spring 2020, there were reports of drug traffickers going as far as imposing state curfews, similar to curfews imposed by gangs in El Salvador. Those gangs were primary reason for police raids of favelas that barely relented, even after a Supreme Court Justice order prohibited police raids in favelas until the pandemic declines.[49] With a planet gripped by a pandemic, new viral economies of scale needed to be envisioned, but one "that multiplies opportunity, not one that rations it."[50]

Systems smashing needed to occur when investors were told by financiers to "wait out" the pandemic to make more money once the economy picked up again and returns to form. Well-endowed private universities like Harvard University and money-making sports teams like the Los Angeles Lakers were obliged to give back U.S. government handouts, bowing to public pressure. Despite its practice of buying back its stocks, hard-hit industries like commercial airlines hoped for bailout to recoup pandemic losses, but even this measure proved to be a challenge when no one is flying. The U.S. Federal Reserve bought up corporate stocks and slashed interest rates to zero. Captains of industry received a no-strings-attached slush fund as usual. Critics of Keynesian intervention poured scorn on generous stimulus packages, which added to the hefty tab of public debt and overheating the economy. While small businesses took a major hit from the post-COVID falloff, big banks netted loan packages, but the government forked over its bonanza of gifts to mega-corporations with little oversight.

Tax loopholes and corporate protections against potential lawsuits were tucked inside the major coronavirus bill. This legislation gave the wealthy the avenue to turn a profitable windfall from total economic meltdown. The number of billionaires soared past 30%, some of whom reaped the rewards of that surplus wealth to launch their private spaceflight businesses (a running joke on social media was that the uber-rich were leaving the rest of us behind on earth to die with COVID-19). Multinational companies with a "too big to fail" mentality received coronavirus aid on top of their usual tax credits. The stimulus bill came with no conditions for tax avoidance and sideswiped economic reparations for slavery and segregation. A survey for the Color of Change and UnidosUS found only 12% of minority businesses received federal assistance. Without prioritizing underserved communities, big corporations acquired cash reserves meant for small businesses. Puerto Rico's people suffered long delays in obtaining relief in a redux of what happened after major disasters, because the Internal Revenue Service delayed approval due to old colonial laws in the unincorporated territory.

Canada's sure-footed COVID-19 response burnished its credentials as a country that cares for its citizenry. After being hit by SARS, Canada implemented the Quarantine Act of 2005 that grants the health ministry the ability to zone anyplace for quarantine. This authority would force people into treatment even if they did not want to. Despite Canada's nationalized healthcare system and digital network, the country did not respond in the same way as South Korea. Canada's mitigation campaign vowed to protect its visible minorities and taking a tentative approach. The policy had been implemented through its prefect of public health, Theresa Tam, who initially missed the mark for stopping early warning signs of COVID-19. The physician soon received commendation for her technocratic approach. Meanwhile, Trudeau announced no bailouts for Canadian firms that operate tax havens and do not pay an equitable share of taxes.

Canada at first did not give much thought to the colonial manifestations of COVID-19. For First Nations, nothing could shed more ideals of Canadian liberal innocence and colonial paternalism than the remains of hundreds of children discovered in Indigenous boarding schools in summer 2021. This discovery set off another moral reckoning with the country's history. The Supreme Court of Canada refused to hear the appeals of the Squamish and Tsleil-Waututh nations alongside environmental groups to stop the Trans Mountain Pipeline based on the Species at Risk Act and ecological risks. It primed the pump for a government-owned company to clear and mow trees. The government's call to protect First peoples from COVID-19 deflated under these economic developments, which went hand in hand with the Dakota Access Pipeline in the United States derailed by the Standing Rock

Sioux (after courts found the U.S. Army Corps of Engineers did not consider the environmental impacts on tribes). Despite Canada's munificence and strong social safety net, its First Nations were still jeopardized by capitalist expropriation and effluence.

The pandemic did little to dim capitalist impulses, even though it tamped down on every single industry, including the influential biofuel sector. The COVID-19 disaster cued us all to the fact that although the planet's inhabitants were in the same sinking boat, passengers inhabited separate levels with some cast adrift or left to die first. Denmark and Poland declined to bail out companies with overseas tax shelters with the proviso that if businesses so desired COVID-19 funds, they must pay domestic business taxes and stop dodging their responsibilities. With "surplus scarcity" from global demand tapering off, commodities markets roiled when a spat between Saudi Arabia and Russia led global oil prices to post their biggest single-day drops since the tail end of the Gulf War in 1991, which sent shares of megacompanies Chevron and ExxonMobil tumbling due to a glut of crude.

Price wars in 2020 fizzled out with an OPEC-led agreement by top oil producers. This pact downed petroleum production and output by 10%. Business gurus admitting that there was suddenly "too much" oil is a bizarre statement, precisely when for years many economists predicted the death knell for global oil supply and reserves. As 136 countries agreed to settle on a minimum global corporate tax rate in Fall 2021, the "Pandora Papers," leaked by the International Consortium of Investigative Journalists, exposed the money laundering and tax havens of hundreds of leaders and celebrities. Economists fleetingly related these old market travails to the new "corona-capitalism."

Corona-capitalism did rework the common end of profit maximization. To coax more subjects into taking their COVID-19 shots, governments incentivized vaccination. They offered lottery prizes, manipulating the psychology behind consumer "choice" to mitigate vaccine apathy and skepticism. The WHO asked that this race to the top end, to spread the wealth. It wanted leaders of rich countries to help one-fifth of the world to achieve first vaccination before giving boosters to their own citizens. Giving muted responses or no response at all, wealthy countries strove for domestic herd immunity at 70% by any means necessary. Perks and giveaways came in the form of free cars (Russia), cannabis (the United States), soccer game tickets (England), beef raffles (the Philippines), beer (Israel), dessert (Malaysia), and cash (Cambodia).[51] All the stops were given for well-off citizens, while the poor suffered.

Some positives did come with the pandemic. Smart city planners in the world's busiest cities closed roads to allow for bicyclists and pedestrians to cut back on congestion, offering utopian visions of white urbanist fantasies rooted in "environmental racism" and "purple-lining," city planning that controls mobility through the socioeconomic spectrum.[52] The vast majority of police summons for social distance violation in New York occurred in low-income neighborhoods withering from poor air quality, but the cops were not at crowded public squares in wealthier parts of the city.

The deathly sickle of coronavirus gave complement to the capitalist god's hammer. The deferral of profits wrought by the novel coronavirus hurt the bottom line of companies, but it emptied faster the wallets of workers who paid out-of-pocket for medical expenses. For many wage laborers, they had dealt with many jobs lost and shed before in times of crisis, but the pandemic was a juggernaut. Pandemic-induced economic slowdown meant pruning of jobs in a capsizing market system. Even for knowledge workers teleworking from home, COVID-19 managed to bulldoze its way through their personal finances and professional lives. That one virus could jeopardize capitalism as it stood at the end of the decade signaled a new player on the scene that could not be left unheeded. Stopping market trade and triggering circuit breakers, COVID-19 pulled the rug on the business-as-usual mindset. This "do-over" lubricated the gears of change in the system. However, global players kept to their usual games.

Japan ploughed forward with plans to host the 2020 Summer Olympics, despite reeling sharply from the multiplier effects of COVID-19. It postponed the games to the following year. With the global sporting event rescheduled, the Land of the Rising Sun promised to rouse spirits in a pandemic-depressed world (it was more afraid to lose a billion invested dollars in the event). Rich countries like Japan had thought that they were impervious to the aftershocks of the pandemic, until it stared them right in the face. Among high-income nations, Japan held the lowest uptake of vaccination and highest distrust of inoculation. With vaccinations starting rather late, the summer tournament began as hundreds of new national cases rose sharply with no abatement. Toyota, Japan's premiere company and the Olympics' major sponsor, pulled commercials for the games, after it was revealed two-thirds of Japanese took umbrage with the tournament and after Japan declared a state of emergency due to high COVID-19 positivity. Citizens doubted the International Olympic Committee organizers and the Japanese government could keep tournament participants safe. They distrusted governing bodies who encouraged travel, preferring to boost the economy over parrying a pandemic. The shared fates among individuals found two positive symbols when high jumpers from Italy and Qatar tied and decided to share a gold medal. Sharing was indeed caring, especially in the worst of times.

In other matters, capitalism also took precedence over care, putting people in harm's way. Approved government proposals in the United States urged a moratorium on housing rent payments and to defer but not outright cancel student debt collection. Amid the need to bend the infection curve, ordinary people asked to be rescued from drowning in debt traps within healthcare, education, and housing. One pediatric infectious disease doctor in New York intimated that he preferred loan forgiveness and debt write-offs over pandemic hazard pay, and this comment prompted a lawmaker to introduce a bill to downsize student loans for healthcare workers on the frontline. Without debt relief, medical staff stood no chance to succeed in a COVID-shattered economy. Their educational finances were in the red, something eclipsed only by the new debts that they accrued under an unrelenting pandemic.

The pandemic did not dial back the clock of "civilization," nor did "corona-time" totally tear up the rhythm of global capitalism to shreds. In April 2020, China's leader, China promised to mobilize a medical and humanitarian agenda for the new age of pandemics. It lunged toward new relations of development and dependency. From instant news briefings to sudden death announcements, the standardized regular "work hours" of China's notorious 996 work culture had been interrupted by the "real time" of viral transmission.[53] *Pandemic time* overlaid time-sensitive worries about the traditional work schedule. The pandemic's pulsations did little to melt away the dreams of capitalism and goals of global domination.

With so many working people living on borrowed time, the concept of "disaster capitalism" transmogrified into "coronavirus capitalism."[54] Hurting from back-to-back disasters, Puerto Rico could not buy medical supplies from abroad, restricted to purchasing items only from the United States federal government. Hampered by a federal law called Buy America Act, agencies in the Commonwealth of Puerto Rico and the District of Columbia—both classified as a territory in the stimulus package, breaking legal precedence—needed to prioritize U.S.-made products even when they were in short supply. Puerto Rico also suffered high outstanding debt load in the billions, leading it into bankruptcy. Debt from the pandemic only warped this sour economic relationship between the United States and Puerto Rico.

Boricuas have always dealt with the recrudescence of colonialism "terrorizing" the island.[55] With disease and debt killing so many, theorist Sandra Ruiz demands a *decolonial* model of space-time, one built by and for the people, a form of living and worlding that cannot be arbitraged by the debt structures of capitalism. Like the many transmutations of coronavirus, there exists the possibility of a knowledge revolution and brokering new viral intercourse for colonized communities.

Community

The power of community stood paramount in the fight against the scourge of COVID-19. Ghana's finance minister urged China to ease African countries' debt burden, and the President of Mining Forum in South Africa tweeted that the novel coronavirus had caused the South African economy to lose billions of rand. He added that the Chinese government must cancel the debt the country owes as a "sign of remorse" for the curse it unleashed. Describing uncoordinated country-specific measures as myopic and counterproductive, Ethiopia's Prime Minister Abiy Ahmed published a public letter to the global community entitled, "If COVID-19 is not beaten in Africa it will return to haunt us all."[56] Spotty responses to health as a "worldwide public good" necessitate a global fund to provide budgetary support and structural ballast to African countries, so they can institute stopgap measures to the pandemic's moribund effects on sovereign wealth. He concludes, "COVID-19 teaches us that we are all global citizens connected by a single virus." For Ahmed, this is a viral world, where a dangerous virus can be the main connector for global citizenship.

Stopping short of cancelling all debt or injecting cash into foreign reserves via "special drawing rights," the G20 wealthiest nations agreed to suspend bilateral loan repayments for one year for the economies in the International Development Association, which includes countries like Tonga, Samoa, and Fiji. This time-bound solution defers an international balance of payment. With COVID-19 tipping the scales of power, countries had tackled the harmful expenditures and pressurized demands of borrowing from the International Monetary Fund (IMF), which gave out coronavirus emergency loans. International bodies like IMF however do not represent global societies and their diverse needs.

All told, the transformation of societies by COVID-19 was impressive, if not total. Hotels were requisitioned and repurposed as touristic lodgings to supplement hospitals at capacity. When hospitals reached full capacity, they were unable to triage a deluge of patients, let alone treat them. People died alone in hospitals as visitors were banned to halt infection. With funerals made illegal, Iran, India, and other principalities built mass graves that can be seen from space. Skating ice rinks temporarily housed cold dead bodies. How does one balance serving others while protecting oneself and the community against capitalist control? The answer lies somewhere on the edge of society and socialism.

Advocating for open-ended "knowledge socialism," the authors of *Pandemic Education and Viral Politics* advocate new social cooperatives: " 'Solidarity', 'community', 'collective responsibility and action' are the key words ringing out as a response … [to] decades of market-speak … to reshape the world in terms of new social solidarities."[57] A viral world built on social solidarity inspired people to speak collective truth to power.

With quarantined Chinese residents connected through WeChat and WhatsApp, the *xiao qu* units ranged from a few dozen to hundreds. Wuhan included over 7,000 groups that shared information and bought food in bulk, while partying virtually together. These hyperlocal mutual-aid societies spread to other localities that spanned the continents in a stunning display of viral/communal bonding. A galaxy of thick worldly relations was built on top of institutional effacement and erasure.

Local community groups seized control of "the situation" from feckless governments. For instance, take the turn of events after Haiti's President Jovenel Moïse was shot dead in his own home and the country fell into disarray.[58] The President's rule by decree after dissolving parliament and suppression of citizens—none of whom had been delivered one shot of COVID-19 vaccination—led to the country's demise. Protests after the assassination caught fire from the rising political temperature in a country that over a year before experienced demonstrations over missing PetroCaribe aid. Apparently embezzled by the president's administration, Moïse's entanglement with international players and dealings with disreputable gang leaders led to his downfall. There was now no one to trust—not the United States, which supplies arms to Haiti, nor the United Nations, which once introduced cholera to the island and had yet to fully compensate for it. With an authority vacuum from the prime minister stepping down (and other top officials dead from COVID-19), organized popular sectors lead the way in safeguarding rural and urban communities, especially after another devastating earthquake that left thousands dead.[59] Only local movements engaged in direct action could truly "save" Haiti, practicing solidarity economies based on communal *konbit* traditions and cooperatives that emphasize food sovereignty over and against the ambitions of vainglorious men.[60]

As one part of his many power grabs, Moïse had given over vast tracts of arable land to rich tycoons like André Apaid, Jr. in early 2020. The businessman led the coalition that forced from power Haiti's first democratically elected president (Jean-Bertrand Aristide), a coup that involved collaboration with paramilitaries and the United States. To build sweatshops for Coca Cola, Apaid financed armed gangs to kill supporters for Fanmi Lavalas, a social democratic politician that wanted reform.[61] Moise's assassination was preceded by the killings of human rights activists like Antoinette Duclaire who spoke out against such corruption. The hail of bullets that brought an end to Duclaire's life only doubled down on the need for justice for community leaders.

While the Diné (known widely by outsiders as the Navajo) suffered greatly from COVID-19, they did not shrink from the moment to play up their communal strengths. The tribe even sent masks to India as that country hit a deadly flashpoint. President of the Diné nation, Jonathan Nez, aired a town hall on Facebook, blasting the U.S. federal government for neglecting the concerns of Native Americans. Indeed, the White House originally wanted to give nothing to tribes in its COVID-19 stimulus bill. At the same time, Nez wanted to head off narratives of helplessness and suffering for the Diné:

We have overcome tough times and we're utilizing resources to help our people out there. Governments can't do everything. I'm hearing about people hauling water for their grandparents, people helping get water and hay for their elders out there. That's Diné right there ... we've got to think of our future ... We can't let our elders leave us earlier.[62]

Despite its strict stay-at-home mandate, the county where the Diné lived was ranked 13th in the world for COVID-19 infection rates. These numbers were proportionally highest within the United States, outstripping even New York City. In New Mexico, which contains a good portion of the Diné reservation, Native peoples consist of 10% of the state's population but 60% of the infected, according to the CDC's COVID-19 Race Tracker (May 23, 2020).[63] The nation had faced worse and leveraged people power to address hauling water from a public tap due to the fact that up to one-third of its residents were without running water.

Delays in coronavirus aid were deferrals of justice. A federal judge ordered the U.S. Treasury Secretary to distribute close to a billion dollars of relief funds to Native communities after months of unjustified delay. As the first Indigenous Secretary of the Interior, Debra Anne Haaland reminded the federal government that by law and "trust responsibility" it must provide adequate health care to Native peoples, even though this group receives only a third of what is spent on the average American.[64]

That tortuous government-to-government relationship means little, when South Dakota's governor faced a stand-off with Sioux tribes over checkpoints on state highways to prevent people entering Tribal land. A similar situation unspooled in Canada, where the Nunavut community of Rankin Inlet blocked the road to the Agnico-Eagle Meliadine gold mine to stop the spread of COVID-19. The Haida Nation asked tourists not to visit in order to protect its citizens as well. Tourists and mining companies defied the wishes of Tribal communities.[65]

Despite not issuing stay-at-home orders for the state, South Dakota's governor set immediately to the task of removing these "illegal" and "interfering" community safeguards. She persisted in removing legal fortifications that defended Indigenous health and sovereignty. By year's end, those Native-governed areas had contracted the highest COVID-19 cases per capita in the world. Cheyenne River Sioux Tribe's Chairman declares that they are defending both the "right to live" as a people and their sovereignty:

Before any white man can travel or reside on our lands, they must get consent from the Indians first ... that these lands, these roads, they are ours, because we were never paid for it. So we have every legal right to do that. And it doesn't matter, you know, what comes today, tomorrow. We're still going to be here.[66]

Legal conditions set by the colonial state posed a hindrance to Native tribes' ability to protect themselves against an intractable pandemic. Such policies border on genocide after centuries of genocidal conquest: a tragedy that Tribal communities have come to know too well. Maternal death rates spike most for Native women. A secret policy of conducting involuntary coronavirus screenings was undertaken by a women's hospital in Albuquerque, New Mexico, picking out test subjects based on appearance alone or residential zip code. This catch-all "Pueblos List" did not accord with actual hot spots or CDC guidelines to test based on symptoms not identity.[67] An expectant mother that "appeared" Indigenous, absent of any symptoms, was designated a "person under investigation," and those residents waiting for their pending test results were pulled apart from their children in a repeat of history where Native youth were separated from their families to facilitate the act of forced assimilation into white culture.

The interhuman transmission of COVID-19 fell into the intergenerational trauma and legacy of forced removal. Jen Deerinwater, a journalist who is a disabled, Two Spirit, and a citizen of the Cherokee Nation, describes the longtime practice of constricting Indigenous people's movement, socially distancing those deemed "useless" or "unworthy" from mainstream U.S. society, and exposing them to disease. She writes, "Pandemics and germ warfare have been used to kill us, and there are signs that this could happen again."[68] Deerinwater infers that the U.S. government is again sacrificing Native populations.

Messages of "going back to normal" masks ableist colonial language that buries concerns of local tribes. Doctors without Borders, which sends medical professions into international conflict zones and does not typically operate in the United States, sent a team of physicians and midwives to the Diné Nation. By then, the nation suffered more per capita cases of COVID-19 than any U.S. state (those patients seriously infected needed to be airlifted to hospitals outside the reservation). In the final frame, the viability of the Diné people involved more than logistical approaches to public health and medicine, but a grounded awareness of community needs and Indigenous worldviews. Family doctor and frontline worker Michelle Tom worried about the repercussions of the novel coronavirus on her tribe yet finds hope in the tribe's continued survivance and regeneration: "Our languages, our culture, our people … can continue to live forever, as long as there are Diné people."[69]

Taking the people's future survival into their own hands, resourceful seamstresses in First Nations made over 18,000 masks and sent out care packages to first responders, community members, clinicians, and hospital workers. Using materials and donations from across the country, the volunteer group was a subsidiary of the Diné & Hopi Families COVID-19 Relief Fund (Relief Fund), founded in March 2020 to mobilize Diné and Hopi female leaders and provide over 4,000 Native households with food and water. Diné

Seamstresses United COVID-19 Dooda expanded from its original small chapter and now drew members from the Diné and Hopi reservations in other states and members from the Blackfeet, Lakota, Dakota, and Nakota nations.

Demonstrating their labor of love, the seamstresses met the demand for masks and gowns, which were necessary to keep their community and other people safe. Indigenous seamstresses dwelled on the pandemic frontlines, and soon many others were laboring there. As nations closed in and communities worked on themselves, the danger of coronavirus drifted over physical distances, forcing people to collaborate and overcome social separation and physical distancing.

Notes

1 Tracy Samilton, "Detroit Unveils Water Restart Plan Because of Coronavirus Threat," *Michigan Radio*, March 9, 2020, www.michiganradio.org/post/detroit-unveils-water-restart-plan-because-coronavirus-threat

2 The easing of restriction on men who have sex with men also came same time as easing restrictions from donors from malaria-prone places in Africa and European countries with risk of Creuzfledt-Jakob Disease.

3 Nick Martin, "Against Productivity in a Pandemic," *New Republic*, March 17, 2020, https://newrepublic.com/article/156929/work-home-productivity-coronavirus-pandemic

4 CBS News, " 'Shoot Them Dead': Philippine President Orders Police, Military to Kill Citizens Who Defy Coronavirus Lockdown," *CBS News*, April 2, 2020, www.news9.com/story/41967605/shoot-them-dead-philippine-president-orders-police-military-to-kill-citizens-who-defy-coronavirus-lockdown

5 Ted Regencia, 'Kill Them': Duterte Wants to 'Finish off' Communist Rebels," *Aljazeera*, March 6, 2021, www.aljazeera.com/news/2021/3/6/kill-them-all-duterte-wants-communist-rebels-finished

6 Chad Terhune, Dan Levine, Hyunjoo Jin, and Jane Lanhee Lee, "Special Report: How Korea Trounced U.S. in Race to Test People for Coronavirus," *Reuters*, March 18, 2020, www.reuters.com/article/us-health-coronavirus-testing-specialrep/special-report-how-korea-trounced-u-s-in-race-to-test-people-for-coronavirus-idUSKBN2153BW

7 Steven Borowiec, "How South Korea's Coronavirus Outbreak Got So Quickly Out of Control," *Time*, February 24, 2020, https://time.com/5789596/south-korea-coronavirus-outbreak/

8 Peter Banseok Kwon, "Building Bombs, Building a Nation: The State, Chaebŏl, and the Militarized Industrialization of South Korea, 1973–1979," *The Journal of Asian Studies* 79, no. 1 (2020): 51–75.

9 President Moon criticized his predecessor, Park Geun-hye, for her handling of the MERS epidemic. The introduction of a disease associated with camels came by way of a businessman who visited the Arabian Peninsula.

10 Choe Sang-Hun, "South Korean Leader Said Coronavirus Would 'Disappear.' It Was a Costly Error," *New York Times*, February 27, 2020, www.nytimes.com/2020/02/27/world/asia/coronavirus-south-korea.html?searchResultPosition=2

11 Steven Kashkett, "Czech Republic Has Lifesaving COVID-19 Lesson for America: Wear a Face Mask," *USA Today*, July 14, 2020, www.usatoday.com/story/opinion/2020/07/14/how-czech-republic-beat-covid-require-everyone-wear-face-masks-column/5426602002/

12 Haleigh Atwood, "The End of Ice," *Lion's Roar*, October 2, 2019, www.lionsroar.com/the-end-of-ice/

13 S. Nathan Park, "Confucianism Isn't Helping Beat the Coronavirus," *Foreign Policy*, April 2, 2020, https://foreignpolicy.com/2020/04/02/confucianism-south-korea-coronavirus-testing-cultural-trope-orientalism/

14 Porsha Hall and Mary Anne Adams, "Creating Havens for Black Lesbian Elders during COVID-19," *Journal of Lesbian Studies* (2023): 1–13; Hazel T. Biana and Rosallia Domingo, "Lesbian Single Parents: Reviewing Philippine COVID-19 Policies," *Journal of International Women's Studies* 22, no. 12 (2021): 135–147.

15 Frances Nguyen, "This State Says It Has a 'Feminist Economic Recovery Plan.' Here's What That Looks Like," *The Lily*, April 22, 2020, www.thelily.com/this-state-says-they-have-a-feminist-economic-recovery-plan-heres-what-that-looks-like/

16 Malaysia is listed at 104 out of 153 countries for women's political empowerment and economic production/ Michael Sullivan, "Don't Nag Your Husband during Lockdown, Malaysia's Government Advises Women," *NPR*, April 1, 2020, www.npr.org/2020/04/01/825051317/dont-nag-your-husband-during-lock-down-malaysias-government-advises-women

17 Sam Walker, "In the Coronavirus Crisis, Deputies Are the Leaders We Turn to," *The Watertown Works*, April 4, 2020, www.watertownworks.com/in-the-coronavirus-crisis-deputies-are-the-leaders-we-turn-to/

18 It commended the physician for informed straight talk and stoic calm, despite having been lacerated for her shoddy handling of the MERS outbreak.

19 Isobel Asher Hamilton, "11 Countries Are Now Using People's Phones to Track the Coronavirus Pandemic, and It Heralds a Massive Increase in Surveillance," *Business Insider*, March 26, 2020, www.businessinsider.com/countries-tracking-citizens-phones-coronavirus-2020-3

20 Seulki Lee, "South Korea's First Feminist Party Launches on International Women's Day," *The Jakarta Post*, March 3, 2020, www.thejakartapost.com/news/2020/03/03/south-koreas-first-feminist-party-launches-on-international-womens-day.html

21 Whitney N. Laster Pirtle, "Racial Capitalism: A Fundamental Cause of Novel Coronavirus (COVID-19) Pandemic Inequities in the United States," *Health Education and Behavior* 47, no. 4 (2020): 504–508.

22 Stevie Ruiz, *Earth Stewards: Reclaiming Hidden Labor Practices in Environmental Spaces* (Chapel Hill, N.C.: University of North Carolina Press, 2025).

23 Layla Brown-Vincent, "The Pandemic of Racial Capitalism: Another World Is Possible," *From the European South* 7 (2020): 68.

24 Kevin Dukes, "Transgender Woman Shot to Death in Ambulance while Being Treated in South Charlotte," *Lovelyti*, March 19, 2020, https://lovelyti.com/2020/03/19/transgender-woman-shot-to-death-in-ambulance-while-being-treated-in-south-charlotte/

25 Alexandra Juhasz, Nishant Shahani, and Jih-Fei Cheng, eds., "Foreword, Preface, and Introduction," *AIDS and the Distribution of Crises* (Durham, NC: Duke University, 2020), 4, 16.

26 Mary Papenfuss, "Norway College Urges Students to Return from 'Poorly Developed' U.S. amid Pandemic," *Huffpost*, March 15, 2020, www.huffpost.com/entry/nor way-students-us-collective infrastructure_n_5e6ec485c5b6dda30fcbba2a

27 In 2021, the Labour Party won a landslide victory in parliament, riding to success on a platform of reducing inequalities, such as lowering taxes for low-to-middle-income earners and increasing taxes for the rich. With the largest party working with the Centre Party and Socialist Left, the country with the largest sovereign wealth fund and the biggest producer of gas and oil in Europe hoped to move in a new direction, economically and environmentally.

28 Rob Wallace, Alex Liebman, Luis Fernando Chaves, and Rodrick Wallace, "COVID-19 and Circuits of Capital," *Monthly Review*, May 1, 2020, https:// monthlyreview.org/2020/05/01/covid-19-and-circuits-of-capital/

29 Janine Jackson, "'Our Food System Is Very Much Modeled on Plantation Economics'" *Fair*, May 13, 2020, https://fair.org/home/our-food-system-is-very-much-modeled-on-plantation-economics/

30 Matt Sparke and Dimitar Anguelov, "Contextualising Coronavirus Geographically," *Royal Geographical Society* (April 30, 2020): 498–508.

31 Zsombor Peter, "Malaysia Rounds up Hundreds of Undocumented Migrants amid Coronavirus Fears," *Voice of America News*, May 3, 2020, www.voanews. com/east-asia-pacific/malaysia-rounds-hundreds-undocumented-migrants-amid-coronavirus-fears

32 No author, "The COVID-19 Crisis Is Fueling More Racist Discourse towards Migrant Workers the Gulf," *Migrant Rights*, April 5, 2020, www.migrant-rights. org/2020/04/the-covid-19-crisis-is-fueling-more-racist-discourse-towards-migr ant-workers-in-the-gulf/

33 Ibram X. Kendi, "We're Still Living and Dying in the Slaveholder's Republic," *The Atlantic*, May 4, 2020, www.theatlantic.com/ideas/archive/2020/05/what-freedom-means-trump/611083/

34 Vito Laterza and Louis Philippe Römer, "COVID-19, the Freedom to Die, and the Necropolitics of the Market," *Somatosphere*, May 12, 2020, http://somatosphere. net/2020/necropolitics-of-the-market.html/

35 Nick Hanauer, "Our Uniquely American Virus," *The Prospect*, April 14, 2020, https://prospect.org/coronavirus/our-uniquely-american-virus/

36 Kim Willsher, Julian Borger, and Oliver Holmes, "US Accused of 'Modern Piracy' after Diversion of Masks Meant for Europe," *The Guardian*, April 3, 2020, www. theguardian.com/world/2020/apr/03/mask-wars-coronavirus-outbidding-demand

37 Paul Constant, "Coronavirus Didn't Bring the Economy Down—40 Years of Greed and Corporate Malfeasance Did," *Insider*, April 10, 2020, www.busi nessinsider.com/pitchfork-economics-coronavirus-not-hurting-economy-corpor ate-greed-is-2020-4

38 Jordan Fabian, "Trump Told Governors to Buy Own Virus Supplies, Then Outbid Them," *Bloomberg*, March 19, 2020, www.bloomberg.com/news/articles/2020-03-19/trump-told-governors-to-buy-own-virus-supplies-then-outbid-them

39 Joe Garofoli, "Gavin Newsom Wants California to Be Its Own Nation-State in the Trump Era," *San Francisco Chronicle*, February 12, 2019, www.sfchronicle.com/ politics/article/Gavin-Newsom-wants-California-to-be-its-own-13611747.php

40 Dan Burrows, "China's Evergrande Crisis: A Real Threat to U.S. Stocks?" *Kiplinger*, September 20, 2021, www.kiplinger.com/investing/stocks/603465/ china-evergrande-crisis-us-stock-market

41 Michael Barbaro, "The Great Pandemic Theft," *New York Times*, September 27, 2022, www.nytimes.com/2022/09/27/podcasts/the-daily/pandemic-fraud.html

42 Andrea Germanos, "Coronavirus Pandemic Triggered 'One of the Greatest Wealth Transfers in History' " *Salon*, June 7, 2020, www.salon.com/2020/06/07/coronavirus-pandemic-triggered-one-of-the-greatest-wealth-transfers-in-history_partner/

43 Joe Concha, "Glenn Beck: 'I'd Rather Die' from Coronavirus 'than Kill the Country' from Economic Shutdown," *The Hill*, March 25, 2020, https://thehill.com/homenews/media/489472-glenn-beck-id-rather-die-from-coronavirus-than-kill-the-country-from-economic

44 Shannon Pettypiece and Peter Alexander, "Trump Says He Wants Country 'Opened Up' by Easter, despite Caution from Health Experts," *NBC News*, March 24, 2020, www.nbcnews.com /politics/white-house/trump-says-he-wants-country-open-back-april-12-easter-n1167721

45 Andrew Liu, " 'Chinese Virus,' World Market," *N+1 Magazine*, March 20, 2020, https://nplusonemag.com/online-only/online-only/chinese-virus-world-market/

46 Chloe Taylor, "Brazil's President Attacks Amazon Rainforest 'Lies' and Thanks Trump for Support," *CNBC*, September 24, 2019, www.cnbc.com/2019/09/24/brazils-president-attacks-amazon-rainforest-lies-thanks-trump.html

47 Tom Philllips, "Brazil's Jair Bolsonaro Says Coronavirus Crisis Is a Media Trick," *The Guardian*, March 23, 2020, www.theguardian.com/world/2020/mar/23/brazils-jair-bolsonaro-says-coronavirus-crisis-is-a-media-trick; David Biller, "Brazil's Bolsonaro Makes Life-or-Death Coronavirus Gamble," *Associated Press*, March 28, 2020, https://apnews.com/b21a2963694c6726d03e027134dafl

48 This comes after the resignation of the influential minster of justice Sergio Moro, who had advanced the prosecution of the previous two presidents for graft, setting Brazil on a path of destruction.

49 G. Slattery and R. Moraes, "In Violent Rio, U.S. Protests Stoke Backlash against Deadly Cops," *Reuters*, June 7, 2020, www.reuters.com/article/us-brazil-protests-race-feature-idUSKBN23E0QF/.

50 Jay Wamsted, "ZIP Code May Not Be Destiny, but It's as Hard to Fight as Gravity," *Education Post*, May 15, 2020, https://educationpost.org/zip-code-may-not-be-destiny-but-its-as-hard-to-fight-as-gravity/

51 Sonia Elks, "Carrot or Stick? How Countries Are Tackling COVID-19 Vaccine Hesitancy," *Thomson Reuters Foundation*, July 6, 2021, https://news.trust.org/item/20210601155421-gr1fs/

52 Alissa Walker, "Coronavirus Is Not Fuel for Urbanist Fantasies: This Moment Should Be about Reassessing Our Broken Cities," *Curbed*, May 20, 2020, www.curbed.com/2020/5/20/21263319/ coronavirus-future-city-urban-covid-19

53 Peter Adey, Kevin Hannam, Mimi Sheller, and David, Tyfield, "Pandemic (Im) mobilities" *Mobilities* 16, no. 2 (2021): 6.

54 Naomi Klein, *The Shock Doctrine: The Rise of Disaster Capitalism* (New York: Macmillan, 2007).

55 Sandra Ruiz, *Ricanness: Enduring Time in Anticolonial Performance* (New York: New York University Press, 2019), 171.

56 Abiy Ahmed, "If Covid-19 Is Not Beaten in Africa It Will Return to Haunt Us All: Only a Global Victory Can End This Pandemic, Not a Temporary Rich Countries' Win," *The Guardian*, March 25, 2020, www.ft.com/content/c12a09c8-6db6-11ea-89df-41bea055720b

57 Michael A. Peters, Tina Besley, *Pandemic Education and Viral Politics* (London: Routledge, 2020), 83.

58 It was found that a July 2021 by a transnational coterie of assassins mostly from Colombia was responsible.

59 Mamyrah Dougé-Prosper and Mark Schuller, "After Moïse Assassination, Popular Sectors Must Lead the Way," *NACLA*, July 8, 2021, https://nacla.org/haiti-jove nel-moise-assassination-social-movements

60 Dougé-Prosper and Mamyrah A. "Solidarity Economy Praxis in Limonade." *Women's Studies Quarterly* 47.3/4 (2019): 190–211.

61 Yves Engler, "Racial Capitalism and the Betrayal of Haiti," *Canadian Dimension*, February 26, 2021, https://canadiandimension.com/articles/view/racial-capital ism-and-the-betrayal-of-haiti

62 *AMIBC*, "Native Americans Ignored amid Coronavirus," *AIMBCI*, April 1, 2020, https://amibc.com/clear-lens/coronavirus/native-americans-ignored-amid-coronavirus/

63 The CDC tracks excess deaths from any cause, putting mortality above its official totals.

64 Chiara Sottile and Erik Ortiz, "Coronavirus Hits Indian Country Hard, Exposing Infrastructure Disparities," *NBC News*, April 19, 2020, www.nbcnews.com/ news/us-news/coronavirus-hits-indian-country-hard-exposing-infrastructure-disp arities-n1186976

65 Sean Carleton, "Coronavirus Colonialism: How the COVID-19 Crisis Is Catalyzing Dispossession," *Canadian Dimension*, March 23, 2020, https://canadi andimension.com/articles/view/coronavirus-colonialism-how-crisis-is-catalyzing-dispossession

66 Democracy Now, "Standoff in South Dakota: Cheyenne River Sioux Refuse Governor's Demand to Remove COVID Checkpoints," *Democracy Now*, May 12, 2020, www.democracynow.org /2020/5/12/cheyenne_river_sioux_coronavirus_ checkpoints_south

67 Bryant Furlow, "A Hospital's Secret Coronavirus Policy Separated Native American Mothers from Their Newborns," *ProPublica*, June 13, 2020, www.pro publica.org/article/a-hospitals-secret-coronavirus-policy-separated-native-ameri can-mothers-from-their-newborns

68 Jen Deerinwater, "I'm Native and Disabled. The US Government Is Sacrificing My People," *Truth Out*, April 26, 2020, https://truthout.org/articles/im-native-and-disabled-the-government-is-sacrificing-my-people/

69 Christina Capatides, "Doctors Without Borders Dispatches Team to the Navajo Nation," *CBS News*, May 11, 2020, www.cbsnews.com/news/doctors-without-borders-navajo-nation-coronavirus/

4

PHYSICAL DISTANCING

Removal, Racism, Refugee

With the entire world creaking under the COVID-19 pandemic, the next viral hot spot was just around the corner. The probability of catching sickness was so high that communities were heartened to practice "social distancing." Derived from health studies, this strange, inelegant term stood out in the public's mind as one of the best practices to avoid infecting oneself while in proximity to others with COVID-19 hanging around. The origins of this popularized term can be traced to a sociological measure of racial prejudice, the Social Distance Scale, which came after the Red Summer of 1919 when White mobs attacked African American migrants in dozens of cities across the United States.[1] Under the tight grip of state racism, social distancing meant racial distancing. The forcible removal of people of color from publicly "protected" spaces in the pandemic's sandstorm reveals the segregationist history behind this concept. The term gained attention again in history with the AIDS epidemic before morphing into its current form in the early twenty-first century for SARS and COVID-19 to mean *physical distancing* in times of a health crisis and the fear of another contagion.

Physical distance was championed by health officials to hold a fighting chance against COVID-19—even while it instilled fear and paranoia in thinking everyone might harbor the disease. Distancing was the first step and key component for flattening the curve. Inability to distance in crowded hospitals meant a surge in newly infected patients, which would incapacitate the entire medical system. From leprosy to HIV, the call to stay away from infectious dangerous "others" tended toward placing demeaning labels onto marginalized people. The pandemic encapsulated the habituation of racism and the removal of migrants and Indigenous groups. By staying apart from

DOI: 10.4324/9781032694535-5

others with an ample amount of physical distance, this simple act chokes off the highly contagious virus and probability of contact between carriers. We needed to flinch away from others to protect the self.

COVID-19 planted overwrought fears about the safety of extended care in hospitals, where one might become infected while obtaining treatment. On an emotional level, physical distancing brought on loneliness and separation anxieties.[2] Media theorist Ruha Benjamin observes, all of this isolation made the case for "a libertarian ethos that assumes what we all *really* want is to be left alone, screen in hand, staring at reflections of ourselves."[3] The pandemic sped up contractual gig work and on-the-fly care, but the demoralizing, depersonalizing ethos of physical distancing joined the growing chorus to "move slower and empower people."[4]

Political theorist Tiffany Willoughby-Herard posted on Facebook a spiritually reflective poem that speaks to the quiet busyness of pandemic life:

I am busy
Moving/thinking/breathing
Feeling/Reflecting/Knowing …
I am still
But also busy.[5]

This lyrical meditation echoes advice for self-care by theorist bell hooks, who conveys the message that one must savor stillness to assist others. The feminist advises Black women to not isolate themselves despite wanting to hide from a hostile world: "We are 'too busy' to find time for solitude … Without knowing how to be alone, we cannot know how to be with others and sustain the necessary autonomy."[6]

Autonomy and community were major themes for marked women. Muslim women wearing the *niqab* looked differently conspicuous in a masked-up world. Veiled women who were interviewed about head and face coverings found life barely improved for them, even after health officials recommended for everyone to wear thick cloth fabrics over thin surgical masks. Commonly held at a distance by gawkers, these women found a bit more tolerance under the pandemic, donning the veil with less fear of it being forcibly removed by authorities.[7] Yet in France, where citizens carry the risk of being fined if caught in public without a mask, women paid a high fine if they wear the *niqab*. Physical distancing policies did not prevent physical violence against Somali refugee women who were just going out. As reported in the Canadian city of Edmonton, Muslim women avoided public transits and parks. To feel safe, especially after hearing about a fatal stabbing in Toronto and a Muslim family ran over by a van in London, women practiced even more physical distancing than needed.[8] Sisters Dialogue, a feminist Muslim advocacy group, planned safe-walk services for women, overriding the downstream effects of physical distancing with social intimacy.

Physical distancing signaled a loss of the human dimension, something that did not work for those people with disabilities and special needs or requiring personal assistance. For low-income school children who require free lunch programs for daily meals, physical distancing meant hunger and starvation. Little protection was offered to minors abused at home, the early signs of which can be caught by social workers or teachers. Rates of domestic and intimate partner violence skyrocketed as part of a "shadow pandemic" according to United Nations Women. As reported by Refuge, the United Kingdom's largest domestic abuse charity, there was a 700% bump in calls to its helpline during lockdown. Domestic abuse survivors feared for their lives staying indoors too long with their aggressive partners; homestay could mean death. Mexico saw close to 1,000 women murdered within the first three months of 2020. Martha Tagle from the Citizens' Movement Party confirmed that "the deadliest pandemic for women in our country, more than the coronavirus, is feminicidal violence."[9]

Physical distancing extends into death as when families were recommended by Ireland's health ministry to not kiss their deceased kin in open caskets with funerals barred in favor of burial videos sent to mourners. In Spain, patients in nursing homes were abandoned by caretakers fearing infection. Not only did it make democracy harder in terms of collective activity, Spain's prime minister called COVID-19 a "cruel" disease since it freezes the all-too-human need to socialize.[10] Indeed, how one socializes within the deadly jaws of a pandemic is linked to a longer history of dislocation and removal. Hence, this chapter examines closely the subjects of removal, racism, and refugees.

This chapter probes how the pandemic language of social/physical distancing perpetuates the ongoing dispossession of First Peoples, the segregation of people of color, and the expulsion of refugees. It examines distancing as more than a public health precept, but something that reinforces and furthers isolation from those deemed unworthy of protection. One example concerns U.S. military spread of COVID-19 to the shores of Guam/Guåhan infecting the local population, once again requiring locals to protect their world against foreign invaders. Another example is the removal of Indigenous activists from their sacred land and the denial of First Nations from receiving government stimulus funds. Discrimination and forms of effacement can be linked to anti-Black racism in China and Islamophobia in South Asia. Within India, the shutdown of the economy propelled a mass wave of internally displaced migrants. Forced migrants and refugees found difficulty in obtaining asylum at a time when countries shut their borders to keep out the new coronavirus. The figure of the COVID-19 refugee twinned other pandemic specters in a period of global im/mobility.

Removal

Collective repulsions against COVID-19 led to the lockup or removal of populations deemed Other within the "social body." Despite perceptions that Pacific Islanders were statistically insignificant as a population for COVID-19 studies, the pandemic's disproportionate impact on them could not be dismissed. When data charts were released from the California and Los Angeles departments of public health, it was discovered that the death rate for Pasifika people was 12 times higher than for Whites and twice the state average.

Communities on the margins struck back on culturally sensitive terms. Dr. Raynald Samoa, an endocrinologist leading national efforts to treat this group responded by explaining that asking a Pacific person to remove themselves from family is culturally unthinkable. Leaving relatives during times of illness, he emphasizes, is "one of the least Pacific things to do."[11] With its emphasis on a new sociality called "bubbles" or "pods," Samoa indicates New Zealand as an exemplar of quarantine in its aggressive testing and early testing, especially of Maori and Pasifika groups. The "Kiwi strategy" did not prevent COVID-19 from being doubly deadly for these groups who made up a plurality of the prison population. In the United States, despite the high imprisonment of people of color, a lack of disaggregation for race and ethnicity made things hard to distinguish who needed the most support.

A pandemic reveals the weakest links of a viral world. As media studies scholar Shiqi Lin observes,

> Far from being isolated from the rest of the world, we can say that a quarantined camp like the city of Wuhan or the Diamond Princess cruise ship is, in fact, quite emblematic of our fortified world at this moment.[12]

As the first cruise ship to discover COVID-19 cases, Diamond Princess with its 600 infected needed to be docked at Japan for weeks, even while other ships like Ruby Princess kept going out to sea, which allowed SARS-CoV-2 to tunnel into countries like Australia. Lacking real medical facilities onboard and relying on offshore state-of-the art hospitals, the ships got caught up in the blame game. The U.S. Coast Guard told loitering cruise ships with foreign flags that they must take care of its passengers. This memorandum cordoned off ships found loitering around Florida and shackled multinationals that registered in overseas nations.

For a long time, U.S.-headquartered companies like Carnival, Royal Caribbean, and Norwegian avoided taxes through offshore tax havens. The U.S. Coast Guard insisted that these companies should rely on their respective registered countries like Panama, Liberia, and Bermuda to save them. After the United States suspended all sailing trips and set no sail orders,

Holland American sought a port for its cruise ship after four people died and 200 sickened. Several countries made no allowances for docking, a sort of punishment for a profit-driven global industry that grinded on for weeks, even after overhearing the tragedy of Diamond Princess. As a "nation of floating castaways," crew members and passengers were marooned off the coasts of foreign countries and some were briefly stranded at sea.[13]

The pandemics' oscillation extended the state's power to remove or excise people at will. In Ciudad Juárez, hundreds of workers at *maquiladora* factories protested forced labor with COVID-19 floating around, demanding closure of the foreign-run export plants along the U.S.-Mexico border. Sickness had befallen workers, but they were harangued or dismissed without compensation if they walked out on work. Mexico closed more than a dozen *maquilas* when the country, though many companies skirted COVID-19 precautions (the Pentagon asked Mexico to reopen factories for weapon manufacture).

Ecuador and Brazil emerged as the early epicenters of Latin America due to the expulsion of technical and scientific experts from national leadership. A data scientist from the University of São Paulo commented on his role as a COVID-19 researcher:

> I look at the data and make analyses for the government. But as a citizen, I'm frustrated. The government is trying to control the epidemic without the elements of how to control it because they don't know how serious it is.[14]

The government created its own data against those produced by knowledge workers in order to control the message.

There is a fallacy of thinking the pandemic's vertigo as completely shaking up our social core and DNA. The pandemic loaded the dice against the poor, generating prognoses of a not too bright future for them. It did unglue some of the privileged from a tranquil innocent past, but wealth inequities persisted. The wish for science or governments to save everyone from the novel coronavirus is a universalism that elides discriminatory social designs. Black people *already* live in the post-COVID future, says Ruha Bejamin, since "the plight of Black people has consistently been a harbinger of wider processes … which then get rolled out on an even wider scale."[15] Before the outbreak, there were stories involving detestable moments of Black patients dying on hospital floors while waiting to acquire any form of medical treatment.

Under the fulsome reign of a powerful disease like COVID-19, death by racism or the "racial death gap" carried even more weight. The pandemic turned racism into a signpost of group exposure to "premature death," leaving its big mark on an "America-sized outbreak." As common dominators in the pandemic's infernal affairs, racial policing operated as the bellwether to a pandemic racial regime. Blackness and Black bodies are kept out the public's view (through media exclusion, spatial segregation, or imprisonment), while being rendered hypervisible by state surveillance. Reports showed a disproportionate people of color in New York City were arrested for "loitering" in open-space parks meant to help alleviate crowding and prevent sickness. Two years from retirement, phlebotomist Deborah Gatewood in Detroit died from COVID-19 symptoms after being denied a test four times by her own employer. To map "health disparities" that turn her death into a faceless statistic minimizes "racism's economic irrationality."[16]

State mandates to shelter-in-place paralleled the hard work to find housing for the unsheltered, while some housing insecure communities reclaimed vacant homes to escape SARS-CoV-2 (a U.S. government report found half of all American families without shelter were Black).

Public recommendations that social groups, no matter how mammoth or minuscule, should not congregate altered the social fabric beyond recognition. Health media campaigns stayed adamant on people covering their mouths while coughing. Individuals needed an optimal six feet apart from one another, giving wide berth to atomized respiratory droplet nuclei from saliva found within "viral clouds."[17] COVID-19 is detectable and durable in aerosols according to a National Institute of Health study. A Belgian-Dutch study found that traces of virus shedding (lyses) can be picked up from running or biking from the slipstream of others. Other means for keeping up socialization and learning were required.

Education went from being in person to asynchronous distant learning within a matter of days. Low-income students living in crowded homes with no Internet fell into the gulf of the "digital divide." Alongside learning loss, they received less information about COVID-19 to protect themselves. Disadvantaged groups across the social spectrum were removed by intent or by proxy as the novel coronavirus rolled across the globe. The pandemic revealed society's underside and exposed its fault lines.[18]

Encouragement for videoconferencing via Zoom video came over regular face-to-face meetings, despite the invasion of privacy and "Zoombombers" with offensive images or derogatory messages. Gripped by new "panic-gogy," Zoom shut down and blocked the accounts of pro-democracy activists in Hong Kong to comply with Chinese law. Reporters broadcast disconcerting news about the world from the comfort of their homes. Elbow-touching or head bowing now held cachet instead of the usual European handshake or hugging. Prince Charles, successor to the British crown, needed to forgo the latter for a greeting of clasped palms to greet guests as is common in Southeast Asia. But this gesture did not prevent the future King from later testing positive for COVID-19. The Vatican broadcast online masses from empty churches, while prayers were prohibited at mosques in Saudi Arabia, except the major ones in Mecca and Medina.

Physical distancing did not mean emotional distance. Staying a comfortable distance took on relevance in post-COVID life, as a "social vaccine" to protect oneself and protect others while being in communication and community. Under the pandemic's penumbra and necropolitical schemes to wipe out certain populations, what was needed more than ever was social solidarity.

The viral connectivity articulated the world as one and as many. It is crucial then to discombobulate the different viral worlds that people live in. Small nations are keen to watch events in other regions, all more so when the activities of bigger countries impact them acutely. No less significant, these governments' actions serve as the barometer for measuring planetary ups and downs. Austria was one of the first countries to lock down public life, and one influential Austrian businesswoman puts it this way: "We're a small country, but we can learn from everybody and we do not think that we know everything … there is an inborn arrogance of large countries … small countries tend to learn much more from each other."[19] The removal of Indigenous nations and small island developing states (SIDS) from the international decision-making on COVID-19 means few viable methods of confronting adversity in our pandemic-entangled worlds.

Julián Castro, a Latino U.S. presidential candidate in 2020 scoffed at the idea that everyone suffers the planetary condition. He said, the Latine community "seems to have the worst of all worlds."[20] Latine and migrants were on the frontlines as farmworkers, nurses, and services workers, as well as small business owners. These "human shields" bore the lion's share of pain and responsibility for humanity's survival.

COVID-19 rules generated ramifications beyond disease management. Some in the U.S. media asked if the novel coronavirus is "China's Chernobyl," comparing the 1987 nuclear reactor meltdown in the Soviet Union to the Communist Party of China.[21] Indeed, pandemics are only as bad as governments are. On March 27, 2020, the U.S. Environmental Protection Agency announced it would waive its enforcement of legally mandated public health standards and environment protection. Against the backdrop of a pandemic, the agency's decision to relax environmental standards and enforcement of laws made no sense. The biggest polluters, oil and gas companies, stood to gain the most. This relinquishment of government duties and the decrease of monitoring, fines, or penalties set a dangerous precedent in a year like no other. The president of the National Wildlife Federation called it a state-orchestrated assault on the environment and an abdication of responsibilities.[22]

The next day after this announcement, the Bureau of Indian Affairs called to "de-establish" the Mashpee Wampanoag Tribe. Cancelling out land put in federal trust, this act of Tribal termination (not done for half a century) dealt a blow to the People of the First Light. Reeking with another foreign disease brought to their shores, their latitude in protecting reservation land was put at risk. Trump administration's jettisoning of the Wampanoag's autonomous territorial status and land recognition raises another instance of settler colonialism.[23] The Confederated Tribes of the Chehalis Reservation, the Tulalip Tribes, Houlton Band of Maliseet Indians, Akiak Native Community, Asa'carsarmiut Tribe, and the Aleut Community successfully filed a lawsuit to halt government dispersal of coronafunds to corporations that manage and oversee Alaska Native communities, reasoning that they were not traditional tribes in the same vein as the plaintiffs.

Governments did not put much of a referendum on for-profit entities, as they continued their profiteering with a pandemic synchronized to "crisis colonization."[24] According to Ojibwe activist-scholar Winona LaDuke, this crisis-to-crisis environment stems from the militarization of the world and the U.S. colonization of Indian Country. LaDuke cites the example of the Diné being forced from self-reliant economies into concentration camps in New Mexico, where they were exposed to starvation if not disease.[25]

U.S. militarism remained operational on island nations like Guam. The aircraft carrier U.S.S. Theodore Roosevelt reported the first COVID-19 outbreak at sea, this time in Micronesia. After departing from Vietnam, the naval ship needed diverting to Guam to confront a viral threat onboard. Sailors were lifted out from the nuclear-powered vessel with nearly 5,000 sailors and the ship needing to be cleansed. Captain Brett Crozier sent a (leaked) letter to the Pentagon leaders pleading for help. They left him with no choice other than to leave sailors onboard a ship equipped with high-powered weapons, instead of removing and sending them to facilities to obtain treatment. Along with his request being declined, the Defense Department maintained that the ship must remain operational with the proviso that a core crew of 1,000 stay onboard.

As part of military readiness for any flare-ups in the region, the ship serves to flex American muscle in the Pacific. Crozier put the government on notice for overlooking that physical distancing does not work for a crew that lives and works in close quarters. He said, "We are not at war. Sailors do not need to die. Due to warship's inherent limitations of space, we are not doing this."[26] For breaking the chain of command, the skipper, found positive for COVID-19, was relieved of his duties by the acting navy secretary. The biggest military force on the planet was, in some ways, no match for the pathogenic machinery of the novel coronavirus.

For the Indigenous people of Guam who call their home Guåhan, another story unfolded. According to Tiara Na'puti, an expert on the Commonwealth of the Northern Mariana Islands,

Centuries of continuous colonization are not Guåhan's defining story. Insofar as the COVID-19 pandemic exacerbated U.S. military exceptionalism, the people of Guåhan deserve even more . . . they deserve an end to colonial violence.[27]

Decolonization addresses the forced incorporation of aquatic seascapes and Pacific communities into militarized spread of disease. Despite the perennial threat of enemies like North Korea to attack U.S. sea bases, this other viral threat is abridged by the U.S. military's own introduction of COVID-19 to the islands, under the ostensibly paternalistic guise of trans-Pacific security in areas of geostrategic importance. Was there a way to deal with SARS-CoV-2 without *manu militari* and the harsh hand of the military?

As an "unincorporated territory," Guam/Guåhan falls under the jurisdiction of the U.S. Navy, which had relocated its troops in Okinawa to this Pacific locale. Guamanians were gobsmacked by the big outbreak among naval personnel, believing the United States was not taking the disease seriously on an island overrun with military bases and one recently battered by typhoons. As the governor and public officials began testing positive, Senator Sabina Flores Perez found the military's reckless decision a danger to the local community, insisting that infected sailors should be offloaded only at the naval base and not in the rest of the islands. She adds that sailors enjoy better health benefits than the lower-wage, higher-vulnerability employees at the hotels where the infirm would be housed.[28] The remit of state removal and who should be removed took on greater import. Legally and spatially removed from the continental United States, Guam/Guåhan and the militarized island states of the northern Marianas banded together under a covenant against COVID-19. These microstates united in a way that other bigger countries could not.

In the face of colonial removal and infection, Mississauga Nishnaabeg scholar Leanne Simpson charts the *radical* resurgence, regeneration, and resistance of Native communities. Native presence, she asserts, offers a strategic weapon for hope, where "ancient Indigenous futures" are collapsed into the now.[29] For too long, Natives warned of the environmental dangers posed by assaults on their autonomy.

COVID-19 delivered a message about those Indigenous futures as they relate to pandemic futures. The coronavirus is telling the world what Indigenous Peoples have been saying for thousands of years—the cure for the next pandemic, and even for this one, can be found in the biodiversity of our Indigenous lands. "This is why we need to protect our lands and rights, because the future of life depends on it," emphasizes Levi Sucre Romero, a BriBri person from Costa Rica and coordinator of the Mesoamerican Alliance of Peoples and Forests.[30] To prevent ecological disruption, it is instructive to think about Indigenous dislocation and dispossession.

Mainstream perspectives about environmental disaster often pass over Native cosmologies and lifeways. In October 2020, thousands of Indigenous people rallied in the capital of Colombia, demanding talks with President Iván Duque. Joined by Black Colombian activists, they wanted consultation on major development projects and remediation for the systematic killing of

Indigenous leaders, but the president refused to meet them. The protesters expressed concern with two forms of removal: the central government's lack of engagement with rural Indigenous (taking them away from the political process) and the request for security forces to leave Indigenous lands (removal of external intrusion). Stemming COVID-19 contagion would not do as much without first addressing the twin forces trying to deracinate Indigenous presence. The history of removing Indigenous groups from historical memory, the electoral process, and landscapes emerged when the presidents of Mexico and Guatemala apologized for centuries of colonial domination, despite both countries pursuing infrastructure projects on Indigenous territories as the pandemic took the global spotlight.

Days before the announcement of a two trillion-dollar stimulus package to cushion the pandemic's economic shockwave, Hawai'i's state governor recommitted to plans for building the Thirty Meter Telescope, an international observatory with funding from countries and the University of California. Construction shut down for months in the face of protests by Kanaka Maoli people, who consider the site of the proposed telescope, Mauna Kea, to be sacred. Disease control was pitted against military control, when Pentagon commanders stopped reporting its high viral loads on Hawaii's military bases, supposedly to protect against adversaries who could use such information. Security held more priority than transparency, and no difference was made between community spread and the military spread of COVID-19.

Indigenous peoples stood at the global "frontlines," and they remained undaunted by new terms of survival set forth by COVID-19. The difficult undertakings of saving the world from a biological threat gloss over the enormous risks to life faced by Indigenous communities in the zones of danger, murdered by illegal loggers and poachers. As LaDuke observes, "Native people are on the front lines of resistance to many ecologically devastating projects … we continue vigilant struggles for land, culture, and future generation."[31] Through adaptive "Indigenous thinking," Native frontline communities are engaged in proactive struggles to regain control over endangered ecosystems from capitalism's primitive accumulation. Flying in from helicopters, Christian evangelicals in their zealous quest to proselytize and find new converts in the Amazon basin, carried forth vector-borne diseases into isolated communities such as the Zo'é or the Awá-Guajá. Spreading the gospel drives the spread of plague, and Survival International for Tribes released a communiqué that said Indigenous people are experiencing genocide from such incursions.

The death-carrying impulses of settler colonialism tick on. In 2019, Brazil's president issued what critics admonished as a "land grabbers decree," a policy which allowed farmers that squatted on government reserves to own these public land.[32] In February 2020, Bolsonaro's administration hired an ex-missionary to head the state agency responsible for protecting uncontacted tribes.[33] Right in the middle of the global pandemic, he pushed a bill to allow commercial mining on Indigenous reservations, which violated the country's existing environmental laws. This piece of legislation made good on Bolsonaro's campaign promise of providing guns to ranchers to wipe Tribes out, while eliminating FUNAI, Brazil's agency for Indigenous affairs. Vowing not to give one more "centimeter" of Indigenous land, he claimed that the Yanomami reserve, the largest protected space in Brazil, was too big while spitting on environmental agencies for even fining violators.

The long history of forced removal led Indigenous communities to decolonize the meaning of COVID-19. Jade Begay who is Diné and Creative Director of the Tesuque Pueblo of New Mexico, released this statement:

> It is imperative for us to decolonize from individualism and reconnect with ways of community care ... Unfortunately, we are seeing some toxic individualism play out in response to the recent COVID-19 pandemic ... This is all decolonial work: getting back to community and even matriarchy, honoring the interdependence of all beings, and valuing the collective over our own ego.[34]

Begay's calls for "Indige-nueity" fits with the broadscale mission of revitalizing Indigenous know-how, language, identity, and communal ways of life. Leaning into interdependence and matriarchy differs from much of the "helpless" discourse of vulnerable communities caught in the pandemic's enveloping vortex. Decolonization of community care follows the aims of the group that Begay belongs to, the NDN Collective, an organization dedicated to promoting social equity, healing power, and a better just future for youth but also elders who are the keepers of knowledge.

As the world went up in flames, community protection and eldercare offer a sturdy defense against the expulsion and policing of Native bodies. While spying, monitoring, and surveillance by state agencies stayed constant or increased, pandemic racism inspired viral acts of antiracism.

Racism

"I can't breathe," George Floyd cried out in a chilling phrase that shot around the world. Choked to death under the knee of a police officer, the cold-blooded murder of an unarmed Black American man under custody in broad daylight whipped up international anger and protests. Fed-up "agitators," as they are called by the conservative set, were expressing pent-up frustration around the constancy of police brutality. The globally circulated video of Floyd's death drew comparisons to the asphyxiation of Eric Garner, Byron Williams, Elijah McClain, and so many others who died uttering the exact same final words.

Their deaths produced global repercussions and exposed problematic relationships. Minneapolis police, like many other departments around the United States, had been trained by Israeli Forces in knee-on-neck technique, a staple practice long used in Palestine, as reported by Amnesty International and the United Nations.[35] Despite testing positive for COVID-19 in an autopsy, Floyd passed away, according to the medical examiner, from cardiopulmonary arrest and neck compression due to homicide. Activists blamed his death to over-policing of oppressed communities of color and called for boycotts and sanctions in both the United States and Israel. Minneapolis Police Chief Medaria Arradondo delivered this universal message, "In my mind, this was a violation of humanity."[36]

Protestors became livid with rage and marched in open defiance of city curfews made in response to COVID-19. Their anger boiled over and public demonstrations broke out all around the country. Political improvisation and demands to defund the police were met with weapons and tear gas, used as agents of riot control. Chemical irritants provoked the painful coughing, sneezing, and wheezing up phlegm after gasping for air (and spreading SARS-CoV-2 further). Minneapolis bus drivers refused to transport protestors to jail for the police. Without regard for physical distancing or using face masks, Los Angeles police used UCLA's Jackie Robinson Stadium as a "jail field" (also a COVID-19 testing site), while the Bureau of Prisons sent armed men to patrol the streets and block protests in Washington D.C., the nation's capital.[37]

Despite protests, the litany of horrific killings of Black people did not stop. Bodies were reported hanging from trees in California, including a boy in Texas. A pregnant woman named Tshegofatso Pule had been hung in Johannesburg. Twitter followers urged the government to hunt down the killer with the same gusto that they did in pursuing illegal alcoholic traders during lockdown. U.S. Immigration and Customs Enforcement detainees held a hunger strike in honor of Floyd. Far from coming out on the side of police, public health experts gave broad support to BLM protestors, recognizing institutional racism as the root of much evil. Rather than stick to the usual line of scientific neutrality, medical experts came out in droves, fingering the public health issue of racism as the reason for COVID-19 health disparities.

In a show of political solidarity with the Black Lives Matter movement, international flash mobs defied lockdown restrictions. These rallies popped up in the Netherlands, Brazil, South Korea, Canada, Germany, New Zealand, Hong Kong, and Palestine. Protestors in Taiwan and Australia added the issue of Indigenous incarceration to underscore the ways Aboriginals are racialized and policed. Police communication systems were hijacked by the global cyberhacking group Anonymous, threatening to out police secrets. Korean pop music fans jammed the signal of police radio airwaves, while drowning out racist online threads. Scotland's Parliament unanimously voted to suspend all exports of "weapons of oppression" like riot gear and tear gas to the United States, while Ghana invited African Americans to return to safety and settle in the African homeland.[38]

Essential workers across all industries walked out in a national strike to protest racism. Murals depicting Floyd's face featured prominently in Britain, Syria, Kenya, Spain, and the West Bank. Marchers in Greece flung Molotov cocktails and firebombs at the U.S. embassy in Athens. Thousands signed petitions to remove edifices to the father of modern India, Mohandas Gandhi, for his anti-Black racism, while Ugandans petitioned to remove landmarks honoring colonialists. The Dutch Prime Minister finally admitted his country's "Black Pete" Christmas minstrelsy tradition was racist, promising to end it. Monuments to Spanish conquistadors and Christopher Columbus took their final bow. Whether taken down by the hands of protestors or by state decrees, the statues of imperial figures like Queen Victoria, Theodore Roosevelt, Woodrow Wilson, and Cecil Rhodes were whisked away. In the United States, students pushed to make Ethnic Studies and the teaching of Critical Race Theory a requirement in schools despite state bans. Protests for racial justice rolled on, even though the bloodletting did not stop.

The global crisis was not a "natural" disaster but a man-made one and, as such, bore human faces. Statues honoring enslavers or imperialists in the United States and United Kingdom were taken down or dropped into rivers; the statue of Canada's first prime minister was splashed in red paint to symbolize the blood of so-called "boarding schools" where First Nation children were sent off to be assimilated and sometimes killed. Royal monuments to Belgium's King Leopold II (the "Butcher of Congo") were draped in a hoodie with the words, "I can't breathe."[39] Despite police bans on public gatherings as a matter of health safety, protestors in Paris registered their horror at Floyd's death as one way to also remember Adama Traore. The victim of policing died in 2016 from a chokehold, a practice which France said will finally end in 2020. Organized and spur-of-the-moment protests were never isolated incidents; they crisscrossed others like those demonstrations generated over the death of Regis Korchinski-Paquet, a Black Canadian woman who fell from her balcony while police were investigating a domestic incident at her home. Britain's Labor Party head and Canada's Prime Minister suggested that these unfortunate deaths might open the floodgates toward a more just society.

The United States came to be a symbol of a fascist world. Leaders like Turkey's President Recep Tayyip Erdogan pointed to the U.S. leader as the problem even when he himself practiced fascism, facing nationwide protests after installing and removing a regent of Bogazici University. His anti-COVID-19 rhetoric called for police crackdown on university students as well as LGBTQ+ paraders denied permits to march in the capital of Istanbul. An Iranian foreign minister spokesperson took to Twitter to highly edit a

U.S. press release about political protests in Iran, a rapid response to the U.S. Secretary of State comments about Iran's treatment of Jews, gays, and women. In response to the State Department's stinging dig that China's Communist Party was pulverizing Hong Kong's "freedom loving people," a Chinese foreign ministry surrogate deployed a Black Lives Matter slogan to chide the Americans. The tweet gave this short but caustic rejoinder: "I can't breathe."[40]

A global wave of hate rode atop a pathogenic enemy, compelling bystanders to wake up to the multiple undeniable threats to Black health and safety. Place-based racialization of a pandemic mapped onto a global conjuncture of power and pain. Demands for justice remain bracketed by "a corresponding rise in racialized containment."[41] Black Americans once again conveyed how institutions meant to protect "the [white] public" are "policing the air out of us."[42] "Public safety" sounds hollow and proves worthless when racial sickness is inherent to American society. One critic edifies this point, "Black people are sick without optimal living standards because America is sick."[43]

Monitored by Predator surveillance drones diverted from the U.S. border to circle above BLM protests, demonstrators and journalists were showered with a hail of rubber bullets (made of metal), pepper balls, and other projectiles by state troopers, who did not bother to mask up.[44] The face shield worn by police took on a menacing counterpoint to the kind worn by frontline workers and protestors, who at rallies were hit without provocation by batons. They lost eyes and teeth and other body parts. Their constitutional right to protest met the state's renewed "right to maim."[45] In a time of "herd immunity," justice warriors contended with the "qualified immunity" protections for police and the "diplomatic immunity" of foreign officials (The Gambia demanded investigation into the son of a diplomat shot dead by police in Georgia). With the death of David Dungay Jr. while held in police custody in Sydney, Australia, and so many other Aboriginals, "I can't breathe" became the rallying cry for anti-racist protests everywhere.

President Donald Trump announced military force to subdue racial rebellions. Then came the incursion of Homeland Security agents within local vicinities like Portland, who arrived without marked insignia. Racism drove the pandemic to greater heights.

White conservative Christians sought godly retribution against the godless Chinese communists for the horrid diseases that they put out in the world. Malthusian ideas of human overpopulation orbited around a sinful lost world which remains unsalvageable, one sullied by the crimson stain of COVID-19 and "fertile" darker populations. Firmly moored to a "model of viral collapse," religious fanatics proclaimed that the end time is "not in the future, it is *here and now*."[46]

Proclaiming himself the "law and order" president on Twitter, Trump sought to "dominate the streets" and spewed questionable speech such as "when the looting starts the shooting starts," echoing a racist police chief during the Civil Rights era. His tweets prompted Snapchat to stop promoting his content due to its glorification of violence and Twitter to hide Trump's personal account and that of the White House. The recourse to civility and the broadsides against "violent" hoodlums by the president washes over the history of violence against people of color.

Online memes accused colonizers and corporations as the real thieves. A neo-Nazi posse went undercover to astroturf "disorderly" conduct, while anti-government militants and former U.S. veterans associated with the "boogaloo" movement did a drive-by shooting near protests in Oakland and ambushed courthouse guards.

A bipartisan congressional bill was introduced impugning China exclusively for COVID-19, but the Democrat heading the effort withdrew support for his own resolution, realizing that it could be used to stoke more race-baiting. As the catalyst for a "racial pandemic," COVID-19 appeared to carry side effects like racism. The spread of disease tends to bring out the worst human inclinations—a tale as old as time. Recall the smear campaign against gay people, migrants, prostitutes, and Africans for AIDS. Racist spats underlain epidemics, doing more harm by driving a bigger wedge between cultural/viral insiders and outsiders. In response to fears of Asian contagion, the president of the Oakland Chinatown Chamber of Commerce made this striking comment: "They look at me and think I'm some kind of virus."[47]

More than bearers of physical disease, visible minorities are construed as disease, a subhuman infestation. The *Wall Street Journal* published an editorial rehashing Orientalist lingo to label China "the real sick man of Asia," forecasting a "de-Sinicizing" of supply chains now turned into viral infection chains.[48] Chinese have historically been unduly vilified in the United States as a diseased race, one specifically banned from immigration or naturalization for decades. Popular assumptions made about cleanliness, morality, and what they ate informed the passage of laws like the Chinese Exclusion Act.[49] Linking foreign disease to "foreign bodies" triggers vaccine-skepticism and the belief that eradication of disease is tantamount to social extermination.[50]

The "dirty" Chinese trope became code for blaming migrants for outbreaks of syphilis, bubonic plague, smallpox, yellow fever, and cholera. Racial ascription of disease ("Asian cholera") obfuscated historically the denial of Chinese from segregated hospitals in colonial territories like Hong Kong to protect the health of Whites.[51] When tuberculosis broke out in Chinatown districts in the United States, the public isolated and faulted the ghettoized Chinese, under the belief that it was an Asian-specific disease. It was beyond belief that Whites could catch it easily, and a labyrinth of segregationist policies paved the way for an opportunist disease and its indiscriminate spread in the territory.[52] While by the late nineteenth century,

Asian immigrants were "already perceived as a virus," the difference today is that digital media allows people to record racist incidents and fight against attacks.[53]

This citizen reporting was vital to rooting out malice and the fallacy that certain groups hold a monopoly on disease. There is no geographic basis to disease as it visits upon a place and fans out.[54] In the late 1950s, the Asian flu pandemic was found to be possibly derived from a virus first identified in southern China and mutated from wild ducks. Avian influenza or "bird flu" or H1N1 virus, purportedly isolated from a goose in China, threatens livestock and people every year due to the global explosion in poultry production. China put a nationwide five-year ban of poultry from the United States due to outbreaks of Avian flu there, which it lifted amid the COVID-19 pandemic. Meanwhile, Brazil froze beef exports to China after finding an atypical form of mad cow disease. This pathography calls for an equally "viral network" of experts to fight state machines run on unwarranted fear.[55]

Wearing surgical masks took on the properties of "racial hygiene" in a viral world. A "civil" form of surveillance induced Asian people to veil/mask themselves, becoming model citizens to ward off hate under the world-bending force of COVID-19.[56] While one Australian tabloid printed the header "Chinese Virus Pandamonium," a French newspaper splattered the words "Yellow Alert" on its frontpage, marking another iteration of "Yellow Peril" fear. Racist "humor" was only one aspect of the cascading hate crimes and insensitivities pouring in from all corners of the globe. A prestigious music conservatory in Rome suspended instruction to all its "Oriental students," a sting of racism that adds insult to injury for those victims beached and hurting from the pandemic. Hotels and taxis turned away Asian travelers. Elderly Asians and women were hospitalized or killed. Graffiti with disgusting slurs and repulsive messages popped up everywhere. People were called "coronavirus" to their face or confronted with the slur "go back to China." They got mocked, punched, taunted, spat on, scratched, dragged, acid attacked, and hair pulled. Members of an Asian American family "mistaken" for being Chinese were stabbed, including the children, at a general store. The Texan man hoped to murder a toddler and a six-year-old during this stabbing. Given this spate of unceasing rancor, the "stay at home" order translated into "safer at home" for many. Cyberbullying and hate speech on Twitter spiked 900%. Racist remarks, part of the viral social media landscape, left a lot to be desired in the pandemic "attention economy."

Plagues bearing the words "Wuhan Plague" were glued to street walls and the exteriors of businesses in Atlanta, Georgia (see Figure 4.1). The seal contained the image of Winnie the Pooh (a common social media jab at Xi Jinping) holding a bat in chopsticks ready to eat it. The bear and bat share an animality that racializes Asians and dehumanizes them. Feeling unsafe

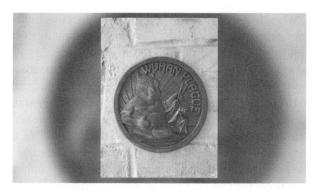

FIGURE 4.1 "Wuhan plague" photo (Krystle Rodriguez).

even while sitting mostly at home, media scholar David Oh expresses, "I was a liability, a racialized contagion … a human contagion. I'm not seen as a person … Though I've been fortunate to not catch COVID-19, I know I symbolize it, anyway. It's dehumanizing."[57]

Evacuated of one's humanity, a victim of corona-racism becomes reduced to social pollution and cultural rot. This surge of racial violence was nothing new in places like Australia and the United States with a long history of expunging Asians. These angry outbursts to masking orders were misplaced, reflects Japanese American actor-activist George Takei. Having survived a concentration camp, he wrote: "I didn't spend my childhood in barbed wire enclosed internment camps so I could listen to grown adults today cry oppression because they have to wear a mask."[58] Military veterans who comprised part of the San Francisco Peace Collective volunteered to patrol streets to protect residents. The viral hate that traveled with the pandemic stretched through Italy, the United Kingdom, Kenya, Ethiopia, South Africa, and Brazil. Anti-Semitism and racial disgust exploded and went nuclear in this tidal wave of viral hate.

With hundreds of hate incidents recorded per day, Asian communities took a stand against hate. In online campaigns against viral racism like #ChinkVirus, Asian Americans reported incidents with the hashtags #WashTheHate, #RacismIsaVirus, and #IAmNotCovid19. Harkening back to World War II days, when some Asians would distance themselves from the Japanese, T-shirts were sold bearing the not too subtle message, "No, I'm not Chinese" (it was unclear who was selling these items online)."[59] Shirts sold with the message #IAmNotChinese found popularity but wearing them did not prevent cases of "mistaken" identity.

Anti-Asian racial violence bubbled up in parts of Asia, due to antipathy toward China's economic influence and the Chinese comprador class. Restaurant entrances and restrooms with "No Chinese"' signs brought back racist anti-Asian practices of yesteryear. The University of California, Berkeley received negative press for cycling a form of xenophobia. The school's health services apologized for an infographic listing "normal" reactions to the pandemic. Symptoms included "fears about interacting with those who might be from Asia and guilt about these feelings."[60] The presumption that all people of Asia are Chinese and, secondly, that all Asians look alike turned heterogeneous communities into a faceless monolithic. The threat of stereotypes reared its ugly head when fear-based projections hit other "Orientalized" and viralized groups like Thais, Koreans, Cambodians, Vietnamese, Japanese, Hmong, and even South Asian Jews. An Indian man in Israel, a member of the Bnei Menashe religious community, needed to be hospitalized after being taunted and kicked by two men who thought he was Chinese, shouting "Corona! Corona!"[61]

Corona-racism was real and social media revealed that. African citizens talked online about having to prove their health status to procure visas to travel to Europe. Users shared videos of Africans without symptoms of sickness being evicted from their homes in Yuexiu district of Guangzhou, the location of China's Little Africa. Houseless residents slept on the street as Chinese authorities forcibly outed and tested African communities for the novel coronavirus. Five infected Nigerians that broke quarantine impelled local authorities to increase monitoring of an expatriate community that had fallen under suspicion. As the world watched people lash out at the Chinese for COVID-19, Africans were dealt a hand of indignities by some Chinese. A news outlet reported a Nigerian attacking a Chinese nurse who blocked him from leaving a quarantine hospital. A note photographed on a window at McDonald's said Black people were not allowed to enter the restaurant. Reports of Black people on short visas denied housing or kicked out on to the streets drove the U.S. consulate to send a security alert to African Americans, warning them to avoid Guangzhou. Fearing reprisals from police, one woman on WeChat wrote, "As a Black person living in China right now it's pretty scary … Don't use the African/Black community as a scapegoat for the virus."[62]

China's Foreign Ministry spokesperson tried to quell social unrest with this diplomatic response: "Since the beginning of the coronavirus outbreak, China and African countries have always supported each other and have always fought against the virus jointly … the Chinese government treats all foreigners in China equally."[63] Nigeria's Foreign Affairs Minister and speaker of the House demanded answers from the Chinese embassy, as did concerned leaders from Ghana and Kenya, who decried how stones were cast against their nationals. China's ambassador to Zimbabwe and the Foreign Ministry insisted that they treat all people fairly, calling the one-off incidents sensationalized news. Corona-racism, they claimed, existed but it was more understated.

Sensationalized videos released on the Internet snapped into focus increasing physical attacks and public maulings against Muslims in India. Attackers impugned them as carriers of COVID-19, equating them with the disease after attendees at the missionary Tablighi Jamaat gathering in New Delhi tested positive. BJP officials labelled the meeting "Talibani crime" and "CoronaTerrorism" with social media users fanning the flames with the viral hashtag #CoronaJihad.[64] A cartoon on Twitter featured a caricatured Muslim with the label "corona jihad" pushing a Hindu person off a cliff.[65] The viral world, for some, was an anti-Muslim world.

These images reinforced border security officers' claim of "infiltrators" coming through Nepal with the express purpose of spreading SARS-CoV-2. The federal government sent a memorandum to vent concern about Muslim-dominated areas, which the chief minister of West Bengal rejected as anti-Muslim agenda. This embittered campaign included the Citizenship (Amendment) Act passed in December 2019, which defined the path to citizenship for the first time expressly through religion and which excised Muslims. Meenakshi Ganguly, South Asia director at Human Rights Watch spotted a contradiction: "India's prime minister has appealed for a united fight against COVID-19 but has yet to call for unity in the fight against anti-Muslim violence and discrimination."[66]

Another commentator finds that the Hindu caste system oppresses the "untouchables" or Dalits and reflects how "we had always been 'socially distant' from the destitute and vulnerable—only now it is worse."[67] India's Supreme Court found that the government was anything but bound to providing reservations for Dalits and hillside Tribal groups like the Adivasis, though these provisions are enshrined by India's constitution. In May 2020, a two-judge bench of the apex court based its decision on stereotypes, calling these reservations "human zoos" for "primitive" cultures.[68]

Corresponding "racism epidemics" pummeled Africa, Latin America, Europe, and Asia. Lockdown commands hit Israel, coterminous with state orders for all African migrants in the country to leave. The Population and Immigration Authority ordered these foreign "infiltrators" to exit its shores, and the Trump administration directed swift removal of all asylum-seeking migrants at the border without due process. In the whirlwind year of 2020, cross-cutting "viral" issues of racism, nationalism, and xenophobia intersected with that of forced migration and refugees.

Refugees

As the aerodynamic novel coronavirus wormed itself into Europe, this disease exacerbated the deadly impasse for refugees also trying to enter Europe. In this house of pandemic horrors, doomed castaways fell into the waiting arms of the novel coronavirus upon landing on the continent. Goals of safety and protection remained undimmed by COVID-19, and refugees insisted on their right to asylum due in part to the virus. Before or after the virus, economic migrants and refugees faced incredible danger.

Pandemic border closures pointed out signs of worsening conditions for global migrants. Despite being accused of bringing the virus into countries, migrants brought recharged demands for free mobility under the pandemic's dire terrain. A resurgence of infection occurred as people fled to Europe, and refugees became part of transmission chains that encompassed all people. These "pandemic migrants" put a dent in governments' inaction around migrant insecurity. Step by step, the pandemic chipped away at the heart of anti-immigrant societies braving the ravages of nationalism. South Africa announced that it would build a fence wall and tighten border controls with Zimbabwe to keep out its possibly infected irregular migrants, although South Africa held many more cases than Zimbabwe. Checkpoints delivered on a government promise for years to keep out unauthorized workers from its neighbors and "protect" a shrinking economy. Such are the reminders of Apartheid, when the country maintained segregated reserves and checkpoints for Black residents and worker migrants entering White-controlled areas.[69]

Dwindling spaces of refuge deepened physical distancing for migrants, signaling troubling times for those people most in need of help. As the largest stateless population in the world, the Rohingya were denied asylum and temporary work permits in Malaysia. Blamed for the country's first COVID-19 outbreak, the Malaysian government expelled boats carrying Rohingya refugees massing along its border. As governments turned their backs to outsiders to erect more barriers within national walls, a loaded language for speaking about pandemics informed the improper reception of forcibly removed stateless people. Cases of refugees denied entry spiked, even with a virus chasing and hounding them.

Physical distancing as a practice remained a luxury for the more than one billion people living in makeshift shantytowns and informal settlements. In these sprawling "slums," locals mix regularly with irregular migrants to form multilayered social webs, potent sources of shared infection. What these webs tell us is that we are co-conspirators in this endeavor called life and we must learn "the conditions we breathe in are collective and unequally distributed, with particular qualities and intensities that are felt differently through and across time."[70]

For those forced to work under horrid conditions, time dragged on forever. For farmers working on tight schedules, and for urban guest workers, their time was disrupted. In March 2020, India's Prime Minister Narendra Modi announced a nationwide lockdown to protect the country's residents from COVID-19. Amid a pall of desperation, rural laborers fled in huge numbers from India's cities, since they were now removed from their source of regular work. This mass exodus added another layer of regulated fear. As seen in videos of police beating people, the "people's curfew" came with canes and other heavy-handed methods by police. Daily wagers who lost their jobs in the city needed to return to distant home villages. However, national bus lines and railways had been shut down. Many died or starved due to what had been noted as the "biggest human migration on foot" after Partition."[71] A viral video uploaded by the *Times of India* shows a smattering of returnees to the city Bareilly in the state of Uttar Pradesh, sitting on the ground while sprayed and doused in chemicals by health workers. In a country already grappling with swine flu epidemic, the war against COVID-19 turned on the demobilization of "pandemic refugees."

Without enough problems to handle, Modi's government deregulated wholesale trading (ending major subsidies and minimal support prices for small farmers). The rigidity of this policy angered half a billion peasant farmers who aired grievances, even as India became the new fulcrum of the pandemic (and the place where the highly contagious Delta variant of COVID-19 first surfaced). Grain growers in the states of Punjab and Haryana protested this law designed to "help" farmers, many of whom were Sikh. The Modi government made accusations to the effect that farmers have been infiltrated by Khalistani separatists. The same held true in Indonesia, where an omnibus law passed to boost a pandemic-battered economy. Intending to cut bureaucracy and "modernize" trade, this controversial bill lowered protections for the environment and worker's pay. Joined by students and labor unions, cast out Indigenous groups and workers fought their removal from the economy. Protestors found themselves arrested on sight. Reporters were defamed, locked up, or killed, with 2021 being the deadliest year for journalists.

Influenced by news about countries with more robust healthcare systems like Italy and the United States, India locked down a billion people in what was the largest social engineering project. While its neighbors Bangladesh and Sri Lankan used the term "holiday" to avoid mass panic, India rushed into central command mode, denying any community transmission. China switched on to lockdown mode, opting for tiered controls for half the country without any national transport links severed. A 39-year-old man walking by foot from Delhi to Madhya Pradesh (a 300-km trip) died after complaining of chest pains and exhaustion, while a 62-year-old man returning from a Gujarat hospital by foot collapsed and died outside his house. Migrants turned away at the borders on their way to Rajasthan were killed after being mowed down by a truck.

Prime Minister Modi apologized but said "tough measures were needed to win this battle."[72] Speaking to worshippers at Kumbh Mela (a weeks-long Hindu religious festival with millions of people), Modi spurned his own lockdown policies. His government did not stop the millions of pilgrims, but

Muslims had been blamed for spreading the novel coronavirus during one academic conference. Modi staged mass rallies during an election campaign in West Bengal. In response, the prime minister of Nepal had started calling COVID-19 the "Indian virus." As SARS-CoV-2 surfaced in India, the nation's leader offered that the virus spread from India was more lethal than what comes from China or Italy, due to Nepal's open borders with its large neighbor.

We can crudely juxtapose the "shelter in place" decree made to U.S. citizens against the "remain in Mexico" program for migrants.[73] For many Americans, the cabin fever and bored restlessness of being cooped up in one's home for months are a far remove from the jarring feelings of uprooted people without housing. All federal government offices were closed, *except* for immigration courts, due to COVID-19. Magistrates and lawyers conducting in-person court proceedings reported becoming sick. Immigration judges then postponed Migration Protection Protocol hearings in protest of the Fed's unhalted practice of busing migrants from Tijuana (the Mexican municipality with the largest number of infected) to San Diego for hearings, and then taking them back across the busiest land port of entry in the world. Other cramped migrant shelters with high human density, like the ones in Juarez, had temporarily seized up due to a chicken pox outbreak. Health experts recommended asylum-seekers stay with family members, while awaiting court orders and paperwork processing. In short, the ailing migrant processing system simply fell to pieces.

Customs and border patrol stopped following recommendations by the Centers for Disease Control and Prevention to give flu vaccinations at the border, even after the deaths of migrant children due to infectious diseases, which caused more casualties. The special legal protection long accorded to unaccompanied migrant children no longer applied as they were deported immediately. The first person to die in immigration custody from COVID-19 was Carlos Ernesto Escobar Mejia, who came to the United States after fleeing death squads in El Salvador. He died in a detention center run by a private prison corporation, which denied any complicity. Despite begging for treatment for infirmity and masks in quarantined units, Mejia was refused medical attention at a hospital when his symptoms worsened. Other detainees grumbled about painful bleeding and burns from disinfectant spray.

The adage "a disease knows no borders" does not square with the fact that gatekeepers manipulate borders to wield power. Trump announced turning away of all refugees even if they show no signs of affliction, and the United States began to charge asylum-seekers to file claims, no longer making this sorting mechanism free for poor migrants. After shutting down the U.S. border to Canada and Mexico, the alien specter of a marauding band of invaders led Trump to propose siphoning off money for fighting COVID-19 to build his costly southern border wall. Its construction was protested by the Kumeyaay and Tohono O'odham nations to protect their sacred sites.[74]

Moving through the pandemic borderlands, unauthorized migrants needed to wrestle with all sorts of depredations. Ineligible for government aid, they teetered on a precipice. Many migrants stayed as employees in hospitality services, an industry stung by the fallout from COVID-19. The San Diego Immigrant Rights group doled out the aid where needed: "When the most vulnerable in our community are at risk, our whole community is at risk."[75] Guatemala's minister of health took no comfort from the fact that 75% of all deportees on one flight to the country contracted COVID-19. As the first to halt migrant deportations, Guatemala begged the United States to stop sending migrants its way, despite an agreement it made a year earlier to hold them. The health minister called out the "Wuhan of the Americas" for dispersing the disease across the hemisphere.[76] With the United States strengthening its fortress against migrants, Haiti's ambassador to the United States, Hervé Denis, made a biblical reference to describe the political headwinds. The authority to manage human flow followed a lopsided battle between a superpower and a smaller island nation: "We are a poor country. This is always the situation. This is David and Goliath. So what can we do? We are not even David."[77]

When Ghana, Uganda, Rwanda, and Mali banned travel from European countries, it looked like a turning of the tables for African countries that had long endured historic humiliations from European powers and their maltreatment of overseas émigrés. Kenya took precaution to an unusual degree by prohibiting all travel from European countries with reported COVID-19 cases. The Democratic Republic of Congo, long stigmatized as the geographic origin of Ebola and HIV, imposed quarantine on travelers from France, China, Germany, and Italy. Tunisia and Mauritania deported Italian citizens, while Cameroon reported higher-than-expected cases of Italians escaping to the west African nation to little avail. (When the Omicron variant of COVID-19 turned up in South Africa, those European nations responded by barring travel from southern African nations). Despite these moves to protect national health by banning travel, an Ethiopian health official implored, "The international community should stand in solidarity."[78]

This solidarity appears impossible in an enfeebled global health system where countries like the United States refuse to work closely with the World Health Organization. The former decided to go alone in the COVID-19 fight, and thus left refugees to face the problem alone.

"I am a Coronavirus refugee," declares Sina Farzaneh on the microblogging platform Medium. Outlasting two lockdowns, one in Shanghai and one after his return to San Francisco, the traveler shared the personal phases of dealing with COVID-19 quarantine: survival, security, and self-importance. It brought home the *im/mobilities* that can arise for subjects-on-the-move and how viral states "keep migrants in situations of prolonged social exclusion."[79] Out-of-work residents in the First of May Refugee Camp faced water cannons fired at them by Rio de Janeiro's police, who ejected migrants from a plot of land now reserved for Brazil's state-run Petrobas oil company. The pathologizing of itinerant migrants continued within the viral world.

Despite scarcity in the "developed" world, online memes gave sobering reminders that people in richer nations should appreciate what forced migrants from low-income countries experience all the time, but to a worse extent.

Shoppers bombarded stores and stripped bare shelves like scavengers. Watching people hoard toilet paper and food, keen observers on social media reminded First World denizens to never look down on Third World refugees again. Despite the run on stores in the United States, availability of these consumer items was never at risk, since supply chains were domestic (hoarding and panic shopping act as a form of psychological security and comfort in crises). True to form, angst-ridden Americans bought more guns, while Asian Americans stocked up on firearms to protect themselves from racist attackers. Sorely lacking information and clear instruction, individuals and stores stocked up on consumer items like hand sanitizer to sell for a higher cost, with price gouging subsequently banned. In Taiwan, the Ministry of Economics plastered posters warning of harsh penalties with jail time. It came out with this direct message: "Don't' stockpile. Don't believe gossip."[80]

During 2020's pandemonium, the quandary of unprotected or warehoused people who had left their homelands became swept aside temporarily, even though the issue never really went away. Waves of people fled the feud between Turkey-backed rebel groups in Syria and the government of Bashar Al-Assad backed by Russia. Quarreling among nations drew narrowing viral circles around fleeing migrants, intransigent populations with nowhere to escape. Held in confinement and routed as suspected carriers of disease, over 30 million people needed to find safe refuge in a COVID-lashed world suddenly turned hostile to *all* outsiders.

To make matters even worse, refugee hosting or accepting countries like Germany, Austria, Italy, Australia, Canada, and Greece shut their borders; the European Union closed down all travel for a month. The United States unilaterally pared back all nonessential travel from China and from Europe. China passed an immigration law against "fake refugees," closing borders to fleeing Hong Kong residents. Pandemic policies *nuclearized* the global migration underfoot.

Nothing could stop the lethal arc of the novel coronavirus' path, which reignited another international refugee crisis. Countries no longer could afford to host border crossers, but refusing to do so put them more at risk. Turkey closed its borders to the European Union but let refugees march through its territory to the rest of Europe (Turkey held off refugees as part of a 2016 deal with Europe in return for aid). Nongovernmental organizations like Doctors without Border (*Medicins Sans Frontieres*) endorsed the evacuation of migrants languishing at refugee camps in Greece, where many fled after Turkey shut them out. Turkey reopened its borders to Greece ahead of the curve. Refusing to loosen controls, Greece stepped up blockades to migrants and solidified its controversial pushback policy and illegalization of rescue missions. With 1,000 people sharing one tap of water, the Moria camp on Lesbos Island was a potential coronavirus bomb.[81]

At the forefront of this downward spiral in the Eurozone was Italy. Although it was the first country to enact a full ban of flights from China immediately upon discovering its very first infection cases, it became the continent's COVID-19 epicenter. When global news media began reporting that the country suffered the highest number of deaths of any nation, even more than China, some chalked it up to the fact that its population was much older.

For all its outward cosmopolitanism and ecumenicalism, Italy opposed accepting displaced migrants. Meanwhile, small island nations like Trinidad and Tobago leaned into humanitarianism to accept refugees, while still closing its borders for outside travelers. Italy was now at the frontline to protect elders from disease amid warding off migrants perceived as potentially diseased. As Italy fell victim to COVID-19, what was forgotten was the country's long-standing practice of restrictive citizenship, straightjacketing who can become Italians. Restrictive nationality boiled down to Italy's populist coalition government taking on an anti-globalist stance.

Exclusion breeds anxiety and discord, in spite of the desirable effects of friendship like when the mayor of Florence urged residents to "hug a Chinese" in the early pandemic days. Yet, Italy's act of sending search-and-rescue flotillas awhirl with "boat people" back into the sea furthered death's grip. Worse still, Italian fishers risked jail and their lives to save migrants out at sea. Heroes abounded in times of turmoil. These unsung heroes toiled away on the frontlines as the world fell quiet, but their time of recognition had come.

Notes

1 Olivia B. Waxman, "The Surprisingly Deep—and Often Troubling—History of 'Social Distancing," *Time*, June 30, 2020, https://time.com/5856800/social-dis tancing-history/
2 To deal with people starving for affection, the Icelandic Forestry Service encouraged people to hug trees, embracing Nature's curative power to heal by embracing it.
3 Ruja Benjamin, *Race after Technology: Abolitionist Tools for the New Jim Code* (Hoboken, NJ: John Wiley & Sons, 2019).
4 Ibid.

5 Tiffany Willouby-Herard, Facebook post, March 19, 2020, www.facebook.com/tiffany.herard

6 bell hooks, *Sisters of the Yam: Black Women and Self-Recovery* (London: Routledge, 2014), 143.

7 Anna Piela, "COVID-19 Is Increasing Religious Tolerance. Here's Why," *Fast Company*, February 8, 2021, www.fastcompany.com/90602111/covid-19-is-increasing-religious-tolerance-heres-why

8 Jillian Kestler-D'Amours, "Why Are Muslim Women Living 'in Fear' in This Canadian City?" *Aljazeera*, July 13, 2021, www.aljazeera.com/news/2021/7/13/why-are-muslim-women-living-in-fear-in-this-canadian-city

9 Maya Oppenheim, "Mexico Sees Almost 1,000 Women Murdered in Three Months as Domestic Abuse Concerns Rise amid Coronavirus," *Yahoo*, April 28, 2020, https://news.yahoo.com/mexico-sees-almost-1-000-135946687.html

10 Angelo Amante, Parisa Hafezi, and Hayoung Choi, " 'There Are No Funerals:' Death in Quarantine Leaves Nowhere to Grieve," *Reuters*, March 19, 2020, www.reuters.com/article/us-health-coronavirus-rites-insight-idUSKBN2161ZM

11 Josie Huang, "In LA County, Pacific Islanders Are Dying from Coronavirus at a Rate 12 Times Higher than Whites. These Leaders Are Fighting Back," *LAIst*, April 30, 2020, https://laist.com/2020/04/30/pacific_islanders_coronavirus_death_rate_california.php

12 Shiqi Lin, "CUT! Community, Immunity, Vulnerability in the Time of Coronavirus," University of California Humanities Research Institute, March 2020, https://uchri.org/foundry/cut-community-immunity-vulnerability-in-the-time-of-coronavirus/

13 Patrick Greenfield and Erin McCormick, " 'No One Comes': The Cruise Ship Crews Cast Adrift by Coronavirus," *The Guardian*, May 1, 2020, www.theguardian.com/environment/2020/may/01/no-one-comes-the-cruise-ship-crews-cast-adrift-by-coronavirus

14 Orion Rummler, "Brazil and Ecuador Emerge as Latin America's Coronavirus Epicenters," *Axios*, April 23, 2020, www.axios.com/coronavirus-latin-america-brazil-ecuador-ff4e1b94-0715-479e-92b3-c3ce42f85007.html

15 Benjamin, *Race after Technology*, 26.

16 Iyko Day, *Alien Capital: Asian Racialization and the Logic of Settler Colonial Capitalism* (Durham, NC: Duke University Press, 2016).

17 Celia Lowe, "Viral Clouds: Becoming H5N1 in Indonesia," *Cultural Anthropology* 25, no. 4 (2010): 625–649.

18 These fault lines are not just cultural or ideological, but military, which is why September 9, 2020 marked the first UN International Day to Protect Education from Attack.

19 Sam Jones, " 'Arrogance' Blinded Big Countries to Virus Risk, Says Austria Adviser," *Financial Times*, May 3, 2020, www.ft.com/content/87495a18-f7a1-4657-a517-ba2b16c146dc

20 Suzanne Gamboa, "Julián Castro: Latinos Grapple with 'The Worst of All Worlds' amid Coronavirus Pandemic," *NBC News*, April 27, 2020, www.nbcnews.com/news/latino/juli-n-castro-latinos-grapple-worst-all-worlds-amid-coronavirus-n1193666

21 Olivia Humphrey, "Is Coronavirus China's Chernobyl?" *China Channel*, March 24, 2020, https://chinachannel.org/2020/03/24/corona-chernobyl/

22 Ellen Knickmeyer, "Citing Outbreak, EPA Has Stopped Enforcing Environmental Laws," *Associated Press*, March 27, 2020, www.pbs.org/newshour/economy/cit ing-outbreak-epa-has-stopped-enforcing-environmental-laws

23 WBUR Newsroom, "Secretary of Interior Orders Mashpee Wampanoag Reservation 'Disestablished,' Tribe Says," *WBUR*, March 28, 2020, www. wbur.org/news/2020/03/28/mashpee-wampanoag-reservation-secretary-inter ior-land-trust

24 Nick Martin, "This Is Crisis Colonization," *The New Republic*, March 30, 2020, https://newrepublic.com/article/157091/crisis-colonization

25 This was later used as a prime example by Hitler for his extermination death camps. See Winona LaDuke and Sean Aaron Cruz, *The Militarization of Indian Country* (East Lansing, MI: Michigan State University Press, 2013).

26 Deirdre Shesgreen and Tom Vanden Brook, "Navy Says It Can't Empty Roosevelt amid Coronavirus Because of Its Weapons, Nuclear Reactor," *USA Today*, April 1, 2020, www.usatoday.com/story/news/politics/2020/04/01/coronavirus-navy-sailors-roosevelt-guard-weapons-more-sick/5104785002/

27 Tiara Na'puti, "Archipelagic Rhetoric: Remapping the Marianas and Challenging Militarization from 'A Stirring Place,'" *Communication and Critical/Cultural Studies* 16, no. 1 (2019): 4–25.

28 Kate Lyons, "Anger in Guam at 'Dangerous' Plan to Offload US Sailors from Virus-Hit Aircraft Carrier," *The Guardian*, April 1, 2020, www.theguardian.com/world/2020/apr/02/anger-in-guam-at-dangerous-plan-to-offload-us-sailors-from-virus-hit-aircraft-carrier

29 Leanne Betasamosake Simpson. *As We Have Always Done: Indigenous Freedom through Radical Resistance* (Minneapolis: University of Minnesota Press, 2017), 21.

30 Emilee Gilpin, "COVID-19 Crisis Tells World What Indigenous Peoples Have Been Saying for Thousands of Years," *National Observer*, March 24, 2020, www. nationalobserver.com/2020/03/24/news/covid-19-crisis-tells-world-what-indigen ous-peoples-have-been-saying-thousands-years

31 Winona LaDuke, "Traditional Ecological Knowledge and Environmental Futures," *Colorado Journal of International Environmental Law & Policy* 5 (1994): 139.

32 Dom Phillips, "Brazil Using Coronavirus to Cover Up Assaults on Amazon, Warn Activists," *The Guardian*, May 6, 2020, www.theguardian.com/world/2020/may/06/brazil-using-coronavirus-to-cover-up-assaults-on-amazon-warn-activists

33 Sue Branford, "Spreading the Word of God and Coronavirus: Outrage over Evangelical Group Trying to Contact Isolated Amazon Tribes amid Pandemic," *Common Dreams*, www.commondreams.org/views/2020/03/18/spreading-word-god-and-coronavirus-outrage-over-evangelical-group-trying-contact

34 Jade Begay, "Decolonizing Community Care in Response To Covid-19," *NDN Collective*, March 13, 2020, https://ndncollective.org/indigenizing-and-decoloniz ing-community-care-in-response-to-covid-19/

35 Alison Weir, "Minneapolis Cops Trained by Israeli Police, Who Often Use Knee-On-Neck Restraint," *Israel-Palestine News*, June 2, 2020, https://israelpalest inenews.org/minn-cops-trained-by-israeli-police-who-often-use-knee-on-neck-restraint/

36 Christina Maxouris, "Holly Yan and Ralph Ellis, "Cities Extend Curfews for Another Night in an Attempt to Avoid Violent Protests over George Floyd's

Death," *CNN*, May 31, 2020, www.cnn.com/2020/05/31/us/george-floyd-prote
sts-sunday/index.html

37 The stadium is leased to the university's baseball team under the U.S Department of Veterans Affairs.

38 Jon Stone, "Scottish Parliament Votes for Immediate Suspension of Tear Gas, Rubber Bullet and Riot Shield Exports to US," *Independent*, June 11, 2020, www. independent.co.uk/news/uk/politics/scotland-us-exports-tear-gas-rubber-bullets-riot-shields-blm-protests-a9560586.html

39 Eric Schultz, "Belgians Target Some Royal Monuments in Black Lives Matter Protest," *NPR*, June 5, 2020, www.npr.org/sections/live-updates-protests-for-racial-justice/2020/06/05/871278150/belgians-target-some-royal-monuments-in-black-lives-matter-protest

40 Jen Kirby, "George Floyd Protests Go Global: Foreign Leaders Are Also Reacting to the Turmoil in the United States," *Vox*, May 31, 2020, www.vox.com/2020/5/31/21276031/george-floyd-protests-london-berlin

41 Yousuf Al-Bulushi. "The Global Threat of Race in the Decomposition of Struggle," *Safundi* 21, no. 2 (2020): 149.

42 Douglas Haynes, "Policing the Air out of Us: Douglas Haynes," *Orange County Register*, June 14, 2020, www.ocregister.com/2020/06/13/policing-the-air-out-of-us-douglas-haynes/

43 UCI Office of Inclusive Excellence, "The Fire Next Time: Anti-Black Racism and the Struggle to Live in the United States," *UCI OIE*, June 4, 2020, https://inclus ion.uci.edu/2020/06/04/the-fire-next-time/

44 These actions were condemned by Amnesty International for failing to follow international law and respecting the right to peaceful protest.

45 Jasbir K. Puar, *The Right to Maim: Debility, Capacity, Disability* (Durham, NC: Duke University Press, 2017).

46 Jean Baudrillard, *L'illusion De La Fin* (Stanford, CA: Stanford University Press, 1994), 38, 119.

47 Kristine Phillips, "'They Look at Me and Think I'm Some Kind of Virus': What It's Like to be Asian during the Coronavirus Pandemic," *The Daytona Beach News-Journal*, March 30, 2020, www.news-journalonline.com/zz/news/20200 330/they-look-at-me-and-think-im-some-kind-of-virus-what-its-like-to-be-asian-during-coronavirus-pandemic

48 Walter Russell Mead, "China Is the Real Sick Man of Asia," *Wall Street Journal*, February 3, 2020, www.wsj.com/articles/china-is-the-real-sick-man-of-asia-1158 0773677

49 See Nayan Shah, *Contagious Divides: Epidemics and Race in San Francisco's Chinatown* (Berkeley, CA: University of California Press, 2001).

50 Simon Schame, *Foreign Bodies: Pandemics, Vaccines, and the Health of Nations* (New York: Ecco, 2023).

51 Ka-che Yip, "Segregation, Isolation, and Quarantine: Protecting Hong Kong from Diseases in the Pre-War Period," *Journal of Comparative Asian Development* 11, no. 1 (2012): 93–116.

52 Jeannie N. Shinozuka, "Deadly Perils: Japanese Beetles and the Pestilential Immigrant, 1920s–1930s," *American Quarterly* 65, no. 4 (2013): 831–852.

53 Rachel Chang, "Racism against Asian Americans Isn't Unique to the Coronavirus Pandemic—Everyone Else Is Just Becoming More Aware Now," *Hello Giggles*,

April 29, 2020, https://Hellogiggles.Com/Lifestyle/Racism-Asian-Americans-Coronavirus/

54 Nükhet Varlik, *Plague and Empire in the Early Modern Mediterranean World* (Cambridge: Cambridge University Press, 2015), 95–96.

55 Theresa MacPhail, *The Viral Network: A Pathography of the H1N1 Influenza Pandemic* (Ithaca, NY: Cornell University Press, 2015).

56 Thy Phu, *Picturing Model Citizens: Civility in Asian American Visual Culture* (Temple University Press, 2011).

57 David C. Oh, "Ethical (Re)Positioning: Asian American Doctors and the Struggle against Structural Racism and Covid-19," Texas A&M University, November 2022, https://oaktrust.library.tamu.edu/bitstream/handle/1969.1/188225/David%20C.%20Oh%20%28QAB%20Entry%20%235%29.pdf?sequence=1&isAllowed=y

58 George Takei(@GeorgeTakei), "I Didn't Spend My Childhood in Barbed Wire Enclosed Internment Camps so I Could Listen to Grown Adults Today Cry Oppression Because They Have to Wear a Mask at Costco," *Twitter*, May 9, 2020, 7:00pm, https://twitter.com/GeorgeTakei/status/1258939947723169792

59 Kimmy Yam, "Black, Asian and Hispanic House Caucus Chairs Unite in 'No Tolerance' for Coronavirus Racism," *MSN*, March 31, 2020, www.msn.com/en-us/news/politics/black-asian-and-hispanic-house-caucus-chairs-unite-in-no-tolerance-for-coronavirus-racism/ar-BB11YZqf

60 Lauren Fries, "UC Berkeley Had to Apologize for Saying Anti-Chinese Xenophobia Is a 'Normal Reaction' to the Coronavirus," *Business Insider*, January 31, 2020, www.businessinsider.com/uc-berkeley-called-out-anti-chinese-xenophobia-normal-reaction-coronavirus-2020-1

61 Times of Israel, "Indian Immigrant Beaten in Tiberias in Apparent Coronavirus-Linked Hate Crime," *Times of Israel*, March 16, 2020, www.timesofisrael.com/indian-immigrant-beaten-in-tiberias-in-apparent-coronavirus-linked-hate-crime/

62 Jenni Marsh, Shawn Deng, and Nectar Gan, "Africans in Guangzhou Are on Edge, after Many Are Left Homeless amid Rising Xenophobia as China Fights a Second Wave of Coronavirus," *CNN*, April 12, 2020, www.cnn.com/2020/04/10/china/africans-guangzhou-china-coronavirus-hnk-intl/index.html

63 Ibid.

64 Human Rights Watch, "Covid-19 Fueling Anti-Asian Racism and Xenophobia Worldwide," *Human Rights Watch*, May 12, 2020, www.hrw.org/news/2020/05/12/covid-19-fueling-anti-asian-racism-and-xenophobia-worldwide#

65 Apoorvanand, "How the Coronavirus Outbreak in India Was Blamed on Muslims," *Aljazeera*, April 18, 2020, www.aljazeera.com/indepth/opinion/coronavirus-outbreak-india-blamed-muslims-200418143252362.html

66 Human Rights Watch, "India: Protests, Attacks over New Citizenship Law," *Human Rights Watch*, April 9, 2020, www.hrw.org/news/2020/04/09/india-protests-attacks-over-new-citizenship-law

67 Ayesha Mahmood Malik, "We Had Always Been 'Socially Distant' from the Destitute and Vulnerable—Only Now It Is Worse," *The Review of Religions*, April 28, 2020, www.reviewofreligions.org/21768/we-had-always-been-socially-distant-from-the-destitute-and-vulnerable-only-now-it-is-worse/

68 Anurag Bhaskar, "When It Comes to Dalit and Tribal Rights, the Judiciary in India Just Does Not Get It," *The Wire*, May 3, 2020, https://thewire.in/law/when-it-comes-to-dalit-and-tribal-rights-the-judiciary-in-india-just-does-not-get-it;

Times of India, "SC Wonders How Its Two-Judge Bench Usurped Powers of CJI," *Times of India*, November 10, 2017, https://timesofindia.indiatimes.com/india/sc-wonders-how-its-two-judge-bench-usurped-powers-of-cji/articleshow/61597 707.cms

69 Sharad Chari, "Detritus in Durban: Polluted Environs and the Biopolitics of Refusal," in *Imperial Debris*, ed. Ann Laura Stoler (Durham, NC: Duke University Press, 2013), 131–161.

70 Kristen Simmons, "Settler Atmospherics," *Society for Cultural Anthropology*, November 20, 2017, https://culanth.org/fieldsights/settler-atmospherics

71 Shoaib Daniyal, "Not China, Not Italy: India's Coronavirus Lockdown Is the Harshest in the World," *Scroll.in*, March 29, 2020, https://scroll.in/article/957564/not-china-not-italy-indias-coronavirus-lockdown-is-the-harshest-in-the-world

72 Soutik Biswas, "Coronavirus: India's Pandemic Lockdown Turns into a Human Tragedy," *BBC News*, March 30, 2020, www.bbc.com/news/world-asia-india-52086274

73 Max Rivlin-Nadler, " 'Remain-In-Mexico' Paused as Asylum-Seekers Stranded in Crowded Shelters during Pandemic," *KPBS*, March 24, 2020, www.kpbs.org/news/2020/mar/24/remain-mexico-program-paused-asylum-seekers-are-st/

74 At this point in time though Latin America had very low numbers at that point and some had not found their first cases yet. The U.S. Army Corps of Engineers tried to override Native sovereignty over sacred lands for national security reasons.

75 Kate Morrissey, "San Diego Fund to Help Unauthorized Immigrants out of Work due to Coronavirus Pandemic," *San Diego Union Tribune*, March 27, 2020, www.sandiegouniontribune.com/news/immigration/story/2020-03-27/san-diego-fund-to-help-unauthorized-immigrants-out-of-work-due-to-coronavirus-pandemic

76 *The Guardian*, "Guatemala Calls US 'Wuhan of Americas' in Battle over Deportees," *The Guardian*, April 15, 2020, www.theguardian.com/world/2020/apr/15/us-deportation-flights-guatemala-coronavirus

77 Monica Campbell, "US Deportation Flights Risk Spreading Coronavirus Globally," *PRI*, April 14, 2020, www.pri.org/stories/2020-04-14/us-deportation-flights-risk-spreading-coronavirus-globally

78 Joe Penney, "African Nations Turn the Tables, Imposing Travel Restrictions against U.S., Europe, and China to Stave off Coronavirus," *The* Intercept, March 15, 2020, https://theintercept.com/2020/03/15 /african-nations-turn-the-tables-imposing-travel-restrictions-against-u-s-europe-and-china-to-stave-off-coronavirus/

79 Megha Amrith, "Ageing Bodies, Precarious Futures: The (Im)mobilities of 'Temporary' Migrant Domestic Workers over Time," *Mobilities*, 16, no. 2 (2021): 251.

80 Jessie Tu, "Taiwan's First Female President Is Delivering a Stunning COVID-19 Response," *Women's Agenda*, April 3, 2020, https://womensagenda.com.au/latest/taiwans-first-female-president-is-delivering-a-stunning-covid-19-response/

81 Reuters, "MSF Urges Greece to Evacuate Migrant Camps due to Coronavirus Risk," *Reuters*, March 13, 2020, www.reuters.com/article/us-health-coronavirus-greece-migrants/msf-urges-greece-to-evacuate-migrant-camps-due-to-coronavirus-risk-idUSKBN2102M1

5

FRONTLINE LABOR

Service, Solidarity, Socialism

The COVID-19 pandemic put a spotlight on an entire class of working people and professionals. Now suddenly thrust into the public eye, these "essential workers" and "frontline laborers" were celebrated as humanity's defenders against the novel coronavirus. Wrenching sympathy for blue- and pink-collar workers as well as medical workers, this attribution lionized hidden figures as our unsung heroes. Heretofore were busy individuals whose acumen and lives often went unremarked, but whose undercompensated contributions to society held up modern life. "Menial" hands were now hailed as public models of goodness and virtue in a viral world.

Previously sidelined, their forced pandemic labor resembled a form of modern-day serfdom, as many frontliners were compelled to work against their will or in bad conditions. The "they" included custodians, nail salon technicians, nurses, transit conductors, farmworkers, plant operators, maintenance crews, warehouse workers, construction workers, food preparers, parcel deliverers, store stockers, security guards, and gas station operators. Their newfound labelling as frontliner inadvertently caricatures a diverse heterogenous demographic, their hardships minimalized in performing occupations of last resort, ones often involving backbreaking repetitive tasks. Glorifying the virtues of the wage worker, Odisha state in India tried to give "coronavirus warriors" official martyr status, but this state "honor" reinforces the incommensurability of service and equity.

Within the new physical distancing economy, the marked contrast between "us" and "them" follows a familiar pattern: *we* were caring for our redistributed selves, while *they* were caring for us. Carrying the heaviest load for global economies now suspended in motion, a proletariat class risked their lives just so others can work safely or from home. They walked the

DOI: 10.4324/9781032694535-6

line between necessary "work" to feed themselves and mandated "service" to the public. The supposed difference between the two categories is best characterized as an illusion—a mirage finally broken by COVID-19, such as even when countries like France offered fast-track citizenship as a reward for the life-giving work of immigrant frontliners. As one *deliverista* from New York City stresses,

> While others are inside their homes, we are placing ourselves at risk to contract COVID-19. This truly worries me. I have four kids and a wife at home who are taking all measures to stay inside, but what purpose does it serve if I just put them at risk from being on the streets?[1]

The language of "frontline" capitulated to the death-drive of pandemic capitalism. Overlooked were the lifeworlds of people with disabilities, the elderly, and the idled migrant workers who made up most of the world's service class. Measuring time in terms of pandemic productivity, business magnates paid scant thought to their frontline futures. Farmworkers felt the wasting away of their minds and bodies, not least due to policies that coerced them into toiling continuously under grueling conditions that traverse legal boundaries and borderlands.[2]

A separation of fates was borne out by class. A sizable proportion of the managerial sector now did their jobs remotely. These digital nomads absconded to cheaper places to live, exacerbating residential inequalities based on income. Far fewer people of color in the United States could work bunkered at home. Only one out of five Latine/Black people could do so, compared to over one-third of Whites, according to the U.S. Bureau of Labor. These sobering statistics betray a grim reality, one which flies in the face of the refrain that disease is a "great equalizer" and that "a virus does not discriminate." The first teenager in the United States to die from COVID-19 was turned away from an urgent care facility for not having insurance.

Though blockaded from attaining Italian citizenship, African fruit and vegetable pickers maintained the country's food supply as the country faced down its biggest nonmilitary threat. Italian nationals avoided harm in their private abode, while a reserve army of peons kept the wheels of public life spinning. These frontlines are transnational, as the Philippines, the world's biggest supplier of nurses, faced incredible staff shortages domestically. For the first time, the government tried to ban nurses from leaving the country and raised salaries to little avail. On the home front, medics were sent as "volunteer" trainees without protective equipment to rural areas in the grips of a drug war. Pandemic martial law and the fears of the unknown it induced laid the footwork for the son of former Philippines dictator Ferdinand Marcos to pull off a landslide win for the presidency in 2022.

As an unyielding novel coronavirus coursed through the least advantaged populations, the question of who was most "exposed" to COVID-19 sharpened into focus, especially those frontline "soldiers" sent into battle without armor. Under a mandate of preserving law and order, the United Kingdom warned that anyone who deliberately coughs at these key workers will face assault charges and spend a year in jail. Latina physicians, serving as cultural brokers between clinics and communities, felt invisible. Some admitted to not being considered as "essential" to the medical establishment, relegated to shadow work behind the scenes.[3] The risk of death while working with COVID-19 was huge, but immigrant workers had always been put in life-threatening situations.

Workers did not ask or volunteer to die. As Luis Jimenez, a migrant worker explains, "We're willing to risk the virus. But I didn't come here to die. I came so that my family in Mexico will live."[4] The synopsis that "we're all in this together" is rendered meaningless and moot when it involves labor exploitation and coercion. Legal scholar Shaun Ossei-Owusu muses on COVID-19 politics of (expendable) labor and why "we" should be careful with the gratifying language of (worker) solidarity and (public) service: "Collective pronouns—the 'we' and 'our' and 'us' of public discourse—are dangerously comforting … when the dust settles … there will be a tale to tell of who mattered and who was sacrificed."[5] We must always wonder where sacrifice ends and service begins and, ultimately asking, service for whom. Thus, this chapter explores service, and its implications for solidarity and socialism.

Continuing my investigation of the pandemic's relational effects, this chapter examines the shifting cartographies of power/knowledge engendered by working people. With the prominent attention given to "frontline labor," this attribution seriously altered conventional perceptions of wage workers as a "new" hero and the service that they provide. A greater push for social services and protections for poor people augmented "communist" fears in societies transformed under collective burden-sharing amid a pandemic. With the focus on frontline workers as sacrificial martyrs, the chapter inquires what exactly service means in the context of a raging pandemic. Sex workers (Brazil), domestic caregivers (South Africa), meatpackers (the United States), and agricultural workers (Canada) are discussed together to track how the world's "frontliners" were exploited as well as empowered. Ensuing sections on solidarity and socialism discuss the interdependency among everyday people, demonstrating what mutual aid could look like. Solidarity was forged when the Navajo nation donated masks to South Korea, while Cuba sent medical aid to distressed places like Italy. The opposite of this socialist strategy of support was rampant individualism, as witnessed in countries like Sweden and the United States. Despite corporate rulers, frontliners and the working class showed who truly ran the (viral) world.

Service

"Muere, bacteria, muere!" an ensemble of nurses in Oaxaca, Mexico, sang in harmony. Their performance came courtesy of an old video from 2016 celebrating Global Handwashing Day, one that took on greater resonance in 2020. The three friends found instant fame as the world was changing under COVID-19, going "viral" on social media for providing a valuable public service in the global fight against a disease the women did not even anticipate, since they were originally talking about bacteria.[6]

At work with sick patients all the time, medical practitioners encounter many brushes with death as hospitals transfigured into a frontline. These battle zones of a pandemic emerged in 2015 when the countries of Guinea, Sierra Leone, and Liberia suffered an outbreak of the West African Ebola virus in 2013 with a grisly toll that topped 11,000 people. The medical personnel who died in the long slog against Ebola were celebrated as national heroes. In Nigeria, an army of contact chasers who visited homes stymied a major outbreak. If viral clusters made it out totally undetected from the transcontinental hub of Lagos, it spelled total disaster for the whole of Africa. This catastrophe did not happen due to medical service providers. Their feats of courage prevented SARS-CoV-2 later from completely permeating African countries, even when prevention plans faltered.

Panic buying of protective masks for COVID-19 though by the public threatened the supply of hospital equipment. Turning scarce the stream of medical necessities, ordinary citizens walked around with covered faces, while nurses needed to go without. When a U.S.-based manufacturer offered to quickly make millions of the much desired "impenetrable" N95 mask, the government refused this offer from the last major domestic mask manufacturer. A whistleblower report from a federal vaccine chief led to his firing for early warning about COVID-19—his service to others interpreted as a crime. From a chronic depletion of supplies to a shortage of staff, overrun hospitals started to look like war zones, with corpses left to rot in the open. Amid government inaction and a declining number of hospital beds, doctors were compelled to make the wrenching choice of who lives and who dies. As public guardians, they had been personally taxed to not only sacrifice themselves and families, but they shouldered the added burden of doing a human calculus, due to the insurmountable hurdle of treating an influx of patients.

Frontliners were caught in a place between delaying others' death and working until they dropped dead from exposure or exhaustion. This positioning "led to a sense of entrapment or feeling stuck, which, in turn, deeply shaped their sense of futurity."[7] What then about the social life behind this labor?[8] As first responders and paramedics fell sick or died while attending to patients, some walked off and left their jobs, due to lacking medical grade equipment. Other staff were dismissed for speaking out about the logjam in hospitals to the media (one nurse used GoFundMe to raise money for equipment like shoe covers but was suspended by administrators). Hospital caregivers needed to wear old gowns or substitute them with flimsy garbage bags. Nurses faced rebuke for objecting to usage of old masks decontaminated with hydrogen peroxide. Workers were suspended for refusing service without masks. Medical television shows and sex fetish companies donated their masks and equipment to real-life medical teams.

Cleaning service. Community service. Religious service. Military service. Erotic service. Innumerable forms of service exist. During a pandemic, service typically means medical service, which is why medics all around the world, from China to Bulgaria, received a rousing applause as gratitude from crowds in the street for their public service. Other forms of service count in equal measure. In the United States, medics cheered on anti-racist protesters for their civil service against unlawful police violence. Temporary migrant workers from overseas were passed over in governments' cash handouts, which were given to all citizens and permanent residents. This contracted workforce in Singapore, Japan, Thailand, and Hong Kong were purposively singled out. Their omission from aid also hurt their home countries depending on overseas remittances. States arbitrated the definition of frontliner.

Public health officials in Hong Kong exerted pressure on the public to wear face coverings to shield against SARS-CoV-2, which ran contrary to earlier ban on face masks in November 2019 in response to veiled pro-democracy demonstrators (the law was overruled by the administrative region's high court as unconstitutional). Masks and personal protective equipment do not represent an unassailable fortress to disease, but they form a barrier to closed autocracies that put subjects "in service" to the public. The shortage of such equipment (and failures to address frontliner mental health) led doctors to stress their martyr status (see Figure 5.1). In a photograph in front of Downey Street, doctors in England protested their martyrdom with bended knee in a symbolic gesture toward the Black Lives Matter Movement. LGBTQ+ pride marches around the world pivoted into queer liberation marches in support of BLM, a gesture of solidarity which can be problematic when it is temporary or ad hoc.[9] COVID-19 made it clear—we all need more and deserve better. From these acts of solidarity, we can interpret how medical martyrs, speaking through and to Black anti-racist activists, turned into advocates of racial justice.

Many sex workers who provide a valuable service themselves found themselves without shelter after brothels were shut down. Too petrified to seek help, some workers resumed work, despite the high risk of catching COVID-19. The U.S. government ruled out benefits for employees in the adult entertainment industry such as strippers and pornographic actors. The online

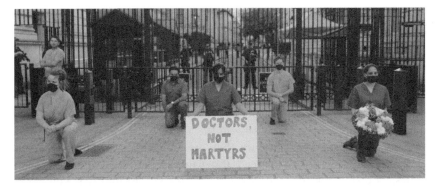

FIGURE 5.1 Photo of doctors holding a silent protest outside Downing Street in London (Getty Images).

application for relief stipulated an applicant cannot sell services and products of a prurient sexual content.[10] "We need a compassionate acknowledgement of our work as legitimate labor," insisted Andre Shakti, a sex worker who lost half of her income to pandemic quarantine and prohibitions. The Pope donated money to aid a group of sex workers who sought the Church's help after their passports had been stolen by the mafia. Father Andrew Conocchia admitted, "We treat these people as if they were invisible. This is a health emergency, but also a social emergency."[11]

Despite hypervisibility as essential workers, frontliners in other fields resented their essentialization during a health emergency. They attested that society required valor from those who did not choose that role for themselves. On May 1, International Workers Day, workers from Amazon, Walmart, FedEx, Target, Instacart, and other big companies led a mass strike and boycott. While small mortar-and-brick businesses suffered gravely as the economy was shutting down, publicly traded online megacompanies received record profits. Google and its parent company raked in high profits, as digital services spiked under lockdown. A whistleblower investigation found that it knowingly underpaid workers in dozens of countries. Amazon's boss, Jeff Bezos, the world's richest person became even richer with almost $30 billion added to his net worth (double the value of his next competitor). The world's (online) largest retailer dropped workers who groused about unsafe work conditions. Others walked off their job at warehouses, demanding the company to close facilities and sanitize them before making employees snap back to work. The grassroots group New York Communities for Change tweeted, "Amazon is putting profits over safety" as it gives money for "hazard pay" but not regular paid sick leave for contract workers.[12] Amazon employees in Staten Island created the first labor union in the United States after a two-year fight.

Under the chorus of a pandemic death march, a new song of service was trumpeted. For the first time in U.S. history, the Department of Homeland Security declared the country's 2.4 million farmworkers as "essential" and "critical" infrastructure workers. Undocumented workers found this special designation hypocritical, as half of them rely on public assistance but cannot access unemployment benefits or attain a clear path to citizenship. Nearly half are without legal status or permanent work authorization permits, and a quarter million come temporarily on the agricultural H-2A visa program. Many do not speak Spanish since they are Indigenous and speak Mixtec or Zapotec, so they did not receive translated information about the virus or physical distancing. *Campesinos* live in crowded dormitories, vulnerable to asthma, and if sick, rarely visit a hospital due to fear of immigration authorities. The United Farm Workers and other community agencies sent letters to growers and public officials about the workers' right to protect their health (including from pesticides), obtain state benefits, and organize through unions.

Despite their appellation as the world's heroes, food workers still fell sick while grinding away at their day jobs. In the food sector, which employs the most Americans, nearly 80% of food workers did not have paid sick days. Food reporter Claire Kelloway indicates that we should "recognize that our debt to food workers does not end when this pandemic does."[13] The Food Chain Alliance advocated ending the "public charge" gag rule installed by the Trump administration to deny migrant claims for asylum or citizenship if they should need public assistance. And yet, COVID-19 turned almost everyone into a recipient of state handouts with no questions asked. Others mostly immigrants of color were "entitled to nothing."[14] The federal bailout package, called Coronavirus Aid, Relief, and Economic Security Act (CARES), barred the undocumented from receiving benefits, effectively shutting out 70% of all farmworkers in California. This ban expanded to U.S.-born children since students with an undocumented parent were denied COVID-19-related school aid. Per one worker, "It's just a slap in the face. We're on the front lines. We're taking risks every day, and we never stop. It's just the money."[15]

Black and brown workers were propped up as human shields. Many frontline workers were people of color, and so the "front line" against COVID-19 followed the color line and what W.E.B. Dubois called the shadow "worlds of color."[16] From these viral worlds, the "frontline laborer" figured prominently in stories flashed across cable channels.

In Hong Kong, medical workers went on strike, assembling a frontline to demand a border checkpoint shutdown with mainland China, which threatened the city's livelihood in terms of both politics and disease. As more ground ceded to the novel coronavirus, employees seen as below-the-radar had been extended the vaunted frontliner status to mail carriers, teachers, and morticians.

Facebook offshored labor to contract workers in the Philippines, who were impelled to work in lower-paid remote offices while full-time "domestic" ones in the United States stayed home with bonuses.[17] Rendering "foreign" contractors as second-class "rearline" employees, Facebook refused to supply even threadbare support to those workers responsible for the "dirty work."

Social burdens are never shared equally. Cleaning crews that fumigated public places reported sickness from the harsh chemicals they used against COVID-19. Migrants recruited from overseas to mitigate job shortages in the Britain's medical field were not entitled to financial or government support under an employer-centered system of sponsorship, which differs from Canada and New Zealand with their public settlement programs. In early 2020, the United Kingdom moved toward the Australian points-based system, tightening the pool of applicants and reducing the status of "invisible heroes and their families."[18] Not all heroes received public accolades.

The pandemic reawakened communities to how infectious kindness and love could be. Memes spread calling for "Love in the Time of Corona," videos were shared of girls dancing or cooking for their working mothers in hospitals, while overworked doctors and nurses displayed the red marks and "battle scars" on their face from wearing tight surgical masks all day. When they went on media to describe their struggles, medical workers turned into powerful storytellers and their stories became viral and witnessed all around the world.

Contrary to a privatized medical screening culture based on risk assessment and the mortgaging of lives, we heard more public messages of care. The gainfully employed however donated their sick days to fellow workers who contracted COVID-19. Oakland teachers pledged to send their COVID-19 stimulus monies to undocumented migrant families. After Turkey's justice minister tweeted that "we should not abandon our animal friends," the interior ministry ordered food and water brought to animal shelters (meanwhile caged prisoners demanded a draft law to release them on a transitory basis due to SARS-CoV-2).[19] Italians, Koreans, Chinese, and Brits under lockdown put out online videos about their experiences. Grocery stores opened their markets late at night to buffer the elderly against frantic shoppers. Youngsters even reprimanded their parents for going out. Intergenerational solidarity was encouraged as was the "right to relate."

Motels and luxury hotels were requisitioned to supplement hospitals or shield the unhoused from the path of COVID-19. Economic systems leaden with power imbalances kept inequality relatively intact amid new pandemic social arrangements, but "moral economies" brought people together. For those folks suffering from the doldrums of home confinement, they took care of themselves, while service (and sacrifice) was imputed to critical maintenance staff who kept everything running smoothly. Poet Audre Lorde once wrote about why self-love matters and why no one should not bank on an easy cure for disease that leaves no room to examine what a life is worth: "Caring for myself is not self-indulgence, it is self-preservation, and that is an act of political warfare."[20] The uncritical illusion of safety is a "heavy-footed hope" that silences people "who were never meant to survive."[21] For the queer Black feminist, living is not a luxury, it is a litany of survival.

Under slipshod pandemic responses, the story of Brazil and the United States converged around another kind of political warfare centered on "bullets, beef, and the bible." JBS is a Brazilian beef company whose economic agenda was backed by government conglomerates. In mid-2019 and in January 2020, its subsidiary JBS USA received millions of government pork contracts funding, more than any other U.S.-based farm, as part of an intended farm bailout program for agricultural producers. With early estimates that 80% of the meat production could shut down, Donald Trump flexed his executive muscle under the Defense Production Act. While Trump did not force whole industries and manufacturers (except General Motors) to make ventilators as first thought, he did classify meat processing plants as "essential" infrastructure, an injunction to make them stay open for the duration of the pandemic.

This directive opposes the wishes of unions on the frontlines of a "class war" between plutocrats and workers, the latter "being forced into labor militancy to protect their lives."[22] Half of all U.S. hot spots in mid-2020 flared in meat-packing factories, which incapacitated workers due to their worse health conditions. But when migrant workers describe themselves as "guinea pigs" and "modern slaves," it becomes evident, per one Liberian refugee meatpacker, "essential worker just means you're on the death track."[23] Without question, the high risk of death or mental health stress for meatpackers preceded the pandemic, but broad awareness of these injurious conditions was uncovered in the post-pandemic industry. When leaders interposed efficiency over ethics, meatpackers transfigured into sacrificial lambs, forced to work on "good faith" that they would not die on the job (two-thirds of all reopened factories underwent outbreaks). Essential meat workers were enlisted in a figurative draft in the war against COVID-19 with consumers treated as economic "warriors" to boost product sales.[24]

With real COVID-19 fears on full display, those laborers recoiled from going to work, which made them ineligible for any government benefits. They exercised the right *not* to work and not get sick. In places under restrictive lock-in, labor rights intersected with the right to access public space, the right to health, and the right to life. The regular five-day week and 9–5 workday took a beating from the pandemic, which required much more flexible hours and time off for employees.

For an occupation like nursing, there is a gendered expectation that women, migrant women of color, and queer femme-presenting people must always bear the burden for others at any time. Sex determinations do little to account for the fact that more women than men live in poverty, being overrepresented in underpaid social/healthcare services, compromising 80% of those workers. In Hong Kong, literary scholar Alvin Wong pontificates on the challenges of mobilizing "freedom in multiplicity" for a frontliner "us"—that include migrants, ethnic minorities, and LGBTQ+ members— who "might feel hesitant to join the frontline protest because the tactics of the protestors might be overtly masculine." Lack of remediation for underpinning social problems ensures a string of *future* crises for the service industry.[25]

The viral world principle of self-sacrifice as public sacrifice remains tenuous for migrants working overseas. Knowing the hidden costs of their labor, seasonal workers from Jamaica headed to Canadian farms even amid a global pandemic. They were hard pressed to sign contracts issued by the Jamaican government, waiving the state of fiduciary responsibility for medical liabilities or financial losses incurred abroad. Officials washed their hands of potential legal damages of migrants being introduced to COVID-19. Canada's government required paid self-isolation for two weeks upon arrival, so guest workers on allotment visas faced not only "emergency" wage cuts but also pressures to work immediately without information on healthcare access. Left to fend for themselves, migrants had been physically distanced from society.[26]

Assistance for those people stuck in the pandemic's messiness was not forthcoming for many groups. Emergency relief funds in the form of direct electronic payments cannot be transferred to migrants without official papers (California sent stimulus checks to undocumented migrants with some help from private donors). To guarantee them regular protection, Portugal temporarily granted all migrants and asylum-seekers full citizenship rights during the outbreak. President Marcelo Rebelo de Sousa called the pandemic "a true war" for the entire country's people, one that requires service to the people and democracy.[27]

War seems the preferred operative term, since the term "frontline" originally derives from the military to refer to field operations that involve enemy contact. For large swaths of the world dependent on foreign workers, the enemy remains immigrants who threaten their national identity. Undocumented essential workers in the United States, most of whom are not covered by health insurance, feared COVID-19 testing due to the greater fear of becoming caught by Immigration and Customs Enforcement (ICE). Even when they were tested, they were refused treatment. A migrant who tested positive went to a hospital with high fever, but staff refused to service her.

> I went to ask for help and they denied me because I am not a citizen … It hurts because I am a human being before the eyes of God. It is horrible that they treat me like this, and I do not have the right to do anything.[28]

The pandemic compounded long simmering issues like migrant rights. These rights can be abrogated by countries that detach health from humanitarianism and that do not feel the need to serve the displaced.

The deportation regime in the United States persisted, while holding thousands in deplorable conditions, even as other countries shut down their deportation programs. Hunger strikes took place in these facilities, which often did not hold regular sanitation staff. Many held in confinement were not told what COVID-19 was, and the detained pleaded to be released, after unsettling news about the deaths of HIV-positive transmigrants denied antiviral medicine as well as child deaths (the Trump administration had previously sparred with a federal court, claiming soap and toiletries were not needed for migrant children). Those migrants with family in the country and not considered a "danger to the community" could have been released with tracking bracelets, but ICE held them without explanation, including a scientist exonerated by a sanctions trial but who was detained indefinitely without any legal justification (his visa had been revoked during the long trial). He explains how detained migrants are not treated as human beings but as objects to get rid of: "I don't think many people in the U.S. know what is happening inside this black box ... Coronavirus is a viral bomb waiting to blow up here."

Cultural theorist Lisa Lowe suggests this viral bomb as reigniting revolutionary feminism on what appears to be the "eve of destruction." She advocates appreciating the work of poor women and feminine reproductive labor, which reflects the "broader range of kin labor, caring labor, and all labors of human contact."[29] Forced to hold up the world once more and bear an "inner martyrdom," women were propped up once more as humanity's security blanket. Feminists called out the problems of this social mandate.[30] A viral post by a Facebook user revealed the gendered emotional and physical labor that runs the pandemic economy: "The economy is not 'closed.' Everyone is cooking, cleaning, and taking care of their loved ones. It's just not valued by economists because it's normally unpaid women's work."[31] While some were "serving" time, others were serving the needs of others.

In an unfolding global crisis, there appears a need to remake the world we live in, recasting our moral imperative by asking first who cares for whom? Who does the work of caring and who pays the price for *not* caring? How does "frontliner" suggest a kind of "able-bodied" persona that ignores the elderly and the differently abled?[32] From "congregational care" to a pandemic ethics of care, movement-builders confronted "the foundation of the current world and the basis upon which we undo its principles towards an unseen and unknown elsewhere."[33]

Writing in the *Corona Times*, anthropologist Rose Boswell dispenses with the ableist gendered trope of women as natural caregivers, nurturers, and cleaners. Even as "essential workers," they are doubly burdened by the duty of care for the public and for the home. But who were taking care of the women? The gender gap in household labor increased with COVID-19, even more so at a time when the task of cleaning and disinfecting fell hard on womyn-identifying people.[34] She adds,

> In South Africa where I live, millions of women are living in an unending disaster movie, where men in power pretend to be heroes ... for such women, the coronavirus is equally deadly, but they have the long experience of the plague of oppression ... I feel that it is time for men to stand up and pick up the mop. It is time for them to pay their maintenance dues.[35]

Obtaining much-needed and deep self-care is by no means simple, since there are many poor women stuck in dire work-life situations. Meanwhile, pandemic "survival circuits" had been built on the backs of women and the day-to-day labor of nannies, nurses, sex workers, inter alia.[36] With the "feminization of survival," a viral pandemic world owed a deep debt to its caretakers as well as a measure of solidarity.

Solidarity

Under the strain of forced isolation, the term "physical distancing" gained currency over social distancing to underscore a fierce commitment to mutual support and solidarity as COVID-19 played havoc on social life. Alcohol distilleries switched gears to churn out hand sanitizers. A man started a free open-source project from his home in the Netherlands to share free sewing patterns, an idea that was picked up after watching his female partner work in a hospital with a dearth of masks. Nail salons voluntarily sewed masks when garment businesses were shut down, while Asian American women without children formed Auntie Sewing Squads.[37]

Viral videos of quarantined Italian, American, and Chinese neighbors sang or played music to each other through their windows to cast a billowy cloud of hope over the pandemic grimness. Meanwhile, Brazilians banged their pots and pans from balconies in protest of President Bolsonaro's inactions, cheering and jeering at the same time. In the eye of the COVID-19 storm, people demanded a better life, and they did so as a form of social solidarity.

What does collective solidarity look in a pandemic? In one sense, it seems no more than an intense form of existing social networks, a recreation of human camaraderie and social complementarity to build new worlds. According to historian Robin Kelley, "Solidarity as worldmaking offers more than short-term alliances or coalitions but a sort of prefigurative politics that demands of us a deeper transformation of society and of our relationships to one another."[38]

Activists with resolve in protecting vulnerable local communities drummed up support from all over to build pandemic solidarity. There was a concerted public effort to protect the elderly, based on early reports from China of high mortality for the old. Taiwan sent 100,000 face masks to the United States and the latter sent 1,000 ventilators to South Africa. A Danish company shipped robots to disinfect and clean Chinese hospitals, while a Japanese company ensured safe transport of medical procurements to China through drones.[39] Chinese companies sent supplies to African countries, while nationals in Africa set on aiding local businesses. Chinese associations in Uganda donated thermometers, goggles, and a quarter million masks.

International amity crossed over into Indigenous solidarity. On the 70th anniversary of the end of the Korean War, South Korea's commemoration committee sent 10,000 masks and hand sanitizer bottles to a Diné veteran group in appreciation for their war efforts as code talkers. Through a GoFundMe online campaign, donations from Ireland poured into the Diné, Hopi, and Choctaw nations as a gesture of mutuality for a good deed done over 173 years ago when the Choctaw Nation sent $170 to Ireland with which it has a special bilateral relationship: an act of selflessness of serving those people in need called *iyyikowa*. Native Americans lent a hand to the Irish during the Great Famine, an act of solidarity amid forced removal onto reservations by the United States. One of the campaign organizers affirmed, "In moments like these, we are so grateful for the love and support we have received from all around the world. Acts of kindness from Indigenous ancestors passed being reciprocated nearly 200 years later through blood memory and interconnectedness."[40]

Despite the fatigue of fighting a pandemic, countless examples of altruism throughout the world proved that kindness can be contagious. Canadian citizens expressed the principles of a new popular movement called "caremongering." Taiwan's Ministry of Foreign Affairs avidly promoted a global campaign with the slogan "Taiwan can help!" As a force of good in the international community, Taiwanese strove to help others as much as it could help themselves.[41]

Solidarity as a matter of "disease diplomacy" means community and global engagement. Through a "digital fence" to rope quarantine rings around its mobile population, Taiwan earned plaudits for crushing the curve. Upon hearing about the novel coronavirus in China via social media, the country dispatched a team to Wuhan and returned to activate its Central Epidemic Command Center (CECC). Steered by Digital Minister Audrey Tang, the youngest in a top government position, the transgender former hacker and her department propelled a technoculture of civil protest and the pro-independence Sunflower Student Movement.

Building up its "nerd immunity" to resist communist falsehoods, tech-savvy Taiwan begin monitoring for localized viral clusters a week after its first reported case.[42] Besides shipping millions of masks to other countries, the island gained admirers who marveled at its multimodal response to COVID-19. Its scintillating campaign used big data and a real-time interactive map, visualizing to the public where masks are sold and store stocks. An integrated communication strategy maintained online telepresence that included a chatbot to answer questions on instant messaging. Using consumers' phone data clouds and information, Taiwan applied the latest information technology to alert police officers of infected residents. This successful pandemic campaign boosted its international reputation, despite exclusion from global emergency meetings and briefings on coronavirus (Chinese nationalists urged the communist leadership to invade Taiwan while the world was busy dealing with COVID-19).

Due to China's global influence, Taiwan goes unrecognized as a full-fledged member of the United Nations and the World Health Organization (WHO). With the pandemic, Taiwan postponed its bid for observer status in the latter, but this issue was pushed by the U.S. at the annual meeting in 2020, where China pledged billions to the organization. New Zealand, Canada, and United Kingdom asked for a probe into the origins of SARS-CoV-2, which was interpreted by the People's Republic of China (PRC) as a probe into its mishandling of the pandemic. China was on the defensive.

The cleavage between China and Taiwan marks a hinge point in the global pandemic response. At the nexus of this triangulation was WHO, which heaped praise upon PRC but had said almost nothing about the Republic of China (ROC)—despite the universal acclaim the latter received from the world. In early 2020, the Taiwanese Foreign Ministry thanked international governing bodies for girding its bid to join the World Health Assembly (WHA), after being blocked by China for electing its pro-independence president, Tsai Ing-wen.[43] Taiwan's ministry conveyed gratitude on Facebook for the outpouring of support from Baltic parliamentary members in Lithuania, Latvia, and Estonia, Czech Republic, and Slovakia. But Taiwan's glimmering image casts a shadow over its half-million undocumented workers who take care of local elderly and the sick.[44] They were relegated to palliative care, while lodged in "container houses" or worker dormitories with no running water.

The pandemic rewound the push and pull between unilateral action and multilateral cooperation. President Trump tweeted a broadside to the WHO, lamenting that the organization was "very China-centric" in its parroting of China's early wrongful claims about SARS-CoV-2. He froze funding to the organization, and China responded shortly after with additional contributions. The WHO muddled through its role as an interstate organ, under strain by voluntary actions on the part of its discordant member-states. It can only give prudent recommendations that can be taken or not (though WHO records reveal that China willingly withheld data). Countries like Indonesia resisted defensive COVID-19 measures (the health minister even said prayer was enough to be safe). Indonesia only declared a state of civil emergency after the WHO requested that it activate emergency protocols. Since the avian flu pandemic, the world's largest Muslim country has been trying to assert its "viral sovereignty" over viruses entering its territorial borders as well as against international actors requesting viral samples.[45] These responses to virus sharing stress the geopolitics of disease.

The WHO defended itself against raw invectives, emphasizing that it alerted the world in early 2020. This alert activated incident management systems of many countries including the United States, which booted up its system the day after. Calling the United States a "generous friend," WHO head Tedros Adhanom Ghebreyesus underlined the need for respect of the United Nations' mission of working with all nations "without fear or favor."[46] UN Secretary-General pleaded for unity to reverse the pandemic, instead of heaping abuse on the global health body responsible for spearheading coordinated action.

In the back-and-forth between the United States and the WHO, the presidents of Rwanda, Namibia, and South Africa rallied behind the WHO's chief, originally from Ethiopia. South Africa's president Cyril Ramaphosa tweeted this riposte to Trump: "The most potent weapon against #Covid19 … international cooperation and solidarity."[47] The chairperson of the African Union Commission struck a chord with Ramphosa's message: "Surprised to learn of a campaign by the US govt against @WHO's global leadership. The @_AfricanUnion fully supports @WHO and @DrTedros. The focus should remain on fighting #Covid19 as a united global community. The time for accountability will come."

Italy asked the world's help when it became the first European nation to experience a major outbreak and the first country in the world to induce a national lockdown. With the numbers of infected rocketing, Italian viral media requests for assistance were answered by Somalia, which sent volunteer doctors to aid the country's former colonizer. China directed an elite medical team knowledgeable in dealing with SARS-CoV-2 to the beleaguered country. Russia delivered a whole medical convoy from its army, a goodwill gesture labelled "From Russia with Love." Actions from major powers can be held suspect, since China needed to repair its global image after COVID-19, Russia needed an ally in the European Union for its invasion of Ukraine, and Cuba needed its altruism to persuade others to end its decades-long sanctions by the United States.

In the global tug of war to control the master narrative, China leaned into its "wolf warrior" diplomats willing to defend the country at all costs, deploying "coronavirus diplomacy" and economic aid to disabuse any perception of pandemic mismanagement. Countering China's struggle for global influence through media spin and its "politics of generosity," Josep Burrell believes there is a war over the COVID-19 story that must be wrangled over to shore up global cooperation. The High Representative of the European Union and member of Spanish Socialist Worker's Party proposes that Europe be "armed with facts" and fortify itself against its detractors from outside and from within. "There is also a battle of narratives within Europe. It is vital that the EU shows it is a Union that protects, and that solidarity is not an empty phrase."[48]

Leftist governments in Bolivia, Venezuela, and Brazil went downhill in the face of mass revolts and political coups. Communist stronghold Cuba held ground as a paragon of self-sacrifice, sending a medical brigade to Italy's badly affected Lombardy region. It deployed "armies of white robes" to Nicaragua, Venezuela, Jamaica, Suriname, and Grenada just as it did when the country help battle Ebola in West Africa and cholera in Haiti. Proclaimed one of the team's doctors, "We are not superheroes, we are revolutionary doctors." Another declared, "We are going to fulfill an honorable task, based on the principle of solidarity."[49] China coordinated with fellow communist country Cuba to cook up a vaccine and allowed tourists to dock on its shores and receive treatment. This cross-country reception contrasts with the situation in Japan, where the cruise ship Diamond Princess stayed afar and could not land, after it was discovered that its members on board were infected with COVID-19. Images portrayed the crew mostly from Southeast Asia stuck on the ship and the harrowing rescue operations of wealthy countries like Canada, Australia, and the United States evacuating their citizens.

Cuba displayed incredible feats against the novel coronavirus, motivated by a political alchemy of socialist-inspired internationalism combined with health humanitarianism. This marriage is best exemplified by Havana's Latin American Medical School (the largest medical school in the world) created in 2005 to train doctors from poor countries. Cuba realized that solutions like training more doctors was necessary to troubleshoot the pandemic's psychodrama.[50] It even developed its own drugs and named its vaccine Abdala after a drama written by revolutionary José Martí. Optimized through Cuban-Chinese joint venture, a potential "wonder drug" called Pan-Corona was created based on materials previously effective in treating HIV/AIDS, hepatitis A and B, meningitis B, and shingles.[51] Cuba's experience with dengue hemorrhagic fever (viewed largely by Cubans as introduced from the United States) coalesced into a fast-track program for innovative drugs on a massive scale, despite a six-decade U.S. economic blockade.

Given Cuba's incredible display of service and solidarity, organizations like the WHO, Organization of American States, and Pan American Health Organization advocated lifting restrictive sanctions on the country during the pandemic. Cuba's state-owned vaccine manufacturers vied to purchase ventilators and other supplies from over 60 U.S. companies, but it encountered the U.S. embargo of Cuba. This embargo also undercut Cuba's medical aid to countries in a "solidarity alliance" like Iran, Vietnam, Venezuela, Bolivia,

Nicaragua.[52] This roused Cuba to accuse its northern bully of "contempt for life" as part of a "genocidal, inhumane policy."[53]

Pressures for change came to fore in the United States, Cuba, Venezuela, Iran, and Nicaragua. Undeterred by sanctions, Cuba went ahead to develop five of its own vaccines intended for local and worldwide distribution. With some named after national heroes, the two major drugs are named Soberana 01 and 02 (coproduced with Iran). Soberana means sovereignty in Spanish. The naming of the COVID-19 drugs attests to a desire by nations to assert their authority. But despite this show of sovereignty, the largest protest in a generation erupted in Cuban cites in 2021, demanding the end of communist rule.

Like authoritarian regimes, global value chains are hard to change. The state of Baja California closed a plant operated by a U.S. firm given its refusal to sell ventilators to hospitals in Mexico. The firm claimed it lent an "essential" service, something refuted by Baja's governor:

> We said to them 'if you want us to consider you essential, you have to provide some benefit to the people of Baja California'…They said 'no,' we are not going to sell you anything, we are just going to continue to use your labor.[54]

As prime site for *maquiladora* factories, border states like Juarez suffered a 26% mortality coronavirus rate compared to 6% for the world. This spelled trouble for migrants toiling to make products for global export, their lives rendered inconsequential or "non-essential" to corporate overlords. At the behest of U.S. *maquila* owners who wanted the same "essential" status that they enjoyed in the United States and Canada, President Trump, along with the Pentagon and automakers, forced Mexico to keep *maquilas* open, as 40% of American assembly parts come from south of the border. Despite labor protests demanding total stoppage (and reports that workers were boxed-in and forced to work), factories were open three days after the U.S. request. They functioned at half capacity, especially after the U.S. ambassador to Mexico delivered this threatening message, "You don't have 'workers' if you close all the companies and they move elsewhere."[55] A pact was sealed among governments and companies at the expense of workers and citizens.

As COVID-19 swept the world, nationalist policies clashed with appeals for global solidarity. Finding himself in an unworkable coalition with more conservative partners, Italy's Prime Minister Guiseppe Conte warned of "nationalist instincts" on an upward trajectory not only in Italy but also on the broader European continent. This trend toward nationalism manifested when fiscally conservative wealthy northern countries led by the Netherlands blocked prospects of a common corona-debt, even though the European Union shared a common currency. Indisposed to issuing "coronabonds" and motioning against regional reciprocity, the indebted nations of Spain and Italy were left to trudge through the pandemic's thicket.[56] This slog persisted, despite the Tax Injustice Network finding that countries most hit by COVID-19 have lost billions of profits over the years to the Netherlands, a tax haven and conduits for shifting corporate profit revenues. Slow to isolate travelers and limit their movement, the woes of Europe and its adjuncts came from a confluence of factors: fractious governments, insolvent public debt, and high unemployment. COVID-19 entered a messy patch for already sickened societies, and their fates seemed almost sealed.

A puttering economy made life rockier. In debt-saddled Greece. Impromptu strikes crafted by steelworkers, shipyard loaders, and chemical textiles workers urged the closing of all companies. Despite their golden status as "essential" workers, strikers could not shake the feeling they were being held hostage, while the rest of the population nests at home. Strikers and unions responded negatively to the obstinate predilection to maintain industrial production and the capitalist mantra of valuing profits (over lives). The Cofindustria, the national chamber of commerce and federation that organizes industrial employers in Italy, increased pressure on the government to keep "key" open sectors deemed indispensable. Wielding enormous sway, the Cofindustria sent a letter to the government to open businesses days after the state announced the shutdown of all nonessential production. The successful request claimed that this closure would lead to stocks to tumble, so Italian leaders complied with owner demands, leaving open sectors of "strategic" importance, such as banks, call centers, and the defense industry.

The world-scale importance of the pandemic marked a foray into social decomposition and recomposition of socialist struggles. The leftist pro-worker newspaper *La Voce della Lotte* (The Voice of the Struggle) made this point:

> In the face of the disaster to which the capitalists have led us ... democratic, bottom-up workers' control can be imposed in the workplace ... to meet social priorities: all non-essential activities must be closed down, all those who will have to continue working must be protected, and the productive apparatus must be converted according to the extraordinary needs of today. We need workers to take control of the whole process.[57]

While global solidarity was expected during a pandemic, it was not always forthcoming. In its stead, we witnessed untold greed and avarice. Mike Davis, author of *The Monster at Our Door*, denaturalizes our "convergent crises," which he posits lay siege to our ability to cope with future biological disaster, from food deserts caused by the overuse of carcinogenic pesticide to the rentier capitalism of Big Pharma. He locates hostilities festering between two *humanities*: elites and professionals thriving under capitalism and poor subalterns and slum-dwellers working in the informal subsistence economy. The urban historian deems workers as the vanguard of struggles of tomorrow, suggesting that "in addressing the pandemic, socialists should find every occasion to remind others of the urgency of international solidarity."[58] Socialism promised to deliver that solidarity.

Socialism

From democratic socialism to market socialism, the power of socialist thought soared with COVID-19. In its all-of-society response to the pandemic, Spain nationalized all private hospitals and mobilized all its healthcare workers and military during its lockdown. The diminishing appeal and shell of a hollowed-out welfare system follows the "neoliberal virus" that infected so many industrialized nations. Winning a landslide with his National Regeneration Movement (Morena) and thumping the *Partido Revolucionario Institucional* (PRI) party, which ruled the country for a century, Mexico's center-left president Andrés Manuel López Obrador celebrated humans as social animals and gave Mexicans freedom to roam and self-monitor. At large rallies with throngs of supporters, the social democrat insisted to "live life as usual." Contending that poor people cannot practice physical distancing since 60% of Mexicans make money through the informal market, the populist president was shown kissing and hugging his legion of votaries, which irked journalists who deemed him irresponsible.

Not a fan of anything close to communism, El Salvador's president Nayib Bukele tweeted a message to Mexico's leader begging him to be more responsible: "In 20 days the epicenter of this pandemic will not be Europe, but North America. Stop looking at this as something normal, please, unless it too becomes the next epicenter of coronavirus."[59] After shutting travelers from Mexico, the former charged the latter for knowingly letting infected persons on airplanes, which caused El Salvador to shut down any flights. Bukele's emotive pleas glossed over his own questionable actions at home. His howling cry against Mexico's leader detracted from domestic efforts to stack the courts, setting up his reelection against the one-term limit set by the country's constitution, which then opened the path to his landslide reelection. The "world's coolest dictator passed a raft of new legislation that included restrictions on abortion and same-sex marriage. The conservative nationalist leader occupied El Salvador's Congress with a cadre of armed soldiers to force a session for controlling gangs and other marginalized groups as part of his "state of exception."[60] This executive show of force almost invoked a constitutional crisis, followed by comments from the media-savvy leader to remove security protection for lawmakers. The country's Catholic cardinal called on the world to help "save democracy."

In Mexico, protecting democracy proved to be tricky with a pandemic. In March 2020, President Obrador declared a State of Health Emergency in Mexico due to COVID-19. This proclamation made good on the left-leaning president's promise to protect workers and commoners as part of his election campaign. Nonessential businesses were ordered to shut down and government offices closed. Mexicans were recommended to stay indoors, putting the onus of responsibility on them as moral actors. The Mexican press took Obrador's words and actions to "live life as usual" out of context, emblazoning photographs of him holding up Catholic saints to stare down the novel coronavirus. Obrador's grand *personalismo* is partially attributed to the conservative fear borne out of redistributive taxes, cash assistance to the poor, and no corporate bailouts: socialist achievements which the media paved over in its laser focus on the man's celebrity status.[61] But despite the leader doubling the minimum wage and promising to respect freedoms of organized association, Obrador was still reticent to support the Matamoros strike in 2019 and its continuation of activism in the pandemic years on the behalf of *maquila* workers.

The political winds tilted toward "coronasocialism" to correct the course. For Latin American countries like Peru marked by endless scandals, a cleaning of house was in order. In Venezuela's "Worker's Paradise," the pandemic's purgatory affected poor workers, who had the highest out-of-pocket healthcare costs in all of Latin America. Marred by corruption and mismanagement, Venezuela's economy under socialist President Nicolas Maduro had been a mess before the pandemic. COVID-19 made the economy run amuck, but Maduro still won a new term in late 2020 in an election that did not meet international standards. Riding on an anti-corruption campaign, democratic socialist Xiomara Castro in 2021 became the first female president of Honduras and the first woman leader in Central America.

Meanwhile, Colombia elected its first leftist president, a former insurgent rebel who promised changes given the depletion of the liberal economic model under "epidemic-capitalism."[62] Another leftist "pink wave" washed over Brazil and Chile as the pandemic tipped the balance toward great equity and community ownership of the mode of production. In June 2021, Indigenous socialist schoolteacher and trade unionist Pedro Castillo defeated Keiko Fujimori to emerge as Peru's new president (only to be impeached). This result came after the dual shocks of the novel coronavirus and the deposition of President Martín Alberto Vizcarra Cornejo the year before. The erstwhile president had been banned from public office for a decade after jumping the line to grab a COVID-19 shot. This ban followed the unanimous vote of no confidence after Vizcarra also tried to dissolve the parliament for its investigations of corruption on the grounds of "moral incapacity." Peruvian democracy was stymied by a splintered congress with no single party holding a majority. A government for the people was needed after snap elections were called in June 2020. COVID-19 took a backseat in a polarized country with the highest per capita death rate in South America.

Stoking hopes for agrarian rights by peasant workers, socialism was the stuff of dreams in Bolivia, especially after the 2019 reelection of Indigenous president Evo Morales. After being charged with terrorism, rape, and sedition by the right-wing government, the socialist leader escaped to political exile in Mexico, returning only with the victory of his Movement Towards Socialism (MAS) in late 2020. Morales joined with agricultural workers and *cocalero* activists to build a socialist movement to circumvent newly elected president, Luis Arce. The new leader of the MAS party distanced himself from the forebearer to strike a more moderate tentative path.

A pandemic could not have come at more opportune time for those seeking social(ist) change. The U.S. House of Representatives impeached Trump in December 2019, as the SARS-CoV-2 began to take hold on the world. The disease tested the president's brand of absolutism, rattling the invincible force fields with which he repelled all charges thrown at him (such as collusion with foreign governments). His charge of communism and socialism against enemies fell flat at a time when social programs were badly needed. The outgoing president however jumped on the "socialist" free money bandwagon, demanding even higher stimulus checks to the chagrin of fellow Republicans. Coupled with cyberhacking by Russia, electoral manipulation in the form of voter suppression exposed the United States as an *unfree* democracy. In the chaos of a health emergency, many asked why lives were put at risk just to vote? What did democracy stand to lose from a president suing to block states from counting votes?

With voters donning masks and gloves, South Korea powered through national elections and pulled off its largest turnout in 30 years. Similar to stunning victories for leftists in countries long ruled by austerity like Finland, the Democratic Party of Korea reigned supreme with a landslide win. This hard-won victory was its biggest majority since 1987—a tell-tale sign of the public's approval of President Moon's response to COVID-19 and his "socialist" policies that included pro-environment laws, housing price controls, and stronger safety nets for the poor. The government's prioritization of wealth redistribution and serious hikes on minimum wages could not prevent the South Korean republic from remaining in the hands of conglomerations like Samsung, which the Moon administration asked to share its pandemic profits with other struggling smaller companies. The push for democratic socialism found success in local elections throughout France, where the movement's climate manifesto energized a pro-environment, pro-worker agenda to boost renewable energy and phase out coal use. Spasmodic concerns with COVID-19 drove a wrong turn back to old habits but also steered us toward new solutions.

During the U.S. Democratic presidential primary race, businessman Andrew Yang plugged his message of universal basic income (UBI). Such an ingenious initiative would be a boon to those workers on the edge of imminent layoffs or furloughs. With no cushion in savings to soften the blow of recession, the average worker without a certified floor of income teeters on the ledge of disaster. With the pandemic's drag on the economy, already-vulnerable workers hit rock bottom. In an attempted show of solidary with suffering people, Republic conservatives temporarily latched onto "lefty" solutions once pushed by progressives. These welfarist solutions demanded renter strikes, free student lunch programs, and mortgage cancellations. The moral hazards of "socialism" became absorbed by its enemies, in the short run, within the mental floss of reactionaries who long suppressed it.

When the pandemic threatened to make one-fifth of the U.S. labor force unemployed, the Treasury and Congress floated UBI proposals in the same amount of $1,000 that the Democratic presidential hopeful Andrew Yang had proposed. Where he once warned of robots taking jobs from blue-collar workers, Yang now recognized the overwhelming might of COVID-19 to change the nature of work. On Twitter, he admitted, "Apparently, I should have been talking about a pandemic instead of automation."[63]

The lofty goals of socialism are incomplete without ecology-in-action. In early April 2020, Spain when became the second hardest-hit country in the world, the socialist coalition government of Prime Minister Pedro Sanchez proposed a basic universal income for all its citizens, to make it unconditional and permanent. To short-circuit COVID-19 infection, the coastal resort town of Zahara de los Atunes sprayed bleach onto beaches with children at play, showing little care for the corrosiveness to health and disintegration of human and marine life. The successes in dealing with the novel coronavirus by "socialist-leaning" countries like Venezuela, Vietnam, Nicaragua, Cuba, and China proved too good to be true. Nicaragua's "Christian socialist" President Daniel Ortega jailed opposition figures ahead of his country's 2021 elections. As longtime head of the Sandinista National Liberation Front (FSLN), Ortega ruled with an iron fist. Even if the numbers released from Ortega's administration were to be believed, what was the point of living free of SARS-CoV-2 if it meant dealing with constant duress?

Critical fragilities laid bare by biothreats like COVID-19 exposed the dangers of not having universal health care and social protections. Not least of these concerns were basic rights for low-income girls and women who were most vulnerable to the pandemic. Into this breach stepped a disease pointing at governments for not ensuring basic social wage, child daycare, elderly care, free school lunches, and public utilities like water or Internet.

With the highest level of economic inequality and poverty in the industrialized world, the United States simply could not weather the storm of an out-of-control disease. Through central planks like universal health care, democratic socialists promised to close the wide gaps in feeble social systems in which trust has irrevocably collapsed. With social pressure points cracking under COVID-19, intersectional feminism was needed to address racism, classism, and sexism together. To develop a movement that protects all people and especially women of color, Chicana feminist Cherríe Moraga advocates not running away from a world on fire, but running toward it. She asserts, "The passage is *through*, not over, not by, not around, but through."[64]

The "cure" for a new disease resides in the latitude to tease out emergent contact zones made by COVID-19 as well as new border-making processes in what sociologist and gender studies scholar Victoria Reyes calls "global borderlands."[65]

But how does positive change happen for the common people, when the economy shifted into reverse? A mass transfer of wealth going to the top income earners and running through the pockets of the rich meant those folks living paycheck-to-paycheck lost out. Taking time off from work to care for children, millions of mothers suffered what had been called the *pandemic penalty* and left the workforce—the most massive single-time pullout of employed women in history. In this "she-cession," women of color and single parents without private babysitters were hardest hit. Stay-home orders spelled ruin for those workers reliant on their job for healthcare coverage, necessary to blunt the astronomical cost of long-term medical care due to corona-sickness. A "COVID consensus" in which we were all told simply to "follow the science" hid a global assault on democratic rights. Only an internationalist perspective on socialism could preserve life, many argued, protecting it from new modes of capitalist exploitation and control by the bourgeois state.[66]

The lack of subsidized childcare meant mothering was rarely factored in stimulus packages or policymaking. When COVID-19 government handouts were extended to everyone without question, this form of state welfare rubs up against the pathology long attributed to Black mothers as "welfare queens." With working mothers of color carrying the weight of the world once again, viral world-making becomes linked to the "lifeworlds of motherhood," which sometimes feels like a world unto itself. To redress this burden, activist-scholar Angela Davis suggests we need a feminist socialism based on "self-care and healing and attention to the body and the spiritual dimension."[67] Shifting the burden of childcare "from their shoulders to the society contains one of the radical secrets of women's liberation" and liberation of global society as a whole.[68]

The novel virus did not stop the bullet train of advocacy for workers' rights and financial renumeration. Long before financial struggles brought on by SARS-CoV-2, millions of workers could not afford emergency care or funds. But the long slog of fighting for fair wages and treatment of workers gained traction with millions quitting their jobs (in what some called the Great Resignation), as the lead-up to the pandemic propelled the workers' movement. It retooled labor demands to vent grievances against repressive market states exploiting a pandemic to stomp on collective bargaining rights. The bogeyman of socialism, triggered again by the viral demands of the largest union of nurses in the United States, demanded better treatment. Protestors used the aerial coronavirus as an opportunity to breathe life into old causes, beckoning a new pandemic ethics. Before COVID-19 cropped up, a rise in labor revolts stressed a postmortem diagnosis of capitalist greed as the common denominator, the main plight that ails us. A viral world mandated a new sociality and socialism that could bring working people together.

Pandemic socialism moves uneasily in the turnstile of multiparty politics. Democratic socialists like U.S. Senator Bernie Sanders and United Kingdom's Labor Party head Jeremy Corbyn fell short in capturing the mantle of leadership. Their political failures did not slow a grassroots movement vying to reshape global relations, according to socialist guiding norms based on workers' rights, anti-imperialism, and universal health care. As the first Indian state to report a COVID-19 case, Kerala summoned the spirit of Third World socialism to become a "beacon to the world." Kerala is a socialist-leaning state ruled by a coalition of parties with institutions that consider the betterment of people. Upon hearing about medical students returning from Wuhan (who were put into isolation quickly before infecting the community), the Left Democratic Front government set up call centers and tested the highest number of people in India as part of a bruising campaign to "Break the Chain."

Still smarting from the 2018 Nipah virus outbreak, which reappeared in 2021, the Marxist government of Kerala paid for the cost of hospitalizing quarantined patients. Instead of buying hand sanitizer from private companies, the Democratic Youth Federation of India made their own sanitizing materials, while the women's cooperative Kudumbashree produced masks for the public. Party leader Pinaraya Vijayan called for "physical distance, social unity." Local activists concluded,

> In a pandemic, a rational person would much rather live in a society governed by the norms of socialism than of capitalism, a society where people rally together to overcome a virus; than to live in a society where fear pervades and where stigmatization becomes the antidote to collective action.[69]

In the first Indian state to report a COVID-19 case, the health minister K.K. Shailaja, a former high school teacher dubbed "the coronavirus slayer," mobilized local self-government and on-the-ground activism to great success.[70] But with the COVID-19 Delta variant raging, Kerala by September 2021 grabbed headlines for the highest number of daily cases in India. Locals were crestfallen by the results despite their best efforts. But they still believed in socialist principles to protect them.

In countries like Sweden, public welfare appeared in a different guise. In this democratic socialist country, citizens ranked high on global happiness and standard of living barometers. Sweden took a light, no-lockdown approach to the novel coronavirus, relying on cultural norms of consensus and the public's high trust in its government. Even when the government banned gatherings with more than 50 people and recommended residents to limit travel, it left open daycare centers, gyms, bars, clubs, and restaurants. The wealthy market economy did not recommend quarantine of the infected, opening possibility of herd immunity, while its neighbors Denmark and Norway went under total lockdown. The Swedish stayed true to an honor system of voluntarism that raised eyebrows. As told in the U.S. media, this whatever-may-be-attitude meant not requiring self-isolation for returning travelers. Swede social customs supposedly include a virtuous circle of following rules and obeying good manners (*folkvett*) unlike the attention-seeking individualism of Americans.[71]

Heated words came from dedicated scientists blasting the government at every turn for its poor response to COVID-19 and by health employees dismissed from their jobs for wearing masks. The chief epidemiologist in the public health ministry of Sweden, Anders Tegnelld, doubted at first whether the novel coronavirus was air borne. The skeptical scientist found himself horrified by the same policies that he endorsed, such as suggesting that children could not get COVID-19 (universities and secondary schools were closed, but schools for primary children remained curiously open). Email exchanges obtained by journalists fleshed out this state objective.[72] With 90% of total COVID-19 deaths occurring in individuals over 70, Sweden's social experiment cast doubt on the state's protective abilities for elders. The pandemic's reality had not been lost on thousands of scholars who signed an open letter urging more precaution, after it was found migrants died twice the rate of citizens in the epicenter of Stockholm. Suppositions that wealthy social democratic nations could not be squeezed by COVID-19 was resoundingly wrong. Sweden was that example. When the country registered the most deaths per capita in Europe, twice the mortality rate of the United States, and seven times its neighbors—it was tempting to modify the classic line from *Hamlet* to declare there was something rotten in Sweden.

This rot struck the nation's core mightily. It punctured the shimmering veneer of Sweden's well-planned market economies. After doing little to dispel danger, the Scandinavian country finally imposed mandatory closures and restrictions of public gatherings before year's end. This welfarist market economy, much adored by outsiders, found its Achilles heel. "Everyone's a Socialist in a Pandemic," screamed a *Chicago Tribune* headline. Joking that "we're turning into Denmark," journalist Farhad Manjoo recounts how SARS-CoV-2 obliged U.S. companies like Uber to finally provide sick paid leave and compensatory benefits to its "gig" drivers (considered independent "contractors").[73] A lifesaver was thrown to workers abandoned on the shoals of the pandemic "post-work" economy. A silver lining was the thought of the United States turning into a "Scandinavian Edens." Given its faults, Sweden made obvious that a strong social safety was not enough to fend off the disease of capitalism. The article ends with a reality check: "We're nowhere near turning into Denmark," since corona-plans of relief are ephemeral, as Republicans only tolerate Medicare-for-All temporarily for only this disease. Pandemic rules for not kicking people off Medicaid expired once the health crisis ends.

Pandemic socialism or panic socialism was no laughing matter, since the costs of saving already troubled societies dealt the heaviest blow to citizens and workers on the lower rungs. Epidemiologist Rob Wallace contends that scientists only play the game of catch-up when it comes to new diseases, cleaning up the mess of science made by their corporate funders and sponsors. Health organizations took great pains to root out the causes of new pathogens. Yet, their heroic efforts continue to confront the dangerous circuits of capitalism responsible for spawning deadly germs like SARS-CoV-2. A frenetic rush to temper the advance of new diseases allows little room to unpack corporatizing influences in the medical field and beyond. When cooks, nurses, janitors, and teachers cannot work due to health hazards like COVID-19, what else remains to save them? Perhaps eco-socialism.

In some respects, the multi-scalar dynamics of COVID-19 prevention offset the ruthless wars and internal squabbles among groups to show "threads that may bind many places, peoples, and times together, though never evenly, and in a place specific way."[74] Within the narrow frame of pandemic individualism, infected societies might try to discipline viral pathogens, but "the little buggers routinely violate protocol."[75] The choice is clear, as indicated by Wallace, "If we must partake in the Great Game," let us choose eco-socialism and "international solidarity with everyday people the world over."[76] Like a supernatural creature from a fairy tale, socialist collectivism shaped up to be that beast, which could not be slayed—for it represented hopes rising up from the ether to present an alternative vision of humanity in a viral world.

Critics of corono-capitalism suggest we all wake up to the inviolable truth, coming to grips with a viral world together by Indigenous liberation, farmer autonomy, and strategic rewilding. Success is not possible if solely glued to the zoological tracking of future disease within agroecological systems. It remains fruitless within the larger evolution of pathogens, because a man-made crisis requires human solutions related to socialism, service, and solidarity. Diseases like COVID-19 will always work on their own time, worlding the planet virally, while humankind if they ignore those threats seems on schedule for an apocalyptic-level disaster.

Notes

1 Heather Gies and John Washington, "'Maybe If I Had Papers, It Would Have Been Different': Undocumented during a Pandemic," *The Nation*, March 25, 2020, www.thenation.com/ article/politics /undocumented-coronavirus/

2 Stevie Ruiz, "Contesting Legal Borderlands: Policing Insubordinate Spaces in Imperial County's Farm Worker Communities, 1933–1940," *Kalfou* 7, no. 2 (2020): 352–372.

3 Glenda M. Flores, "Latina Physicians as 'Essential' Workers," *Contexts* 19, no. 4 (2020): 62–64.

4 David Bacon, "America's Farmworkers—Now 'Essential,' but Denied the Just-Enacted Benefits," *The American Prospect*, April 1, 2020, https://prospect.org/coronavirus/american-farmworkers-essential-but-unprotected/

5 Shaun Ossei-Owusu, "Coronavirus and the Politics of Disposability," *Boston Review*, April 8, 2020, http://bostonreview.net/class-inequality-race-politics/shaun-ossei-owusu-coronavirus-and-the-politics-disposability

6 Jorge Valencia, "'Die, Bacteria, Die': Mexican Nurses Croon in Hand-Washing PSA Video," *PRI*, March 6, 2020, www.pri.org/stories/2020-03-06/die-bacteria-die-mexican-nurses-croon-hand-washing-psa-video

7 Purnima Mankekar and Akhil Gupta, "Future Tense," 78.

8 Salvador Zarate, "Migrant Labor and A Life Under Fire: A Triptych," *Foundry*, June 2021, https://uchri.org/foundry/migrant-labor-and-a-life-under-fire-a-triptych/

9 D. Alex Piña, D. "White Supremacy in Rainbow: Global Pride and Black Lives Matter in the Era of COVID." *New Sociology: Journal of Critical Praxis* 3, no. 1 (2022): 136–146.

10 Alanna Vagianos, "Legal Sex Workers and Others in Adult Industry Denied Coronavirus Aid," *Huffpost*, April 2, 2020, www.huffpost.com/entry/legal-sex-workers-denied-coronavirus-aid_n_5e86287ac5b6d302366ca912

11 That same church in a 2019 memo called gender non-binary identity as a "confused" concept. Matt Baume, "Pope Francis Sends Money to Struggling Trans Sex Workers in Italy," *them*, May 1, 2020, www.them.us/story/pope-francis-makes-emergency-gift-to-trans-sex-workers-in-italy

12 Julia Conley, "'The Strike Wave Is in Full Swing': Amazon, Whole Foods Workers Walk Off Job to Protest Unjust and Unsafe Labor Practices," *Common Dreams*, March 30, 2020, www.commondreams.org/news/2020/03/30/strike-wave-full-swing-amazon-whole-foods-workers-walk-job-protest-unjust-and-unsafe

13 Claire Kelloway, "Food Workers Are on the Frontlines of Coronavirus. They Need Our Support," *Civil Eats*, March 20, 2020, https://civileats.com/2020/03/20/op-ed-food-workers-are-on-the-frontlines-of-coronavirus-they-need-our-support/amp/

14 Lisa Sun-Hee Park, *Entitled to Nothing* (New York: New York University Press, 2011).

15 David Bacon, "America's Farmworkers—Now 'Essential,' but Denied the Just-Enacted Benefits," *The Prospect*, April 1, 2020, https://prospect.org/coronavirus/american-farmworkers-essential-but-unprotected/.

16 The term was devised by Dubois a century earlier, who connected the global exploitation of "colored labor" to a colonial "world of shadows," finding that the problems of the modern world are ones inherited by the darker races.

William Edward Burghardt DuBois, "Worlds of Color," *Foreign Affairs* 3, no. 3 (1925): 423–444.

17 Sam Biddle, "Facebook Contractors Must Work in Offices during Coronavirus Pandemic—while Staff Stay Home," *The Intercept*, March 12, 2020, https://theintercept.com/2020/03/12/coronavirus-facebook-contractors/

18 Prodita Sabarini, "Coronavirus: Migrants in Frontline Jobs Not Entitled to Any Financial Help If They Get Sick," *The Conversation*, April 2, 2020, https://theconversation.com/coronavirus-migrants-in-frontline-jobs-not-entitled-to-any-financial-help-if-they-get-sick-134970

19 Ilgin Karlidag, "Turkey Feeds Stray Animals during Covid-19 Outbreak," *BBC*, April 7, 2020, www.bbc.com/news/blogs-news-from-elsewhere-52199691

20 Audre Lorde, *A Burst of Light: And Other Essays* (Mineola: Courier Dover Publications, 2017), 130.

21 Audre Lorde, "A Litany for Survival," in *A Litany for Survival: The Life and Work of Audre Lorde*, dir. Ada G. Griffin and Michelle Parkerson (New York: Third World Newsreel, 1996).

22 Jeet Heer, "Meatpacking Plants Are a Front in the Covid-19 Class War," *The Nation*, April 29, 2020, www.thenation.com/article/politics/meatpacking-coronavirus-class-war/

23 Makenzie Huber, "'Essential Worker Just Means You're on The Death Track': John Deranamie Is a 50-Year-Old Liberian Man Whose Dream Led Him to a Meatpacking Plant in South Dakota. He Contracted COVID-19 as Part of His Job," *USA Today*, May 5, 2020, www.usatoday.com/in-depth/news/2020/05/04/meat-packing-essential-worker-hogs-south-dakota-smithfield-food-chain-covid-19-coronavirus-inside/3064329001/; JCB, "Pinay Nurse in California Shares Struggles in Battling COVID-19: 'We Are the Guinea Pigs,'" *GMA News*, May 2, 2020, www.gmanetwork.com /news/lifestyle/content/736543/pinay-nurse-in-california-shares-struggles-in-battling-covid-19-we-are-the-guinea-pigs/story/; Oliver Laughland and Amanda Holpuch, "'We're Modern Slaves': How Meat Plant Workers Became the New Frontline in Covid-19 War," *The Guardian*, May 2, 2020, www.theguardian.com/world/2020/may/02/meat-plant-workers-us-coronavirus-war

24 Eric Levitz, "Meatpacking Crisis Shows Limits of Human Sacrifice as Recovery Plan," *New York Magazine*, May 6, 2020, https://nymag.com/intelligencer/2020/05/coronavirus-meat-packing-plants-trump-reopen-economy-workers.html

25 Nour Dados and Lucy Taksa, "Pandemic's Economic Blow Hits Women Hard," *The Lighthouse*, April 14, 2020, https://lighthouse.mq.edu.au/article/april-2020/Pandemics-economic-blow-hits-women-hard

26 Alvin K. Wong, "Thinking Hong Kong's Freedom in Multiplicity," *Hong Kong Protesting*, September 21, 2019, https://hkprotesting.com/2020/07/16/multiplicity/

27 Mia Alberti and Vasco Cotovio, "Portugal Gives Migrants and Asylum-Seekers Full Citizenship Rights during Coronavirus Outbreak," *CNN*, March 30, 2020, www.cnn.com/2020/03/30/europe/portugal-migrants-citizenship-rights-coronavirus-intl/index.html

28 Sabrina Gunter, "Under Trump, Undocumented Immigrants with COVID-19 Are Being Denied Care," *In These Times*, April 6, 2020, http://inthesetimes.com/article/22434/trump-undocumented-immigrants-covid-19-coronavirus

29 Lisa Lowe, "Afterword," in *Revolutionary Feminisms: Conversations on Collective Action and Radical Thought*, eds. Brenna Bhandar and Rafeef Ziadah (New York: Verso, 2020), 217–227, 210.

30 Gasviani, Gvantsa. "Inner Martyrdom: Deconstructing the Sacrificial Female Subject in Post-Soviet Georgia," *Journal of Feminist Scholarship* 20, no. 20 (2022): 19–32.

31 Vera Rubin, Facebook post, April 24, 2023, www.facebook.com/FleshPrisonBr eak/timeline?lst=1171484871%3A575001312%3A1589154462

32 Edward Nadurata, "Who Cares?: Ability and the Elderly Question in Filipinx Studies," in *Filipinx American Critique: An Interdisciplinary Reckoning*, eds. Rick Bonus and Antonio Tiongson (New York: Fordham University Press, 2022), 349.

33 Woodly D., Brown R.H., Marin M., Threadcraft S., Harris C.P., Syedullah J., and Ticktin M. "The Politics of Care," *Contemporary Political Theory*, August 24, 2021, https://doi.org/10.1057/s41296-021-00515-8

34 Abromaviciute Jurgita and Emily K. Carian. "The COVID-19 Pandemic and the Gender Gap in Newly Created Domains of Household Labor," *Sociological Perspectives* (2022): 07311214221103268.

35 Rose Boswell, "If Men Want to Be Heroes, They Should Do the Dirty Work," *Corona Times*, April 2, 2020, www.coronatimes.net/if-men-want-to-be-heroes-they-should-do-the-dirty-work/

36 Saskia Sassen, "Global Cities and Survival Circuits," in *Woman: Nannies, Maids, and Sex Workers in the New Economy*, eds. Saskia Sassen, Barbara Ehrenreich, and Arlie Russell Hochschild (New York: Metropolitan, 2002), 254–274.

37 Hong Mai-Linh K., ed. *The Auntie Sewing Squad Guide to Mask Making, Radical Care, and Racial Justice* (Berkeley: University of California Press, 2021).

38 Robin Kelley, "From the River to the Sea to Every Mountain Top: Solidarity as Worldmaking," *Journal of Palestine Studies* 48, no. 4 (2019): 85.

39 Bernard Marr, "Robots and Drones Are Now Used to Fight COVID-19," *Forbes*, March 18, 2020, www.forbes.com/sites/bernardmarr/2020/03/18/how-robots-and-drones-are-helping-to-fight-coronavirus/#799a5c212a12

40 Alyssa Newcomb, "173 years, $170: Why Irish People Are Donating to Help Native Americans Hit by Coronavirus," *NBC News*, May 6, 2020, www.nbcn ews.com/news/us-news/173-years-170-why-irish-people-are-donating-help-nat ive-n1200811

41 Jessie Tu, "Taiwan's First Female President Is Delivering a Stunning COVID-19 Response," *Women's Agenda*, April 3, 2020, https://womensagenda.com. au/latest/taiwans-first-female-president-is-delivering-a-stunning-covid-19-response/

42 Nicola Smith, "Taiwan Builds 'Nerd Immunity' to Resist Chinese Disinformation Campaigns," *The Telegraph*, June 13, 2020, www.telegraph.co.uk/news/ 2020/06/13/taiwan-builds-nerd-immunity-resist-chinese-disinformation-campaigns/

43 Katherine Schultz and Russell Hsiao, "Why Taiwan's Coronavirus Response Shows Europe It Should Join the World Health Organization," *The National Interest*, March 31, 2020, https://nationalinterest.org/feature/why-taiw ans-coronavirus-response-shows-europe-it-should-join-world-health-organization

44 Despite being the Asian country to legalize same-sex marriage in 2019, Taiwan's liberal government suppressed the self-determination of Taiwan's Aborigines, triggering protestation against President Tsai Ing-wen.

45 Stefan Elbe and Nadine Voelkner," Viral Sovereignty: The Downside Risk of Securitizing Infectious Disease," in *The Handbook of Global Health Policy*, eds. Garret Wallace Brown, Gavin Yamey, and Sarah Wamala (Hoboken, NJ: Wiley-Blackwell, 2014), n.p.

46 Bill Chappell, " 'We Alerted the World' to Coronavirus on Jan. 5, WHO Says in Response to U.S.," *NPR*, April 15, 2020, www.npr.org/sections/goatsandsoda/2020/04/15/835179442/we-alerted-the-world-to-coronavirus-on-jan-5-who-says-in-response-to-u-s

47 BBC Africa, "Africa Live: African Leaders Back WHO Head against Trump Attacks," *BBC Africa*, April 8, 2020, www.bbc.com/news/live/world-africa-47639452

48 Josep Borell, "The Coronavirus Pandemic and the New World It Is Creating," *European External Action Service*, March 23, 2020, https://eeas.europa.eu/headq uarters/headquarters-homepage/76379/coronavirus-pandemic-and-new-world-it-creating_en

49 Nelson Acosta, "Cuban Doctors Head to Italy to Battle Coronavirus," *Reuters*, March 21, 2020, www.reuters.com/article/us-health-coronavirus-cuba/cuban-doctors-head-to-italy-battle-coronavirus-idUSKBN219051

50 Sarah Marsh, "Cuba Credits Two Drugs with Slashing Coronavirus Death Toll," *Reuters*, May 22, 2020, www.reuters.com/ article/us-health-coronavirus-cuba/cuba-credits-two-drugs-with-slashing-coronavirus-death-toll-idUSKBN22Y2Y4?feedType=mktg&feedName=healthNews&WT.mc_id=Partner-Google&fbclid=IwAR34b9eelnNjXTIFTsSPv9hwzqpBkotwZzNtu4l9A D2AVfHtwlcgzU86lkc

51 Helen Yaffe, "Cuba's Contribution to Combating Covid-19," *URPE: Union for Radical Political Economics*, March 20, 2020, https://urpe.org/2020/03/20/cubas-contribution-to-combating-covid-19/

52 Russia W.T. Whitney Jr., "Cuba Develops COVID-19 Vaccines, Takes Socialist Approach." *People's World*, February 4, 2021, www.peoplesworld.org/article/cuba-develops-covid-19-vaccines-takes-socialist-approach/#:~:text=Cuba's%20socialist%20approach%20to%20developing,Cubans%2C%20and%20in%20international%20solidarity

53 Steve Sweeney, "US Blocks Sale of Ventilators to Cuba after Acquiring Medical Companies," *Morning Star*, April 14, 2020, https://morningstaronline.co.uk/arti cle/w/us-blocks-sale-ventilators-cuba-after-acquiring-medical-companies

54 Jorge Duenes, "Mexico Closes U.S.-Owned Plant for Alleged Refusal to Sell Ventilators to Mexican Hospitals," *The Globe and Mail*, April 10, 2020, www.theglobeandmail.com/world/article-mexico-closes-us-owned-plant-for-alleged-refusal-to-sell-ventilators/

55 Eric London, "Hundreds of Mexican Maquiladora Workers Dying after Back-to-Work Orders Take Effect," *World Socialist Website*, May 19, 2020, www.wsws.org/en/articles/2020/05/19/mexi-m19.html

56 Silvia Amaro, "Italy's Death Toll Surpasses 10,000 as Prime Minister Warns of Rising 'Nationalist Instincts,'" *CNBC*, March 30, 2020, www.cnbc.com/2020/03/30/italy-coronavirus-deaths-above-10000-conte-warns-against-anti-eu-sentim ent.html

57 La Izquierda Diario Argentina, "Italy Calls General Strike: 'Our Lives Are Worth More than Your Profits,'" *Left Voice*, March 25, 2020, www.leftvoice.org/italy-calls-general-strike-our-lives-are-worth-more-than-your-profits

58 Mike Davis, "The Coronavirus Crisis Is a Monster Fueled by Capitalism," *In These Times*, March 20, 2020, http://inthesetimes.com/article/22394/coronavirus-crisis-capitalism-covid-19-monster-mike-davis.

59 David Agren, "Coronavirus Advice from Mexico's President: 'Live Life as Usual,'" *The Guardian*, March 25, 2020, www.theguardian.com/world/2020/mar/25/coronavirus-advice-from-mexicos-president-live-life-as-usual

60 Katherine Funes, "El Salvador's State of Exception Turns One," *NACLA*, March 27, 2023, https://nacla.org/el-salvadors-state-exception-turns-one.

61 Edwin F. Ackerman, "The Mainstream Media versus Andrés Manuel López Obrador," *Jacobin*, March 31, 2020, https://jacobinmag.com/2020/03/amlo-coronavirus-mexico-covid-19-response

62 José Tenorio, Manuel Romero, and William Andres Alvarez, "La Máquina de Guerra Nómada del COVID-19: Paisajes Estéticos del Epidemiocapitalismo," *Trans/Form/Ação* 44 (2021): 267–284.

63 Andrew Yang (@Andrew Yang), "Apparently I Should Have Been Talking about a Pandemic instead of Automation," *Twitter*, March 12, 2020, 6:30 am, https://twitter.com/AndrewYang/status/1238095725721944065?lang=ar

64 Cherrie Moraga. "Preface," in *This Bridge Called My Back: Writings by Radical Women of Color*, eds. Gloría, Anzaldúa and Toni Cade Bambara (Watertown, MA: Persephone Press, 1981), xiv.

65 Victoria Reyes, *Global Borderlands: Fantasy, Violence, and Empire in Subic Bay, Philippines* (Stanford, CA: Stanford University Press).

66 Green, Toby and Thomas Fazi, *The Covid Consensus: The Global Assault on Democracy and the Poor? A Critique from the Left* (Oxford: Oxford University Press, 2023).

67 Quoted in Magdalena Górska, *Breathing Matters: Feminist Intersectional Politics of Vulnerability* (Linköping: Linköping University 2016), 298.

68 Angela Y. Davis, *Women, Race, & Class* (New York: Vintage, 2011), 232.

69 Vijay Prashad and Subin Dennis, "An Often Overlooked Region of India Is a Beacon to the World for Taking on the Coronavirus," *People's Dispatch*, March 24, 2020, https://peoplesdispatch.org /2020/03/24/an-often-overlooked-region-of-india-is-a-beacon-to-the-world-for-taking-on-the-coronavirus/

70 David Jenkins and Lipin Ram, "Kerala's Pandemic Response Owes Its Success to Participatory Politics," *Novara Media*, August 7, 2020, https://novaramedia.com/2020/08/07/keralas-pandemic-response-owes-its-success-to-participatory-politics/

71 Hilary Brueck, "Sweden's Gamble on Coronavirus Herd Immunity Couldn't Work in the US—and It May Not Work in Sweden," *Business Insider*, May 2, 2020, www.businessinsider.com/sweden-coronavirus-strategy-explained-culture-of-trust-and-obedience-2020-4

72 Jon Henley, "Sweden's Covid-19 Strategist under Fire Over Herd Immunity Emails," *The Guardian*, August 17, 2020, www.theguardian.com/world/2020/aug/17/swedens-covid-19-strategist-under-fire-over-herd-immunity-emails

73 Farhad Manjoo, "Republicans Want Medicare for All, but Just for This One Disease: Everyone's a Socialist in a Pandemic," *New York Times*, March 11, 2020, www.nytimes.com/2020/03/11/opinion/coronavirus-socialism.html

74 Rob Wallace, *Big Farms Make Big Flu: Dispatches on Influenza, Agribusiness, and the Nature of Science* (New York: New York University Press, 2016), 106.

75 Ibid., 91.

76 Rob Wallace, "Notes on a Novel Coronavirus," New York University Press, March 24, 2020 www.fromthesquare.org/notes-on-a-novel-coronavirus/#.Xn2L BKhKhPY

6

CORONAPOCALYPSE

Monster, Mystic, Machine

COVID-19 brought no shortage of prognostications in what doomwatchers called the "coronavirus apocalypse" or "coronapocalypse." An unfolding pandemic broke the spell of human innocence, waking many billions to new horrors like anti-vaccination disinformation. As something of this world but appearing outside of it, this soul-shattering event soon became steeped in *pandemic fictions* that attained the status of "real." Bringing the question of what is "viral" or virality to bear upon the pandemic conversation, spooked humans clung to conspiratorial ideas as their saving grace until everything tipped over. To regular doom-and-gloom mongers, SARS-CoV-2 consecrated the belief that the human species arrived at the point of no return. The path of this death star became patently clear when locally situated global events had spun into a matted viral thread. They remarked upon the frightening sense that *sapiens* had reached a precipice at the proverbial cliff.

Forthright commentators announced humanity's total obsolescence, suggesting the fact that we could not come together to address a singular threat meant the enemy had already won. This virus was to be our winter's tale, they said, the ignominious end to our kind. COVID-skeptics found the entirety a total hoax, abstaining from wearing masks, some taking such wishful thinking into their graves while intubated. Those residents forced to stay at home indefinitely considered it a kind of morbid "entombment." Despite compulsions of finality in the "coronageddon," critical thinkers attuned to the ghostly vestiges of colonialism, racism, and sexism observed something else. These *pandemic specters* pointed to the encrusted features of societies haunted by history's phantoms.

To posit the pandemic posed a sign of the apocalypse seemed somewhat appropriate, given that the modern world was in dire straits. The novel

DOI: 10.4324/9781032694535-7

coronavirus did more than infect bodies in motion; it seared itself into a collective soul worn weary by the battering ram of super-capitalism. The festering open wound of COVID-19 conjured the memory of Antonio Gramsci. The imprisoned Marxist political activist conveyed this famous message against fascism in its ascendancy in the 1930s: "The old world is dying, and the new extraneous struggles to be born: now is the time of monsters." Monsters are signs of an impending apocalypse, and the struggle and will to survive.

The word apocalypse mostly refers to any cataclysmic event.[1] It has been formative in the Christian myth-story in which God struck down all evildoers on *terra firma* and carries all believers to the heavenly kingdom. From something that portrays the end of humankind emanates "planetary dread" about "generalizable, globally distributed forces ranging from weaponized destruction to viral technological displacement … the dread of a future 'overrun' by those taken to be 'not-us.'"[2] With hope for a global solution vaporizing into the horror show of a coronapocalypse, a vulgar (and viral) sense of apocalypticism began to take root. "Coronavirus is the old movie that we've been watching over and over again," historian Mike Davis indicates, and despite all the news about outbreaks, nothing substantial happens, "so Corona walks through the front door as a familiar monster."[3]

Ghoulish figures haunted the COVID-19 horror story and its stupefying plot twists. U.S. Secretary of state Mike Pompeo branded China an insatiable Frankenstein that needed to be reined in.[4] Interestingly, the foreign minister of Venezuela called Pompeo a "zombie" after he flagged electoral fraud in the country. Maduro's government responded to U.S. interference, suggesting the failed Trump administration was a corpse "dying to struggle."[5] The doctrine of market fundamentalism collided with religious fundamentalism to produce a hellish situation chockablock with monsters. A self-coordinating market and economy is based on humans acting as self-interested rational beings. A multitude of people refused to believe in the science behind vaccines.

Another horror took place with infected livestock. In service to scant "demand" by consumers, slaughterhouses "euthanized" and "depopulated" thousands of hogs and chickens—meaning they were smothered, suffocated, gassed, shot, drowned, and drugged. In this super-sized die-off, farm animals were brutally "destroyed" and laid to "waste," their deaths not registered in the logs of coronavirus-related mortalities. Nor did the 17 million minks "culled" after public officials caught wind that SARS-CoV-2 mutated in Spain and Denmark. New "mink strains" were found on farms in Canada, England, and the United States. Minks were reported to "rise from the dead" like zombies from their shallow graves.[6] The "apocalyptic" sighting of dead sea creatures and the carcasses of beached whales, from the Amazon to Australia, presented a foul gift offering from the devil for the most doctrinaire of "satanic" worshippers. But as "sound" regulatory systems went bust, and absurdity became the norm, preposterous ideas outgrew any logic.

The honorific of frontline workers as superheroes fell into a political trap, as China's state propaganda toted out the story of sacrifice about one nurse who returned to work only days after her abortion, and another stayed to treat COVID-19 patients while being pregnant. In a hyper-capitalist "post-socialist" country that eats its young, consumes feminine labor, and tires out its workers—what is the vampiric effect of "laboring by, for, or with others … [and] are we, sitting at home, ready to labor for our collective life?"[7]

Adding to the ghastly tenor of pandemic work were manifestations of vampiric capitalism.[8] Blood-sucking capitalism could make little amends with its workers as "dead capital" or the "living dead." Incentive structures of capitalism drive narcissistic behaviors exhibited in the early months of lockdown hell. Modern cultures of self-promotion put all social risk onto the individual, thus protective collective solidarity becomes "at best, eccentric and unreal, and at worst, reprehensible and probably anti-democratic."[9] Zombies are communitarian figures that refigure human bonds through more-than-human or "posthuman" relations. Such relations emerge in otherworldly forms, as when Kepuh village in the Java state of Indonesia deployed human volunteers to dress up as pocong. They donned white shrouds and drew on folklore about goblins to deter the superstitious from the street by conjuring the dead. Taming COVID-19 would require more than ghosts in a country with the highest coronavirus death rate in Asia after China. When countries are too busy wrestling with their own social demons, how do they wage battle and find the magic "silver bullet" to pierce the novel coronavirus?

This chapter confronts the pandemic's monsters and other well-known figures of the post-apocalyptic genre—mystics and machines. It comments on the "folk" beliefs that gained prominence during the pandemic, broaching the ghostly specters of a "coronapocalypse." Speaking to the "undead" representation of people of color, queers, workers, and others in the media, my analysis attends to paranoid fantasies and conspiracy theories about COVID-19. Pandemic culture revealed the social anxieties and viral forms of demonization that colluded to produce new epidemic imaginaries and witch hunts of the contagious Other. Here, the viral world appears as a single body with innumerable terrorist/terrorizing bodies that need to be recolonized and killed.[10] The chapter provides examples where the holy war against COVID-19 became a moral crusade against difference and otherness. After the video of George Floyd's murder by police went viral, the abiding sense that Black people are "socially dead" paralleled the false perception of them as superhumans who could not contract by SARS-CoV-2. The real "monster" turns out to be the political system, which perpetuates the boogeyman of race. In terms of mystics and machines, the chapter presents the oracles and military powers that added influence in an uncertain time. Their viral words of praise or promise of salvation unleashed intolerance and military excess.

Monster

In the wreckage left behind by the pandemic, a strange apparition appears to reveal the shadows of society. So-called "zombie fires" burned throughout nonregular burning seasons to choke off air in the northern Pacific. A frightful ghost world appears when one-fifth of the planet's human inhabitants are placed under domestic confinement. Humans were now chthonic denizens in their own underworlds like vampires. Seemingly overnight, metropolitan cities like London, Los Angeles, New York, and Paris—long suffering from congestion and traffic—turned into desolate ghost cities. Lightened without the torrential strain of tourists and commuters, these now semideserted municipalities bespeak the sublime feeling of seeing almost no one in places once teeming with people.

Reduced to hollow shells of their former selves, these barren "ghost cities" provided glimpses into a would-be future when human civilization ceases to exist. The penchant for canvassing Global North "ghost towns" for apocalyptic signs paints a distorted social tableau, since the Gaza Strip, Beirut, Nairobi, Lagos, Bangkok, Manila, Rio de Janeiro, and Saigon enacted some policy of quarantine to varying degrees and successes. In the harried cities of the equatorial south, one must still venture outside to noisy street markets to shop for fresh food and find other necessities. Urban cities were shockingly drained of pedestrians and commuters like apocalyptic wastelands.

A human-induced pandemic turned into a monster's ball. With commercial aircraft carriers idled, the sight of all but empty "ghost planes" carrying hardly any passengers looked like an episode of *The Twilight Zone*. Though not carrying any customer, these planes were required to fly and dump tons of jet fuel only to keep airport terminal spots. This absurd and wasteful practice points to a pathological commitment to economic priorities and stockholders amidst potential to reboot everything. "Ghost ships" like luxurious Holland America Lin's Rotterdam were unauthorized to return home due to travel restrictions by countries. The ships floated around the Caribbean, unable to dock, their passengers left for dead. Protection of customers fell by the wayside as they became vectors of disease. Whole countries turned into hellscapes or cesspools, as when *The West Australian* reported the number of Aussies stranded abroad in India and recommended the Australian government to "Ban Trips from Indian Hell."[11] But for millions of Indians living in the bowels of this so-called "hell," they found no form of respite from the constant witch hunt for corona-monsters.

Given its sheer immensity, social media users resorted to calling the pandemic a zombie apocalypse. The term captures what appeared to be an extinction level event, where survivors take on the guise of reanimated corpses. "It's like someone dropped a bomb in the middle of the city. It looks like a zombie apocalypse," commented a resident of Daegu, after the South Korean city's population went into hiding to avoid the path of COVID-19.[12] An American writer locked in the home mused, "It is zombie time: the virus can't be transmitted when all of its hosts have died. So we are all social-distancing; that is, pretending to have died, lying very still, so the virus ... won't get us."[13] China's Beijing government deployed the zombie metaphor to claim social unrest, like the kind in Hong Kong, could be "contagious" and the Communist Youth League website compared it to a "zombie virus" delivering political ruckus to a vulnerable, infectious society.[14]

This zombie typology sums up fears about the end of the world and undead creatures, skulking about the streets as reanimated beings. Almost all contemporary zombie stories hold something in common: they share similar stories of contagious viruses that prey upon humans, precipitating the moment when the world made by humans comes undone. The undead turn into viral "superspreaders," aching to inhabit and infect humans by rabidly biting them to inject infected fluid into the victim's bloodstream.

A being of unclear origin, COVID-19 appears much like the zombie. It occupies the ambiguous border between the living and nonliving. Looking like an alien vessel, this parasitic thing needs host bodies, feeding on others until it or the host dies off. Zombies depict our palpable fears of grotesquerie in a late capitalist era denying workers a "living wage." They are a petrifying reminder of the unseen monster lurking at the door and the monster residing within ourselves. Once dead and resurrected, the zombie returns to kill without thinking with the central aim of feeding and producing more of "them" who happen to formerly be "us."

No one could easily escape the pall of COVID-19 and its "coronazombies." Stuck in the weird dream state of "corona-somnia," stressed-out students and world-weary workers lumbered through the grind of daily life not knowing when they would either wake up, sleep, or rest. We needed to find new ways of living (and dying) together. This out-of-body experience came in the form of a shapeless void of (endless) quarantine. Some faced a hard time figuring out who was the sinister monster: capitalism or coronavirus? An accrual of viral meanings accompanies pandemic zombie-ism, particularly when certain communities are marked as "socially dead."[15] Within unequitable global relations upon which a virus feeds, zombie mythology speaks to the morbid condition of people rendered as inhuman.[16]

Nothing then is ever "natural" when it comes to racism or pandemics. They are the sum of everything wrong within the viral world. The pandemic exaggerated and extended what came before. Structural racism ensured a quick fast death as well as "slow violence" for the poor.[17] It arrived swiftly as in cities like Louisiana or Chicago, where 70% of early mortalities attributable to COVID-19 were related to Black people, even though they make up a third of the population. Fast death hit 25-year-old Ahmaud Arbery, a Black jogger slain by a White ex-cop and his son in open daylight. His killers were not arrested by police until national protests rose up two months later after a clip was posted online of what many called a modern-day lynching. A Facebook group called Christians against Google with close to 80,000 members attempted to humanize the murderers by calling them "god fearing men," while painting the unarmed victim as a monster scaring White suburbia. Counterposed to post-lockdown videos of people exercising outdoors, the video of a Black man's life cut down ignited another lightning rod for an indefatigable Black Lives Matter (BLM) movement.

There came the untimely death of emergency medical technician Breonna Taylor from a hail of bullets at her home from a botched drug raid by plainclothes police holding a "no-knock" warrant. Part of the normalization of violence against Black women and "sacrificing" of essential workers, her murder added another moniker to the viral media campaign #SayHerName. Police in Tennessee shot dead a transgender masculine-presenting person named Tony McDade, while Iyanna Dior was beaten and graphically videotaped by a group of cisgender men in the same city as George Floyd died—an incident that reiterated the stance that "Black Trans Lives Matter." In spite of Black bodies under constant siege, geographer Katherine McKittrick resists the need to try to count Black deaths.[18] She indicates that we must center Black humanity and well-being. The work of reinvigorating "living blackness" was needed more than ever.[19]

Coronavirus was hardly the only thing floating around; revolution was also in the air. As Black gender historian Saidya Hartman suggests, perhaps we can consider the end of the world as a "sonorous echo of earth released from the order of men ... [a] new state of relation inaugurated by the apocalypse, a state in which Blackness is no longer relegated to nothing and death."[20] For philosopher Denise Ferreira da Silva, the global regime always already marks a "horizon of death" for people of color, but Black thought and politics offer a way out of the order of things.[21] With the end of the world and Man comes "other possible ways of knowing and doing ... without the charge of irrationality, mysticism, or idle fantasy."[22] This infinite recomposition of global relations and relationality is what I have been calling a viral world.

There is little need to employ the zombie as racial fantasy metaphor when living death is the cultural patrimony that one inherits as a woman of color. As scholar-writer Roxane Gay explains, "As a Black woman in America, I do not feel alive. I feel like I am not dead yet."[23] Slavery and its afterlives pull oppressed people back and forward in time, while awakening a potent life force that even a coronavirus or racism cannot dent.[24] Amid prevailing conceptions of Black corporality (physiological reasons used to explain why Black people "experienced" COVID-19 differently than Whites), it remains instructive to not simply remark on Black *dehumanization*, but also grasp the "violence of humanization or the burden of inclusion into a racially hierarchized universal humanity."[25] Insofar as people of color are "without shelter, invited into or locked out of 'the human,'" their treatment questions the "humane" commonsense behind a one-size-fits-all approach.[26]

Resisting the tendency to document Black death ad infinitum, Austin Brown conveys this message in *I'm Still Here: Black Dignity in a World Made for Whiteness*:

> In a centuries old line of Black people who must prove they are human in order to call their murders unjust ... lynchings are still here, but so are we. They haven't been able to destroy us. The fear hasn't kept us from showing up, from experiencing joy, from demanding more from America.[27]

Black critique served as foil against White rage. Despite not being a regular churchgoer, Donald Trump received major support from White evangelicals for his pandemic response. That unwavering support, according to one Black preacher, is backed by the "demonic force" of Whiteness and the president as "a convenient fool for white supremacy."[28] Critics of Trump called him a "moral monster" with racist police derided as "monsters in uniform."[29] This grotesqueness resonates with what political prisoner George Jackson once said: capitalism was unquestionably "the scourge of the people" alongside the "fascist monster," the "corporate monster," and the "Amerikan monster." He called out the "monstrous machine" of the American who "suffers from a disease that forces him to build ugly things and destroy beauty wherever he finds it."[30]

One can spot this monstrous machine in one of the no-mask states which opened early. Georgia fell back into routine under orders from its new governor, the former secretary of state who assumed power in a highly suspect election that included mass voter disenrollment. Black businesses like barbershops opposed the measure by a governor to shake up the power of man who executed the wishes of "a small, white ruling class that has been OK with seeing certain populations as disposable."[31] The governor signed a ban on face masks statewide, nullifying the citywide mask ordinance of jurisdictions with sizeable Black populations like Atlanta. One tweeter warned that the man is predisposed "to kill Georgia's Black, Brown, POC, and low-income populations. This is genocide. They know it."[32] Exposed to early death and also thought to be superhumans unable to feel pain by medical authorities, African Americans have been historically loath to trust institutions that experiment on them like Johns Hopkins University hospital, the main national hub for tracking COVID-19 infections and death in the United States.

Gathering under the pandemic's heft were rumors that Blacks could not contract SARS-CoV-2 due to their high levels of melanin. People were first made aware of this "fact" in a tweet from China's embassy in Cameroon. In the satiric post, Chinese doctors boasted of an African international student's fast recovery from COVID-19 due to his black skin and antibodies. An article titled, "People of Color May Be Immune to the Coronavirus Because of Melanin" claimed melanin levels "play a significant factor in why Africans and other Black people who have been exposed to the virus have not become infected or dead."[33] Based on a study done on animals, the article was written for an Afrocentric blog for "curious melanated minds." One Maasai man in Kenya took it to heart, insisting the disease came from adopting European lifestyles, "This is a foreign disease. It is a white man's disease and we don't believe it can infect a Black man."[34]

As it turns out, the original post causing all this hubbub was an article from a fake news website posted by Kenyan and South Sudanese websites, which then became sent to Black-audience news feeds globally. Written by an unknown author, that original post (dated February 14, 2020) ends with a quote from an African student who claims White people are "always at war with our black skin because they know our melanin is our defense against all that they throw at us" and Black people's victory over COVID-19 meant "we are owners of this universe [and] they will never wipe us off."[35]

As incredulous as the "miraculous melanin" theory might sound, it introduced occult or paranormal elements into the pandemic's overmedicalized discourse as a "racial worldmaking."[36] This world-making encompasses fiction, ideological practices, cognition, and perceptual sense-making around race. One urban myth recapitulated Black people's superpower to withstand the onslaught of the novel coronavirus—despite people of color dying at three times the rate of White people.[37] Against the false conceit that Black people cannot get "the rona," African American doctors brought out factual evidence to the contrary to prove that COVID-19 is nothing to sneeze at. The synergistic energies between Blackness, cultural memory, and disease formed a "political anesthesia," requiring militant self-defense to defend Black bodies.[38]

What is considered miraculous takes on even more special properties during periods of social unrest. Black people, observes South African psychologist N. Chabani Manganyi, hold at their command creative weapons against objectification of their racialized corpus.[39] The surrealism and Black magic exercised by radicals aim to "discover the many different cognitive maps of the future, of the world not yet born."[40]

A viral world is one borne of the need for a future free from bondage and from ignorance. As the author of the *Dark Fantastic* Ebony Thomas illuminates, Black people are never given accurate medical information and must constantly "play in the dark," so for "it is less important that myths *are* true than that they *feel* true."[41] The sense that the "melanated" are endowed with special faculties resorted to "Magic Negro" stereotypes, but it also acts as a strange bulwark to (pseudo)scientific arguments propelled by White medical institutions that have historically used captive Black bodies for experimentation and developing technology. A lack of willing Black participants for early trials of COVID-19 drugs speaks to this history.

An uncurable disease is not the primary agent or deliverer of death. Systems of domination mete out a deadly concoction from the "fatal couplings of power and difference."[42] Affirmation of unapologetic Blackness does unmake the false redemption and moral salvation of "post-racial" magical thinking. This affirmation reinforces the radical claim that the fine-grain properties of Blackness matter when there is the (post)racial subtext that "All Lives Matter," and everyone dies equally from disease.

Zombies indulge in fantasies about fighting infected Others. They are marked for dead and fingered as culprits responsible for disease as well as the ending of the world.[43] As the convenient target for displaced anger and animus around SARS-CoV-2, racists exploited this opportunity to spew more hate. Asians of all backgrounds were verbally and physically assaulted due to their racial association with a "foreign" virus. Social media was full of photos and videos of bruised individuals being punched in the face by strangers. Masked Black and Brown people were chased out of stores for looking like "criminals." A steep penalty awaited those people "coughing while Asian," while several Korean immigrant women working at a spa were murdered in a hate crime that took place in Atlanta, Georgia.[44] Mindless zombies attacking human victims were not phantasms conjured from horror films, as some online speculated, they were real flesh-and-blood people. A shared video on Instagram imprinted the image of a rapper chasing down elderly Asian woman, laughing as he sprayed hand sanitizer on her while she runs away in a bewildered daze. Taped on a Miami beach, the entertainer's malice corresponds with socialite retirees throwing bashes and college students flocking to Florida beaches. The revelry of zombie-like gay partygoers was exposed on social media (@GaysOverCovid). Their debauchery ignited much ire for reckless endangerment of public health, given to the stereotype of the gay man who did not fear death and even courts it.

The zombie's "mimetic contagion" links the physical and psychic realms, offering "diagnostic insights into the pathological infections that ... dissolve into someone—or something—other."[45] Beyond senseless and streaks of violence, the exacting toll of hearing daily body counts meant the pandemic had spiraled—a failure almost by design. Herman Cain, a Black Republican conservative sent tweets after he passed away from COVID after attending a Trump rally. These zombie tweets (put out by his family) held onto the claim that SARS-CoV-2 was not as deadly as the media says. Calling forth indestructible zombie bodies, the pandemic brought out all the undead to play.

The zombie metaphor was invoked in countless films and television shows that popped up during world's baptism by fire. One parodic meme retitled the poster for *I am Legend*, a movie about the last man on earth bent on finding a cure for a plague that turns humans turn into zombie mutants. It reads, "I am Going to Costco," making light of store customers sparring over reams of toilet paper. In a distracted era of streaming television (increased exponentially with lockdown), COVID-19 forced hundreds of millions of people to stay at home, watching hours of online content like entertainment zombies. As COVID-mania peaked, video-on-demand company Netflix suddenly released not only science documentaries but all its *Resident Evil* franchise, helping people make cultural sense of a pandemic (in the film, a vile corporation makes an experimental virus and infects the general population to control humanity). Anglophone movies like *World War Z* and the cult classic *28 Days Later* homed in on the foreboding sense of dread from fictional worlds not far from ours. *Reality Z* from Brazil evinced what a zombie world looks like if it were a reality television show, which the real pandemic sometimes resembled. Older movies about infectious disease like *Flu, Mayhem*, and *Pandemic* returned to the public eye, while *Only* plays on fears of a plague that kills only women, hunted in a "feminist counterapocalypse."[46] End-of-the-world zombie flicks came back with more fervor to address "infected" global systems.

Zombie mythology superimposed on a pandemic social order. South Korean flicks like *Alive* (2020) offered a movie about youth locked in their apartment as the world falls apart. The story touches upon a boy hemmed in and struggling in his isolated apartment to avoid those neighbors infected. This plot resonated with the quarantine of the entire Korean peninsula (with no neighboring countries accepting refugees) in *Peninsula*, where zombies ran fast in a lethal stampede. Within the astonishing run of modern global pandemics, the film suggested the progress of coronavirus was no sprint.

Meanwhile, the zombies of the U.S. hit show *The Walking Dead* hobbled toward their victims in its final season with a slowness matching America's tripped-up response to the novel coronavirus. But perhaps no movie represented the COVID-19 pandemic better than the short film *Quota* (2021), wherein two Black women realize all their fellow employees in an e-commerce factory are turning into zombies from an airborne virus. They are unable to escape after being locked inside by managers who want workers to fulfill holiday shipping orders. The infected women's final moments of bonded sacrifice—blowing up the factory to prevent the virus from leaking out—demonstrate how "racialized women create social connections and social worlds in excess to the conditions that produce them and their labor as non-value."[47] The closing lines of the movie speaks to the horror of zombified labor: "We work ourselves to the bone. And when we die, they replace us."

Pandemic zombies hovered in all shapes and sizes. They could be sourced in the regimented masses working "seamlessly" under lockdown to floundering governments lumbering aimlessly through the pandemic like a waking dream. Footage from Wuhan showed a "zombieland" with people acting "like zombies" with blood pouring from their mouth.[48] Malaysia's health ministry sent out a tweet to dispel rumors that people can become zombies from the novel coronavirus. Insofar as the rich are willing to eat their poor, who else can be given over to feed the voracious desires of a zombified world?

COVID-19 made zombie metaphors a cultural force. Do "zombies vanish when the virus dies in the body of a recovering patient?" asks anthropologist Veronica Gomez-Temesio. In the failed "politics of life" during the Ebola crisis, people in Guinea began referring themselves as "the walking dead," which resonates with the Haitian voodoo tradition of zombieism as well as the transatlantic slave trade. The zombie figure escapes social categories as it "incarnates both the one who, still alive, is considered dead, and the one who, being considered dead, still fights for recognition."[49] Those monsters held captive as subhuman commodity—whether by colonial or humanitarian regimes—straddling the border between life and death. Biomedical recovery, emphasizes Gomez-Temesio, is not the same as social or political recognition, something Indigenous communities are all too familiar with.

The Indigenous Action Media collective released an anti-futurist manifesto that put out this message against the empty metaphor of a zombie apocalypse:

> Why can we imagine the ending of the world, yet not the ending of colonialism? So many are eagerly ready to be the lone survivors of the "zombie apocalypse" … This is the futurism of the colonizer, the capitalist. It is at once every future ever stolen by the plunderer, the warmonger, and the rapist … It is apocalypse, actualized. And with the only certainty being a deathly end, colonialism is a plague.[50]

By refocusing attention to "an ending that has come before," the group unlocks the key to survival for the Enemy Other: "Our world lives when their world ceases to exist." This quote resonates with what Yaqui scholar Marisa Duarte calls the art of storytelling through "Indigenous consciousness." Indigenous worlding forms the "basis of future exercises of cultural sovereignty."[51] A perceived "loss of total meaning" under pandemic regimes came with its harshest blows and the constellation of pain. But it also gave new meaning to the future.

Despite these pandemic futures, the hauntology of COVID-19 dredged up colonial memories in the Global South. In addressing the question of how life still flows amid death and violence, West African artists took back the zombie mythos and returned it to its Vodun roots. Senegalese films like the gothic

Atlantique (or *Atlantics* in English versions) released in 2019 revolves around the story of a young girl (betrothed to a rich man who works in Italy) who falls for a poor construction worker. When her lover mysteriously leaves the country and disappears at sea with others, the refugees' spirits come back to possess their girlfriends to haunt the men's former bosses for garnished wages. Zombie capitalism drove desperate poor people into watery graves. Ending with the phrase "some memories are omens," the film recognizes the ghosts of migrant workers that haunt a world swept up in the pandemic's path.

Not weighed down by "First World problems," stand-out African countries like Senegal, Nigeria, Mauritius, South Africa, and Rwanda fleshed out ways to protect life, proving that healthcare could be done well despite the worst of circumstances. For its part, Senegal protected its citizens from COVID-19, promising USD $1 tests and beds for all sick persons. This protection is commendable for a country ranked second to last place in the first World Economic Forum's Global Social Mobility Index conceived in 2020. The coronapocalypse did not happen in Africa as predicted.

For the devout with strict dogmatic views, they denigrated others for perturbing "natural" hierarchies. In a blogpost called "Is God Judging America Today?" a pastor who leads a weekly Bible study group for members of Donald Trump's cabinet blamed COVID-19 on "depraved" environmentalists and gays.[52] Insofar as gay sexual identity and gender fluidity are construed as diseases, the COVID-19 zombie finds its masochistic twin in the queer zombie.[53] This pandemic was a *multidimensional* apocalypse.[54] Predicting universal doom only hurts "others," as one Australian public health expert warns, "if you predict the Apocalypse, anything less is an improvement."[55] For catastrophizers, only God or a messianic savior could fix things now.

Mystic

From the pandemic's maw emanated divine messages that shined a light on the false gods of capitalism and the deities ruling our "occult economies."[56] For many who spoke to God, COVID-19 was a sign that all was coming to end. With coronavirus occupying the attention of the world, vulnerable communities lurched from one moral crisis to another, and the spiritually inclined needed counsel. Worriers plumbed the ancient wisdom of mystics while others reverted to the holy teachings of messiahs. Bowing before no one, President Trump called on the military to clear antiracist protests and held up a Bible at a burned-out church, a publicity stunt his generals objected to.[57] One evangelical supporter found the act to be one of piety against an ungodly world: "He's establishing the Lord's kingdom in the world … this is a president who wears the full armor of God."[58] On Facebook, an online troll wrote that though she lost her daughter to COVID-19, she was thankful for upholding Christian values by rejecting the medical establishment.

The Messiah was coming back to earth, COVID-19 be damned. Religious conservatives reckoned that SARS-CoV-2 must be a sign of Jesus Christ's second coming with Trump as the messenger.

Under pandemic-induced paranoia, coronavirus conspiracies trickled in about humanity's final hour. With the help of Facebook's polarizing algorithm, a popular Internet community of a sect of social conspiracists called QAnon readied themselves for the "Great Awakening," believing Trump an energy healing light worker or demi-god waging a godly war to save trafficked children from a "cabal of Satan-worshipping baby eaters" and pedophiles like the Clintons controlling the "deep state."[59] Claiming that he himself can never do wrong and able to divine the future, Trump perpetuated these QAnon conspiracies, playing into the paranoid style of American politics, where "at stake is always a conflict between absolute good and absolute evil, what is necessary is not compromise but the will to fight things out to a finish. Since the enemy ... must be totally eliminated."[60]

The vaccine wars looped into culture wars, insofar as many anti-vaxxers were often religious conservatives who are hostile to gays and sexual dissenters. One study found that two-thirds of religious Americans believed SARS-CoV-2 was God's sign for humans to change their sinful ways. Half said God would protect them from infection.[61] One pastor called the disease a "phantom plague," while another evangelical leader spoke of Jesus' return and changes leading up to the last day and how the pandemic was the first birth pains of the apocalypse.[62] There were cosmic rewards for tuning out the novel coronavirus and making peace with earthly death. Examining the Book of Revelations (where the Rapture is not mentioned), theologians who study the Bible recognized that the pandemic was not big enough an event to constitute the biblical plague as foretold. They recommended uplifting messages of consolation instead of doom-laden evangelization.

Primed to believe that a fast-encroaching virus could be thumped by the grace of God, charismatic false prophets viewed the End Days on optimistic terms. Avid supporters of Trump revered him, despite his checkered past, and believed he could save the world. Die-hard acolytes proclaimed that he could even walk on water. Less-religious devotees complimented Trump for helping to negotiate Israel's renewed diplomatic relations with Bahrain and United Arab Emirates, which critics said could harm Palestinian rights within Israeli. Gary Ray, a prophecy writer says he and his fellow *End-Times* writers bloviated this political deal as a divine masterstroke and part of a prophesy: "The key focus that we have in our minds is Israel. That's God's prophetic clock. As things progress in that country, we get closer to when the rapture of the church will occur, and then the tribulation."[63] The pandemic nightmare bore fever-dreams of spiritual and worldly domination.

Clerics like Archbishop Carlos Castillo in Peru bore witness to the wrath of COVID-19, after arriving at an empty church with no one from his congregation of 5,000 members alive. An edifying faith in a "white political ideology" explained disasters like the pandemic as God's will.[64] The archbishop recognized how the pandemic response is based on "egotism and business and not on mercy and solidarity with the people."[65] Folk swindlers like Belarus' leader called COVID-19 fears a "psychosis," and claimed vodka and a sauna could quash the virus. Hindu nationalist politicians like Suman Haripriya of Assam peddled the holy benefits of cow dung in treating COVID-19. China's president remarked on old venerable healing medicines, while Mexico's helmsman put stock in Catholic amulets. A high-profile Sri Lankan shaman died of SARS-CoV-2, after treating the prime minister with "blessed" water, special "healing powers" promoted by the health minister. Venezuela's President Nicolas Maduro posted that a special tea made of elderberry, lemon, ginger, and black pepper was the perfect antiviral brew. "The virus has a remedy. It's easy. But the multinational pharmaceutical companies will say it doesn't work. It's a remedy that our ancestors lived on."[66]

When Italy achieved early notoriety for having a disproportionate share of the global burden of sickness, novelist Francesa Malandri, hibernating in Rome, wrote an open letter to fellow Europeans. She projected their impending future and how the infected like her are now quasi-seers with fearsome premonitions.[67]

> I am writing to you from Italy, which means I am writing from your future. We are now where you will be in a few days.
>
> We are but a few steps ahead of you in the path of time, just like Wuhan was a few weeks ahead of us. We watch you as you behave just as we did.
>
> We're in Italy, and this is what we know about your future. But it's just small-scale fortune-telling. We are very low-key seers.

During the interim period between the opening torch relay for the Olympics and commencement of the games, a doomsday cult in Japan released toxic nerve gas in the subway, killing over a dozen people and injuring thousands to bolster fears of the apocalypse. In Christian mythology, the apocalypse depicts the four horsemen that arrive with the end of the world or the Last Judgement, the first horseman being Christ and the Holy Spirit pursued by the horsemen symbolizing war and famine. The fourth, the "pale rider" draws out pestilence and death. Death is the perfect excuse for humans to ponder all sorts of questions. Worried people the world over reported weird dreams, which psychologists attributed to stress from the "coronasomnia." On the brink of ruination, the pandemic dream state was a *memento mori*.

Diviners motioned to a Great Awakening as the omnipresent coronavirus took hold. A church youth leader in Texas tweeted a biblical passage that refers to a moment when "there is no rain, or command locusts to devour the land or send a plague" as a message to turn people "from their wicked ways."[68] In light of global wildfires and the pandemic—White Christian fundamentalists sized up these events as a message sent from above, that cast aspersions on environmentalists, poor people of color, and non-Christian heathens. Nothing it seemed could be more epic than the plague of locusts swarming in the Sahel and a giant dust plume cloud dubbed "Godzilla" from the Sahara that crossed the entire Atlantic. The monsoon in the Indian Ocean generated the breeding grounds and hotbed for the largest infestation of the ravenous bugs in 70 years, which threatened regional food supplies in East Africa. As COVID-19 turned the world on its head, the bubonic plague returned to the news. Trump even referenced COVID-19 as *the* plague rather than *a* plague, harkening back to occult medieval associations of disease. As the pandemic blazed a deadly trail, winding its way around the world, religion and the occult played a more pivotal role in predicting human affairs.

Divination was used to predict rumbling events on a planet circumnavigated by a coronavirus. A whole new zodiac lunar cycle began in the frenetic Year of the Rat. The first bad omen for China began in earnest after infection spun out of control with millions of travelers during the busiest holiday. A world of hurt brought by the pernicious new coronavirus brought fantasists and soothsayers back to the limelight. Tropical astrologers blamed bad fortunes on the tight conjunction of planets Jupiter (expansion/faith) with Pluto (death/renewal) and Saturn (restriction/lessons) in the sign of Capricorn on December 21, 2020. For them, the Age of Aquarius with its emphasis on science and egalitarianism was officially upon us. It augured changes from elections to banking to education and work for the next 200 years. This alignment called the Great Mutation was the most observable in the sky since medieval times. It was time for humanity to meet the demands of the future.

In the field of astronomy, the Webb telescope provided its first images in 2022 to reveal again how our planet was a small speck in the universe. Further realization of that smallness was another "godwink." When studying an enormous gulf of cosmological space-time, scientists glimpsed into eons past and light years to the beginning of the universe, peering into the birth of the very first stars. From the grand perspective of astronomy and astrology, we can ask if COVID-19 is an intergalactic visitor from the heavens, a godsend to awaken complacent people from a long slumber.

The pandemic offered a mirror to the world to perceive society's collective dream, the dream of humanity that comprises smaller personal dreams.[69] This collective mind fog, which the ancient Toltecs called *mitote*, is a big illusion "where people talk at the same time, and nobody understands each other."[70] This dreamlike state is confused further and corrupted by viral information where one obtains some relief from headache of the poison by gossiping and spreading information "in a never-ending chain between all the humans on earth … through circuits that are clogged with a poisonous, contagious virus." Ours is a viral world built on the hidden wisdom of the ancestors.

Mysticism prevails ever so often when science fails to deliver spiritual comfort to the masses. Sylvia Browne had been one of the most famous oracles, and while she had been wrong, the savant hit it big when social influencers retweeted the deceased writers' predictions from 2008. In her book *End of Days*, she penned these ominous words: "In around 2020, a severe pneumonia-like illness will spread throughout the globe, attacking the lungs and the bronchial tubes and resisting all known preventative treatments." Novelist Dean Koontz was perhaps more on target in his 1981 novel *The Eyes of Darkness*, which mentioned "Wuhan-400," a man-made biological "perfect weapon" brought over from China (a fictional disease that only survives in humans and not in other animals).

Older predictions about a viral world came back into vogue. One of the most famous of seers remains Nostradamus, a French astrologer of the sixteenth century whose tomes have been pried open by ardent followers for answers about the mundane world. Followers drew on the physician's poetic quatrains published in the *Les Prophéties* (The Prophecies) half a millennium ago. Consider this quatrain that some of his apostles considered a red herring for the COVID-19 pandemic.

The sloping park, great calamity,
Through the Lands of the West and Lombardy
The fire in the ship, plague, and captivity;

Wuhan's South China Seafood Wholesale Market is located at the base of two parks. As COVID-19 ravaged and ripped into the West, Lombardy in Italy was its nerve center. The reference to "fire in the ship" could have been COVID-infected cruise boats.

Studying the mnemonics of pandemics, psychologist Steven Taylor remarks that people are always unprepared for the future and all eventualities. They could not mentally cope with COVID-19 just as they could not for SARS and Spanish Flu. "These weren't Nostradamus predictions," he posited, but "predictions of responses based on research on what happened in previous pandemics."[71] Familiarizing oneself with COVID-19 as supernatural, we can better graft the fantastic thinking of White evangelicals to conspiracy theorists and new-age spiritual believers. While famous mystics like Nostradamus could allegedly peer into the future, researchers have already told us what we needed to know but did not care to hear. Writers like Arundhati Roy regarded the pandemic as a time portal we must walk through to reach the next world. She observes we must try to "stitch our future to our past" and acknowledge the rupture with everything we had once thought and believed is foregone: "Historically, pandemics have forced humans to break with the past and imagine their world anew. This one is no different. It is a portal, a gateway between one world and the next."[72]

A coming apocalypse heralded a spiritual awakening and mystics like Walter Mercado who invited us to step into a new world of love. The famed Puerto Rican astrologer and Piscean passed exactly two weeks before the world's first COVID-19 case was uncovered. Before his death, he announced his annual predictions with 2020 bringing humanity together to work on the common good. The television star offered the best curative for the world with his customary kiss off to fans: *mucho mucho amor*.

Strange times can incite more repugnance than love. When tragedy strikes, there are religious figures ready to pin social outsiders as the main carriers of bad luck. One right-wing Christian pastor called coronavirus the "homovirus," submitting homosexuality as the virus that ran aground the "traditional" nuclear family.[73] The paterfamilias of the Ukrainian Orthodox Church contracted COVID-19 after calling it "God's punishment for the sins of men," blaming gay marriage, even though same-sex marriage is not legal in Ukraine.[74] Demagoguery acts out in typical fashion to frame a cryptic disease as divine punishment against social taboos.

Hate-mongers of all stripes hoped to eradicate groups that they despise using COVID-19 as an excuse to do so. They recast those marginalized populations as viral beings deserving of death. New York's governor was not inclined to jump to supernatural causes: "This is not an act of God we're looking at. It's an act of what society actually does."[75] In the wake of COVID-19, Christian fundamentalists tethered "satanic" practices to the cursed nature of the Chinese, in the reprised role of pagan menace. Even as "Chinese" eating practices are prevalent throughout the world that hunt "bushmeat," the jump to blame "savage" practices conceals the "racial scripts" behind modern-day phobias.[76] These Orientalist scripts assume certain human bodies are synonymous with nonhuman threats and "unnatural" threats. Without exception, coronavirus myths made abundantly clear what fools mortals be.

COVID-19 set the viral grounds for humanity to be put on notice. It crushed the eternal pursuit for immortality by foolish humans. South Korea was the first country to officially admit to a second wave of infections in the summer of 2020 after the first viral superstorm early in the year. The crisis provoked fear in a country famous for religious leaders claiming godly messiah status, the most noted being Sun Myung Moon of the Unification Church. The pandemic was no exception in terms of exciting fanatical responses from those soothsayers who flirted with death, believing in their own prophetic powers. South Koreans channeled their fury toward an eccentric religious group considered to be a fringe organization by mainstream religious institutions. Led by a leader facing murder charges, the group gathered in secretive congregations after one of their members had been pegged as a "super spreader."

After COVID-19 rates plateaued, new infections popped up in the church and the numbers spiked. The Korea Disease Control and Prevention Agency reported that over 60% of all confirmed cases were related to the Shinchonji Church.[77] Adherents of the apocalyptic church believe they are the chosen ones of God and also think that their octogenarian leader is immortal, whom no coronavirus could kill. When signs of COVID-19 infections and deaths pointed to the church, a manhunt was launched by South Korea's health ministry to track down the names of sect's members. The usual cloak of secrecy surrounding the cult heightened, when thousands of its members were quarantined by the government, and after its leader gave false data about its meetings to health authorities. South Korea's government found itself at loggerheads with pastors wielding power over their flock, the leaders urging the faithful to organize anti-government rallies based on "a belief that wearing masks or practicing physical distancing are signs of a lack of faith in God's protective power."[78]

Something similar happened when New York's governor closed houses of worship; Orthodox Hasid Jews and Roman Catholics objected to those curbs, sometimes violently. Smartphone apps identified Korean church facilities, and one province in South Korea set up a phone hotline to local evangelical members. Meanwhile, a video passed around social networks shed light on a new COVID-19 cluster at the Grace River Church, which sprayed holy water into the mouths of its devotees, thinking it will defeat the virus. But this virus was allowed to fly under the radar and infect numerous more people. Yet, the community infection of megachurches gave South Korea a head start in turning the corner with COVID-19, as the first big concentration of infections there led to a colossal push for conducting industrial-scale testing and door-to-door monitoring. Controlling the pandemic without national lockdown, South Korea banned all religious services.

Queers were selected for targeted harm and blamed for the end-of-days. On the same day, South Korea relaxed its sweeping measures for physical distancing, close to 40 new infections surfaced within the district of Itaewon, a swanky area known for fashionable expats. The local media put out anti-gay messages that infections came from clubs (after King Club confirmed a patient visited it), adding to the stigma and witch hunt of a minoritized community and stanching treatment. A daily linked to a Protestant evangelical church speculated that the clubs and bathhouses in the catered to gay clientele, even though none of those establishments promoted themselves that way. One man was outed by the media for potentially exposing 1,500 people, after visiting five public places while being asymptomatic. This "gay" coronavirus story was picked up by other local newspapers who luridly detailed the age and occupation of the queer "superspreader."

With COVID-19 doubling as another "gay plague," the AIDS-era specter of the hypersexual, hedonistic male engaging in sex with men returned. The religious belief in hell took on a different resonance when one gay man contemplated suicide from potential public humiliation of being doubly outed as gay and a COVID-19 survivor: "If they found out that I was at a gay club, they would most likely tell me to leave … or make my life there a living hell."[79] Life did not look up with the outbreak of a rare disease called Monkeypox, a strangely named oddity which became declared a global health emergency by the World Health Organization in the summer of 2022. Linking its spread early on to gay men's social networks, this disease related more to smallpox than HIV or the fake "VAIDS," a claim that AIDS was caused by the COVID-19 vaccine.

The governmental assumption that all South Koreans were willing to publicly share their personal information to foil SARS-Cov-2 cracked in the mistreatment of transgender people (the Korean military discharged its first trans soldier, even though the World Health Organization rid the association of transgenderism with illness by removing "gender identity disorder" from mental and behavioral disorders in 2019). Afterward, the Korean Disease Control and Prevention Agency issued a public warning to prevent leaking of private information through new guidelines. These policies implemented anonymous testing and contact tracing, since the country lacks anti-discrimination laws that could protect gender and sexual minorities. According to historian Todd Henry, COVID-19 policies unearthed deep-seated anxieties that many queers "are being put under surveillance … [with] no space or room for LGBTQ+ people to move and navigate Korean society."[80] Same-sex relations between soldiers are punishable offenses, and the military before has used dating apps to track down queer soldiers.

The fear of men not being "real men" anymore became such a big deal that China in 2021 restricted gaming for teenagers to one hour, lest gamers (assumed to be mostly boys) turn into electronics-addicted emasculated zombies who could not serve in the military. This rule comes after it banned television performers in breach of the public moral order, such as "girly" male pop stars. Xi Jinping's government and its state media vowed to "resolutely put an end to sissy men and other abnormal esthetics."[81] To protect its national "health," whether from COVID-19 or emasculation/homosexuality, the war machine was called upon to chase down queer monsters.

Machine

Rather than announce a new world peace where nations worked in harmony together to fight an enemy, coronavirus peeled back the curtain to reveal the machinations behind the global theater of war. In a break from the usual stories of monsters and mystics, a true apocalyptic tale makes full run of brutish machines. In dystopian science fiction, the "machine" can mean robots, but it almost always is a reference to the military-industrial complex. In popular movies like *The Terminator*, the U.S. military invents an artificially intelligent system that "wakes up" to the fact that humanity is the enemy (to itself), and it decides to wipe out or capture humans. The U.S. military decided to soften its basic training or boot camp for new recruits, sensitive to mental health and post-traumatic syndrome with COVID-19 in the background of everyone's consciousness. While new recruits learned how to fight virtually on iPad screens, the United States conducted drone strikes against the Islamic State that wrongly hit civilian families and aid workers in Kabul, Afghanistan. A more "humanistic" approach to war did not dampen war machines and their dehumanizing processes.[82] Instead, the pandemic unleashed more methods of killing.

New designs for mass destruction were hatched within the crucible of the COVID-19 pandemic. In December 2019, a Saudi national with ties to Al-Qaeda took aim at a Florida Navy air base, where he was training, to kill service members. An investigation found Saudi Arabia, along with the United Arab Emirates, transferred U.S. weapons to terrorist groups such as Al-Qaeda. Inspectors, general officers responsible for probing malfeasance in government, were fired for attempting to investigate these arms deals. As the author of *Plagues and Peoples* observes, the "macroparasitism" of human civilizations holds its counterpart in the bacteria and viruses intermingling with "other species":

> Warfare and disease are connected by more than rhetoric and the pestilences that have so often marched with and in the wake of armies … warfare characteristically mingled with and masked this epidemiological process. Trade, which was imperfectly distinct from warlike raiding, was another normal way for civilized folk to probe new lands.[83]

Through the "corona wars," the imperial politics of "civilized peoples" digesting "lower species" of people drove the epidemiological limit for disease to greater heights.

The pandemic pushed imperial forces to its limit. Fears that China would seize control of Taiwan, while the rest of the world was distracted by COVID-19 was based on the increase in China's military drills near the island nation in 2022. Taiwan worried about China waging a biowar that included bacteria bombs and virus attacks. Protestors defied China's anti-coronavirus ban and organizers were charged with "incitement" charges for organizing another annual vigil for 1989's Tiananmen Square massacre (some appropriating the message of #LasVidasNegrasImportan to "We Can't Breathe" and "Youth Lives Matter").[84] When China's National People's Congress passed a national security law on May 20, 2002, this policy set off a firestorm in Hong Kong with police using water cannons to drown out the shouts of protestors. Taiwan and France offered refuge to Hong Kong exiles, while Britain offered path to citizenship to "uphold our profound ties of history and friendship with the people of Hong Kong."[85]

In response to Hong Kong, China deployed uniformed military troops at the border in another war footing. Protection against biopolitical threats meant suppression of free thought and movement. A new insurrection law installed a national security bureau, which coordinated with the local judiciaries and law enforcement agencies to quell the movement for Hong Kong independence. Communist China threatened to turn this former British Crown colony into a modern-day penal colony.[86] While the Hong Kong government never issued a full lockdown, but rather enforced curfews, the vaguely written security law, intentionally broad in scope, gave China's communist leaders the right to arrest anyone for crimes punishable up to a life in prison. This repression put the entire island under a de facto lockdown, imprisoning anyone for secession, terrorism, sedition, or collusion. This penalizing law implicated foreigners and anyone in the world, not just Hong Kongese, thus aggregating greater international power for China. To foil Chinese espionage, the United States ordered the closure of the Chinese consulate in Houston, Texas, which Senator Marco Rubio called a "massive spy center" and "a central node of the Communist Party's vast network of spies and influence."[87] The Chinese in response ordered the U.S. consulate in Chengdu closed.

This Chinese security law preceded Anti-Terrorism Act of 2020 in the Philippines. This House law promised to firm up the Philippines' capability to fight Islamic terrorism, repealing the Human Security Act of 2007 that set legal safeguards like warrants for detained suspects. The United Nations Human Rights Office views this crackdown as exercising broad powers to arrest human rights groups as terrorists. An editorial in the *Philippine Daily Inquirer* took the murder of George Floyd as analogous to the murder of the country: "It portends to be a knee on the national neck. Already, we can't breathe."[88]

The coronapocalypse supercharged a general state of war. This machine of destruction was apparent in Nigeria after protests and a movement to scrap the special unit of the country's police force called Special Anti-Robbery Squad that extorted, kidnapped, tortured, and killed unarmed citizens for decades. A shared online video that allegedly shows the killing of a man by an officer in the Delta state kindled protests that spread from Lagos to rest of the world.

In countries besieged by the novel coronavirus, military reserve forces and naval ships were redeployed as auxiliary aid to civil and medical authorities. Discovering that 79% of COVID-19 deaths came from elderly care centers, Prime Minister Justin Trudeau deployed thousands of soldiers to care homes. For a brief time, it almost seemed COVID-19 breached cracks in the treadmill of military activity and provocation. Even the Islamic terrorist group like the Islamic State issued instructions on handwashing and asked Muslims to avoid travel to much of Europe. Iran permitted use of an anti-corona vaccine from its sworn enemy, Israel. The sound of (short-lived) peace shortly reverberated across war zones, manifesting what one Israeli reporter calls a "coronavirus cease fire."[89]

Israel's hyper-militarist ethnonationalism doomed its pandemic mitigation efforts from the start. The state quarantined all its soldiers to preserve military fighting readiness, while its elite intelligence units and special forces did remote electronic data collection in Palestine. Though Israel sent supplies to Hamas and the Gaza Strip and permitted Palestinian workers to enter its gated borders, it still upheld its new strict nationality law and confiscated more land in Occupied Territories. There were reports of the demolition of clinics meant to house sick Palestinians.[90] The eviction of families from Sheikh Jarrah, a predominantly Palestinian neighborhood in East Jerusalem, set off another flare in the Israel-Palestinian conflict, leading to the Israel War with Hamas in 2023.

Global solidarity with humanity opposes the removal of people from their homes inside a country with one of the longest, most strict lockdowns. Despite the highest rate of COVID-19 vaccinations in the world, Israel could not offer vaccinations for the displaced in Palestine, who were left to devise their own methods of protection. In a political cartoon tweeted with the hashtag #coronapocalypse in #Palestine, an older woman draped in the colors of the Palestinian flag (see Figure 6.1). She is forced to face down COVID-19 at gunpoint with Israeli soldiers at her back, armed behind a wall. Palestinians had been living under lockdown for a long time before COVID-19. The world of Gazans living in what many called an "open-air prison" invited an extreme microcosm of the quarantined viral world.

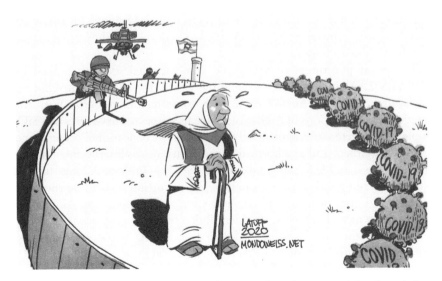

FIGURE 6.1   #Coronapocalypse in #Palestine political cartoon (Mondoweiss).

As the United States gave a million surgical masks to the Israel Defense Forces, which was charged with coordinating national supply chains, there registered a big jump in violent attacks on Palestinians (almost 78%), despite a region-wide lockdown. Human rights groups demanded Israel to lift its blockade of Gaza and the West Bank to allow for medical supplies and personnel to move in occupied territories. Extending its current system and network of security checkpoints, Israel ordered Palestinians to download a phone app giving the military access to their personal data, location, and cameras.

Through software developed in partnership between the city Hangzhou and a subsidiary of e-commerce global brand Alibaba, China mandated all citizens download the analytics tracking device on their phones. This "coronavirus passport" not only assigned a color code to one's health status but determined if one can purchase transit tickets or enter public spaces. In U.S. state of Connecticut, police announced a (scrapped) pilot program with drones that can detect the temperatures and heart rates of pedestrians from afar or identify public gatherings.

Despite their valuable role in giving COVID-19 warnings, social media companies were not always welcome in pandemic information campaigns. President Joe Biden claimed platforms such as Facebook were "killing people" with wrong information, which the U.S. surgeon general characterized as a "serious threat to public health."[91] Anti-vaccine aggression was backed by vituperative attacks on marginalized populations from hate groups. Facebook removed Trump ads for displaying Nazi symbols, and Twitter responded by flagging Trump's tweets or slapping fact-checking labels on his posts for "abusive behavior." The former reality television celebrity misled with smoke and mirrors, claiming a stolen election and priming his followers to retaliate with armed revolt. From France to Venezuela to the United States, everything came to blows.

The apocalyptic threat of terror and war encircled societies zapped by SARS-CoV-2. With COVID-19 lashing the world, the Islamic State-claimed attacks in France and Austria came with some terrorism alerts. With the drawdown in U.S. troops in Afghanistan, locals witnessed massacres in a Sikh temple, the targeted killing of mostly schoolgirls at educational centers, and murder of mothers and newborns in a maternity ward. Internecine violence threatened to derail U.S. peace talks there with the Taliban. A long-running dispute between political factions in government meant no deal on the table as part of an agreement to end America's longest running war. As Taliban began seizing more territories, President Biden rushed a contingent of troops back to Afghanistan to ensure order in the chaotic withdrawal process. Australia too withdrew all its soldiers in Afghanistan and Iraq. COVID-19 anxiety temporarily decreased military pursuits, but saber-rattling by leaders shrugged off permanent peace.

Despite the call for a global ceasefire by the United Nations Secretary-General, declaiming it was time to "end the sickness of war," rival militias never fully laid down arms. After winning the Nobel Peace Prize in 2019 for brokering concord between his country, Eritrea, and South Sudan, Ethiopia's battle-scarred President Abiy Ahmed rebuffed international peace talks in the Tigray War (2020-2022). He rained down military fire upon the semi-autonomous region of Tigray, whose elites conducted its own election after Ahmed postponed national elections due to COVID-19.[92] The United States blocked an agreement by the United Nations Security Council for cooling any disgruntlement, citing its problems with the United Nations' "specialized health agencies," a backhanded commentary on the World Health Organization. A few enemies set aside their differences to fight what United Nations chief António Guterres calls the "true fight of our lives" against the "common enemy that is now threatening all of humankind."[93]

The pandemic struck an active nerve in strained relations between neighboring countries, buttressing fears of military occupation as well as political insurgencies. China and India reignited their border wars, while India and Pakistan remained engaged in the decades-long fight over Kashmir, as India revoked and abolished the region's privileged autonomous status in 2019. India even locked down Kashmir, restricting public movement and communications, after the death of a famed Kashmiri separatist. The pandemic's acceleration barely set back dystopic digitized dictatorships and the global police state.[94]

COVID-19 policies did not have a chilling effect on surveillance technology. Cases of malicious spyware possibly linked to Russia or China attacked thousands of businesses in multiple countries. JBS, the world's largest meat company, paid cybercriminals in Bitcoin cryptocurrency, after an attack shut down its plants. When this computer breach struck, one media critic questioned hacker fears over the cruel logic of allowing corporations to dominate factory pig farming, where the next pandemic-causing foodborne illness might spawn. The path to destruction is not always clear when the viral source of global discontent is hacking or hogs.[95]

Infernal war machines built on lies did their own bidding. France and the United States disagreed over who would sell submarines to Australia. The singularity promised by the awakening of artificially intelligent machines, or AI, founds its precursor in social media, as it was found that half the Twitter accounts pushing for a fast U.S. reopening were bots, including two-thirds of the biggest social influencers. Megacompanies YouTube, Google, Facebook, and Twitter opted not to take down Trump's inflated claims about clinical drugs like hydroxychloroquine, while removing the same misleading statements by Jair Bolsonaro, based on its community policy and expanded rules to protect public health.[96] As a whistleblower revealed from secret documents leaked in fall 2021, Facebook contributed to political polarization and violence in Ethiopia and Myanmar/Burma. Under his watch, Trump boasted release of the United States from binding international commitments to its military allies in North Atlantic Treaty Organization, though some welcomed the breakup of this global force. Trump's successor Biden believed in global cooperation and smart technologies, which could save lives against an apocalyptic threat like asteroids that moved dangerously close to Earth. In 2022, National Aeronautics and Space Administration sent a spacecraft to slam into one as a first-time test to protect humanity from potential hazardous objects. But the nations on earth were too busy fighting to notice these threats.

A war of words heated up at the same time as real military actions and war games did. While COVID-19 chewed up more territories, violent skirmishes erupted between Azerbaijan, Sudan, Armenia, Turkey, Iran, Syria, Iraq, Russia, Saudi Arabia, and other global players. Top leaders never owned up to how pandemic contingency plans missed wide of the mark and that they were spectacularly wrong. They continued to hurl complaints at one another. U.S. prosecutors, ten days before announcing national coronavirus emergency, prosecuted drug trafficking suspects close to the President of Honduras, long considered a "narco-state." Meanwhile, Venezuela's president was indicted on drug trafficking charges by the U.S. Justice Department, a charge that the socialist leader promised to fight by military force.

Corona-fueled war aims threatened peace. Even the death of Mikhail Gorbachev, the last leader of the Soviet Union, could not undim the force of this "new" Cold War. The Non-Aligned Movement (NAM)—countries in the Global South that did not join any major bloc during the Cold War—arranged a summit attended by more than 40 state leaders in May 2020 under the banner of "United against COVID-19." Led by Azerbaijan, NAM came to focus their attentions on global solidarity to put coronavirus in retreat (even as Azerbaijan engaged in a fresh skirmish with Armenia over contested areas). In March 2021, 16 countries marked the 60th anniversary of the NAM, establishing the Group of Friends in Defense of the Charter of the United Nations to protect against isolationism and arbitrary sanctions by individual countries. Promoting multilateralism to solve the world's problems—members included Algeria, Cambodia, Laos, Saint Vincent and the Grenadines, Cuba, China, Syria, and observer state Palestine. As historian Vijay Prashad surmises, "The divide is not between China and the U.S., a division that the U.S. is trying to impose on the world: the divide is between humanity and imperialism."[97] A "post-pandemic world" must be demilitarized and freed from the viral world of imperialism.

While thinking about the fictions of the world ending, we come to know a "post-world pandemic." In popular apocalyptic screeds, earth becomes a technologically advanced dystopia or a postindustrial wasteland. Those stories almost always contain new gadgets of some kind. Innovations in technology were quickly introduced in 2020 to deal with the pandemic. With the science behind coronaviruses boosted from the pandemic, humans today know more than they did about SARS, due in part to headway in high-tech innovations like AI, robotics, and supercomputers, alongside the breakthroughs in genomics and biogenetics. New technology came to the rescue for addressing the panic attack and heartache of COVID-19, a temporary salve for a human problem. Microsoft unveiled a healthcare bot named Clara for the Centers for Disease Control and Prevention in the United States. This online social bot screened patients for risk factors and assisted in a gendered form of service, where machines did the bidding of immobilized humans who could not go anywhere.

As humans ratcheted up social distancing life, the synapses of a global intelligence and online hivemind enabled human intimacy across distance. While a Singaporean healthcare worker built a translator app to help doctors treat foreign workers, a U.S. teenager created a tabulation app with over 40 million users that gives real-time updates on COVID-19 news sometimes months before many governments took notice of the disease. These apps demonstrate the world-building powers of networked global citizens. New digital technologies and technocultures anticipate a pandemic-accelerated knowledge economy, inclusive of rapid-response research and data collection.

Ethical questions crept up whether to allow technology to dig its tentacles deeper into our COVID-afflicted lives, such as utilizing AI to scan patients for coronavirus. In China, they were already being used for X-ray or chest tomography. Technology enthusiasts claimed that the COVID-19 pandemic forced people to become up-to-speed in a tech-based economy. The pandemic put the wheels in motion for cashless e-payments or even cryptocurrency in China, which reverted to paper bills decontaminated for coronavirus and teleconferencing to decrease carbon footprint and inaccessibility. Others gasped at the range of things sociotechnical machines could do better than humans in the pandemic.

Robots are not the evil killers of humanity or job stealers as thought. A team of mechanical automatons cared for patients in Wuhan, serving food, entertaining, and leading exercise in a "smart hospital." The robotic frontliners were remotely controlled by a human team from CloudMinds, a company with headquarters in Beijing and California. Other countries like Italy, Israel, Singapore, and Thailand relied on robots for consultations or cleaning, mitigating the risk to human healthcare workers, while Denmark nearly zeroed its infection through automated meatpacking. A roving robot dog outfitted with cameras roamed around parks, from New York to Singapore, reminding walkers to maintain physical distancing. But Amazon's subsidiary, Whole Foods, secretly upgraded its monitoring technology to squelch union activity in its supermarket stores. Through metadata from heat maps, it assigned a risk score based on machine learning algorithms.

Computing miracles in "outbreak science" led the pack in how to endure the hellfire of COVID-19. Hatched by an infectious disease expert, Blue Dot scours the planet to spit out the first warning signs of trouble, churning out reports based on global intelligence by weeding through reams of texts. Its smart machines calculated health risks based on population movements. With offices located in Canada rather than in the United States, California's governor received a tip from "real-time" data modeling and network analysis, what he called a window into the future in real-time, which is why the state locked down before anyone else. A new initiative called Defeat Disinfo—advised by the former head of U.S. forces in Afghanistan and funded by the Pentagon—set its sights on deploying AI to stop the spread of disinformation, something made worse by COVID-19 deniers. Meanwhile, current technology proved inefficient for handling logistical backlog from the pandemic. Unemployment claims and assistance checks faced bureaucratic snafus and computer glitches. The promise of technology to save us comes down to the fact that the military-industrial complex cannot be the salvation.

Global threats much like COVID-19 emerge anywhere, from earth or beyond. In 2021, U.S. intelligence agencies even declassified reports on unidentified flying objects (UFO), satiating those earthlings wishing a visit from extraterrestrials. Rather than believing the novel coronavirus was otherworldly, we can admit that COVID-19 signaled human problems coming home to roost. Until their verifiable existence is confirmed and alien overlords travel to Earth, what remains is the contest of earthly wills. No pandemic could stop or slow human violence. If "stasis is death" and the general law of the modern world, then speed becomes war, the prized form of politics.

Though COVID-19 threatened the stability of nations, the real obstacle preventing its destructive warpath was the mutual assured destruction of warring states themselves. Inasmuch as countries are forever bracing for the next military war, spending more on munitions than health, many of them found themselves incapable of responding to a "new enemy." As a Singaporean director of infectious disease initiatives observes, the United States can learn from Singapore: "During an epidemic, we fight a war against disease, and health care workers are the soldiers. Everyone must rally around their efforts."[98] This proven strategy included a fund (instantiated after SARS) to provide relief aid to victims and healthcare workers, an economic lifeline topped up with corporate donations. Even Singapore learned its protective garrison island approach could not succeed by neglecting the needs of migrant laborers. As the first country to hit 80% inoculation rate, Singapore enjoyed good company with the United Arab Emirates, Paraguay, and Israel—nations with high vaccination rates. A big question is what price do societies pay for waging an economic war on SARS-CoV-2 while battling against labor and human rights protestors?

The "people's" war on the novel coronavirus exposed the entrails of the modern war machine. It revived anachronistic schisms, putting them on display in the contretemps of today. Mali experienced back-to-back coups by the military against the civilian government, setting off a wave of regional violence that spilled over into Burkina Faso and Niger. Rival armed Islamic militias and separatist ethnic groups raised the temperature of violence, displacing millions and uprooting social institutions. The African continent experienced eight military coups in two years. The resetting of government in Chad, Guinea, and Sudan suggested we were dealing with a "coup epidemic."[99]

A pandemic requiring global unity cautions against a politics of division. But divided countries like United States barreled forward with a spectacle of suffering, the optics of which involved a revanchist fascist culture. Journalist Chris Hedges observes, "The country's infrastructure is rotting. Trump presides over a plutocratic, corrupt, cruel, authoritarian, pathological kakistocracy … Excessive military spending had left the United States incapable of attending to the basic needs of its people."[100] These same fallacies were made during the Vietnam War-era that viewed wars of aggression as "signposts on the road to ultimate victory."[101] The myth of "necessary war" leaves out struggles over scarce resources, putting humanity on a collision course with newfangled disease. COVID-19 instigated what geographer Yousuf Al-Bulushi calls the "decomposition of struggle," breaking global elements of human conflict into smaller bits for us to process.[102]

Peace fell apart further when Russia under the orders of President Vladimir Putin invaded the Ukraine in early 2022. To topple Ukraine's government and thwart its ambitions to join North Atlantic Treaty Organization and European Union, Putin's army threatened to bring World War III. The autocrat justified the "special military operation" on the invented memory of Russia as historically under threat from European nations. Building his case against Russia's fake charges of Nazi-like genocide against ethnic Russians (and viral deepfake videos of him telling soldiers to lay down arms), Ukraine's President Volodymyr Zelensky called Russia's invasion "another virus attack, another disease, by those who suffer from severe annexation and occupation of foreign lands" and arrive "like locusts."[103] The world's richest man Elon Musk allowed the Ukraine military to access Starlink, the billionaire's satellite internet service (meanwhile, Musk said he was willing to let Trump, who was banned for espousing disinformation, return to Twitter upon purchase of the company). As the first large-scale military conflict on the European continent in close to 80 years, a global pandemic almost paled in comparison to the first networked war and its toxic concoctions. Meanwhile, Trump officially moved the U.S. embassy from Tel Aviv to Jerusalem, opening more tensions in the Israel-Palestine conflict region.

Amid all the gamesmanship and wars of attrition, the swift collapse of Afghanistan's government to the Taliban after the U.S. pullout in 2021 marked the "returns of war."[104] The U.S. embassy made the recommendation to U.S. military staff and Afghan collaborators to "shelter in place" in Kabul and to hunker down at home. Nowhere to be found on the day the capital fell to the Taliban, the president of Afghanistan escaped to the United Arab Emirates supposedly with lots of cash stolen.[105] For Afghans, awaiting safe passage out of the country, the viral entanglements of war and disease meant fewer places they can find safety.

If the COVID wars exasperated by the pandemic were to be smoothed over, the offensive "war against people" must end. In late December 2022, a few days short of the New Year, China declared the end of its "Zero-COVID" measures, downgrading the management of the disease. This 180-degree reversal came after weeks of protests from citizens who finally had it after three years of quarantine. Borders were now open to travelers, and the "war on COVID" and people came to an end. But three years of near-total isolation, and the lack of efficacious Chinese vaccines meant many more deaths. Deaths were not the only mortal catastrophe that China was preparing for. In 2023, the government announced a three-child policy, fearing a drop in population due to low birth rates. Decades of the one-child policy promised to collapse the most populous country and retract the "world's factory."

A peaceful solution to this "people's war" require unveiling the hidden wizards operating behind the political economy of war. More hucksters than heroes, they operate as mere mortals who want to manipulate society. They tell us nothing about life-and-death battles that must be overcome to return "home" to places eaten away by ravages of war, disease, and terminal capitalism. As disability activist and artist Patricia Bearne comments, "We are in a global system that is incompatible with life. There is no way to stop a single gear in motion—we must dismantle this machine."[106] Speaking to the world-as-body, feminist writer Aurora Levins Morales' says antidote to disease can be found within all of our bodies:

> The heart muscles of five-star generals is distinct from ... the pancreatic tissue and intestinal tracts of Black single mothers in Detroit, of Mexicana migrants in Fresno, but no body stands outside the consequences of injustice and inequality ... If there is a map to get there, it can be found in the atlas of our skin and bone and blood, in the tracks of neurotransmitters and antibodies.

The charted path to justice hardens and fossilizes though when certain bodies are rendered as monster-like. Political scientist Sahar Ghumkhor remarked on the twentieth anniversary of the War on Terror in 2021 that the West loves its monsters as much as it loves its freedom. The War on Terror is often told like a fairytale, of Muslim women as damsels in distress, and White knights bravely fighting brutes to free them. Monsters repel as much as they fascinate, but ultimately, they mask the violence which made them.[107]

How do we fight internal demons monsters of our own creation?

These creatures cannot be defeated by regular killing machines and fake oracles pretending to predict death. Winning in a demon-haunted monstrous world involves the destruction of creation myths as historian Gerald Horne suggests in *Dawning of the Apocalypse*. The esteemed historian of slavery explains the spawn of empires repeat bloody actions from centuries before until we learn "world reconstruction." Another historian Carlos Dimas says that coronavirus-related diseases will return just like cholera always as part of a never-ending story: "The world of pathogens is continually changing. Yesterday cholera had a hold on society, and today it is a respiratory virus; tomorrow it will be something new or the reappearance of an old disease."[108] Nothing ever stays the same, but nothing comes from doing little to stop it.

How we "end" disease in a viral world depends on whether it means killing ourselves in the process. World-ending practices are part of the unflinching state-societal commitment to "mass death as a veritable norm, bloodthirstiness as a way of life."[109] A viral world of bad monsters and machines arose from COVID-19, one full of scheming mystics willing to exploit a pandemic for political gain. Another viral world is begotten from an appreciation and love for monsters, the question of how and why we use technology (and for whom), and a sense of a future based on spiritual justice. For planet experiencing a "coronapocalypse," we should not fall back on total and cruel violence. Radical solidarity with others is the answer to evil.

Notes

1 Merriam-Webster, "Apocalypse" Comes from Greek to "Uncover, Disclose, Reveal." "Apocalypse." Merriam-Webster.com Dictionary, accessed June 12, 2020, www.merriam-webster.com/dictionary/apocalypse

2 David Theo Goldberg, "Dread: The Politics of Our Time," *University of California Humanities Research Institute*, June 2018, https://uchri.org/foundry/dread-the-politics-of-our-time/

3 Mike Davis, "The Coronavirus Crisis Is a Monster Fueled by Capitalism," *In These Times*, March 20, 2020, https://inthesetimes.com/article/coronavirus-crisis-capitalism-covid-19-monster-mike-davis

4 David Brunnstrom and Daphne Psaledakis, "Pompeo Urges More Assertive Approach to 'Frankenstein' China," *Reuters*, July 23, 2020, www.usnews.com/news/world/articles/2020-07-23/pompeo-calls-for-more-assertive-response-to-frankenstein-china

5 INF News, " 'A Zombie Speaks,' Pompeo Intervened in Venezuela's Internal Affairs and Was Mercilessly Taunted by the Venezuelan Minister of Foreign Affairs," *INF News*, July 28, 2021, https://inf.news/en/world/f6f3fd211c642e90af2e34ab68ffe2fa.html#:~:text=%22dying%20to%20struggle.%22

6 It turns out gases within the decomposition led to those bodies rising to the surface. Jon Henley, "Culled Mink Rise from the Dead to Denmark's Horror," *The Guardian*, November 25, 2020, www.theguardian.com/world/2020/nov/25/culled-mink-rise-from-the-dead-denmark-coronavirus

7 Ian Liujia Tian, "Vampiric Affect: The Afterlife of a Metaphor in a Global Pandemic," *Social Text Online*, June 17, 2020, https://socialtextjournal.org/periscope_article/vampiric-affect-the-afterlife-of-a-metaphor-in-a-global-pandemic/

8 David McNally, *Monsters of the Market: Zombies, Vampires and Global Capitalism* (Leiden: Brill, 2011).

9 Paul Kennedy, *Vampire Capitalism: Fractured Societies and Alternative Futures* (New York: Springer, 2016), 99.

10 Anjuli Fatima Raza Kolb, *Epidemic Empire: Colonialism, Contagion, and Terror, 1817–2020* (Chicago: University of Chicago Press, 2021).

11 Lanai Scarr and Peter Law, "Ban Trips from Indian Hell," *The West Australia*, April 28, 2021.

12 Hyonhee Shin and Sangmi Cha, " 'Like a Zombie Apocalypse': Residents on Edge as Coronavirus Cases Surge in South Korea," *Reuters*, February 19, 2020, www.reuters.com/article/us-china-health-southkorea-cases/like-a-zombie-apocalypse-residents-on-edge-as-coronavirus-cases-surge-in-south-korea-idUSKBN20E04F

13 Lorrie Moore, "Experiencing the Coronavirus Pandemic as a Kind of Zombie Apocalypse," *The New Yorker*, April 6, 2020, www.newyorker.com/magazine/2020/04/13/the-nurses-office

14 Jeffrey Wasserstrom, "Four Masks and a Funeral on the loss of Freedoms in Hong Kong," *The American Scholar*, April 10, 2021, https://theamericanscholar.org/four-masks-and-a-funeral/

15 Lisa Marie Cacho, *Social Death: Racialized Rightlessness and the Criminalization of the Unprotected* (New York: New York University Press, 2012).

16 Orlando Patterson, *Slavery and Social Death: A Comparative Study* (Cambridge, MA: Harvard University Press, 2018).

17 Rob Nixon, *Slow Violence and the Environmentalism of the Poor* (Cambridge, MA: Harvard University Press, 2011).

18 Katherine McKittrick, "Mathematics Black Life," *The Black Scholar* 44, no. 2 (2014): 16–28.

19 Christina Sharpe, *In the Wake: On Blackness and Being* (Durham, NC: Duke University Press, 2016).

20 Saidiya Hartman, "The End of White Supremacy, An American Romance," *Bomb*, June 5, 2020, https://bombmagazine.org/articles/the-end-of-white-supremacy-an-american-romance/

21 Denise Ferreira Da Silva, *Toward a Global Idea of Race* (Minneapolis: University of Minnesota Press, 2007).

22 Denise Ferreira Da Silva, "Toward a Black Feminist Poethics: The Quest (Ion) of Blackness toward the End of the World," *The Black Scholar* 44, no. 2 (2014): 90.

23 Roxane Gay, "On the Death of Sandra Bland and Our Vulnerable Bodies," *New York Times*, July 24, 2015, www.nytimes.com/2015/07/25/opinion/on-the-death-of-sandra-bland-and-our-vulnerable-bodies.html

24 That not-yet dead sentiment drives the story of a delayed Hollywood movie that came out in 2020, called *Antebellum*, which is about an enslaved woman from the era who gets transported to present-day America.

25 Zakiyyah Iman Jackson, *Becoming Human: Matter and Meaning in an Antiblack World* (New York: New York University Press, 2020), 18.

26 Ibid, 20.

27 Michael Stone, "Christian Group Defends '2 God Fearing Men' Who Killed Ahmaud Arbery," *Patheos*, May 8, 2020, www.patheos.com/blogs/progressive secularhumanist/2020/05/christian-group-defends-2-god-fearing-men-who-kil led-ahmaud-arbery/

28 Isabella Rosario, "Jesus Was Divisive: A Black Pastor's Message to White Christian," June 12, 2020, www.npr.org/sections/codeswitch/2020/06/12/699611 293/jesus-was-divisive-a-black-pastor-s-message-to-white-christians

29 Ian Schwartz, "Eddie Glaude: 'I Overestimated White People,' I Didn't Think They Would Put Trump in Office," *Real Clear* Politics, October 31, 2018, www. realclearpolitics.com/video/2018/10/31/msnbc_eddie_glaude_i_overestimated_ white_people_i_didnt_think_they_would_put_trump_in_office.html

30 George Jackson, *Soledad Brother: The Prison Letters of George Jackson* (Chicago: Lawrence Hill Books, 1994), 265.

31 Jay Reeves, "In Clamor to Reopen, Many Black People Feel Overlooked," *AP News*, May 5, 2020, https://apnews.com/5a70d53a228265269c07a5976 4382273

32 Tom Kertscher, "People of Color May Be Immune to the Coronavirus Because of Melanin," *Politifact*, March 10, 2020, www.politifact.com/factchecks/2020/mar/ 10/facebook-posts/melanin-doesnt-protect-against-coronavirus/; Royce Dunmore, "Gov. Brian Kemp Is Slammed as Committing 'Genocide' after COVID-19 Stats on Black People Are Released," *Newsone*, April 30, 2020, https://newsone.com/ playlist/brian-kemp-slammed-genocide-covid-19-stats-black-people/

33 Tom Kertscher, "Melanin Doesn't Protect against Coronavirus," *Politifact*, March 10, 2020, www.politifact.com/factchecks/2020/mar/10/facebook-posts/melanin- doesnt-protect-against-coronavirus/

34 Dauti Kahura, "The Unforeseen Threat," Africa Is a Country, April 2, 2021, https://africasacountry.com/2021/04

35 AF Feednews, "Chinese Doctors Confirmed African Blood Genetic Composition Resist Coronavirus after Student Cured," *Af.FeedNews*, February 14, 2020, https://news-af.feednews.com/news/detail/223e120f939f8d0a06b7ce3cee653 18c?client=news

36 Mark C. Jerng, *Racial Worldmaking: The Power of Popular Fiction* (New York: Fordham Univ Press, 2017).

37 The rate of infection was four times as much in the U.K., and vaccine hesitancy was highest among BAME communities in U.K. (except when distributed by trusted ethnic or minority community sources).

38 Tiffany Willoughby-Herard, "(Political) Anesthesia or (Political) Memory: The Combahee River Collective and the Death of Black Women in Custody," *Theory & Event* 21, no.1 (2018): 259–281.

39 Chabani N. Manganyi, *Being Black in the World* (Johannesburg: Wits University Press, 2019).

40 Robin D.G. Kelley, *Freedom Dreams: The Black Radical Imagination* (Boston: Beacon Press, 2002), 10.

41 Ebony Elizabeth Thomas, *The Dark Fantastic: Race and the Imagination from Harry Potter to the Hunger Games* (New York: New York University Press, 2019), 74.

42 Ruth Wilson Gilmore, "Fatal Couplings of Power and Difference: Notes on Racism and Geography," *The Professional Geographer* 54, no. 1 (2002): 15–24.

43 Dahlia Schweitzer, *Going Viral: Zombies, Viruses, and the End of the World* (New Brunswick: Rutgers University Press, 2019).

44 Lauren Aratani, "'Coughing while Asian': Living in Fear as Racism Feeds Off Coronavirus Panic," *The Guardian*, March 24, 2020, www.theguardian.com/world/2020/mar/24/coronavirus-us-asian-americans-racism

45 Nidesh Lawtoo, *Conrad's Shadow: Catastrophe, Mimesis, Theory* (Lansing, MI: Michigan State University Press, 2016).

46 Joanna Zylinska, *The End of Man: A Feminist Counterapocalypse* (Minneapolis: University of Minnesota Press, 2018).

47 Salvador Elias Zárate, "Invisible Bodies, Devalued Labor: Contract, Reproductive Labor, and the US Sunbelt, 1900-1963" (PhD diss., University of California San Diego, 2017), 19.

48 Oli Smith, "Coronavirus Horror: Social Media Footage Shows Infected Wuhan Residents 'Act Like Zombies': Disturbing Footage Emerged Overnight Showing People Collapsing in the Street in Wuhan, China, as They Quickly Succumb to the Deadly Coronavirus," *Express*, January 24, 2020, www.express.co.uk/news/world/1232814/Coronavirus-horror-China-virus-Wuhan-zombies-epidemic-video

49 Veronica Gomez-Temesio, "Outliving Death: Ebola, Zombies, and the Politics of Saving Lives," *American Anthropologist* 120, no. 4 (2018): 745, 748.

50 Indigenous Action, "Rethinking the Apocalypse: An Indigenous Anti-Futurist Manifesto," *Indigenous Action*, March 19, 2020, www.indigenousaction.org/rethinking-the-apocalypse-an-indigenous-anti-futurist-manifesto

51 Marisa Elena Duarte, *Network Sovereignty: Building the Internet across Indian Country* (Seattle: University of Washington Press, 2017), 144.

52 Brooke Sopelsa, "Trump Cabinet's Bible Teacher Says Gays Cause 'God's Wrath' in COVID-19 Blog Post," *NBC News*, March 25, 2020, www.nbcnews.com/feature/nbc-out/trump-s-bible-teacher-says-gays-among-those-blame-covid-n1168981

53 Lorenzo Bernini, *Queer Apocalypses: Elements of Antisocial Theory* (New York: Springer, 2016).

54 Jacques Prieur. "Critical Warning! Preventing the Multidimensional Apocalypse on Planet Earth," *Ecosystem Services* 45 (2020): 101161.

55 David Isaacs, "Apocalypse Perhaps," *Journal of Paediatrics and Child Health* 56, no. 8 (2020): 1169.

56 Jakob Krause-Jensen and Keir Martin, "Trickster's Triumph: Donald Trump and the New Spirit of Capitalism," *Magical Capitalism* (New York: Palgrave Macmillan, 2018), 89–113.

57 A Department of Defense advisor and former undersecretary of defense for policy resigned from the military's science board.

58 Matthew Teague, "'He Wears the Armor of God': Evangelicals Hail Trump's Church Photo Op," *The Guardian*, June 3, 2020, www.theguardian.com/us-news/2020/jun/03/donald-trump-church-photo-op-evangelicals

59 Ben Collins, "How QAnon Rode the Pandemic to New Heights—and Fueled the Viral Anti-Mask Phenomenon," *NBC News*, August 14, 2020, www.nbcnews.com/tech/tech-news/how-qanon-rode-pandemic-new-heights-fueled-viral-anti-mask-n1236695

60 Matthew Rozsa, "QAnon Is the Conspiracy Theory that Won't Die: Here's What They Believe, and Why They're Wrong," *Salon*, August 18, 2019, www.salon.com/2019/08/18/qanon-is-the-conspiracy-theory-that-wont-die-heres-what-they-believe-and-why-theyre-wrong/

61 Carlie Porterfield, "Two-Thirds of Religious Americans Believe Coronavirus Is a Message from God," *Forbes*, May 15, 2020, www.forbes.com/sites/carlieporterfield/2020/05/15/two-thirds-of-religious-americans-believe-coronavirus-is-a-message-from-god/#446e7cbea2ae

62 Sebastian Kettley, "Coronavirus in the Bible: Preacher Warns of 'Apocalyptic Signs' as 'End of World Nears,'" *Express*, March 17, 2020, www.express.co.uk/news/weird/1256517/Coronavirus-bible-end-of-the-world-warning-COVID19-apocalypse-latest-coronavirus-news

63 Julie Zauzmer and Sarah Pulliam Bailey, "This Is Not the End of the World, According to Christians Who Study the End of the World," *Washington Post*, March 17, 2020, www.washingtonpost.com/religion/2020/03/17/not-end-of-the-world-coronavirus-bible-prophecy/

64 Bryan S. Turner, "Theodicies of the COVID-19 Catastrophe." *COVID-19: Volume I: Global Pandemic, Societal Responses, Ideological Solutions*, ed. by Michael J. Ryan (London: Routledge 2020), 29–42.

65 Franklin Briceño, "In Peru, Thousands of Faces at Mass—None Now Alive," *Associated Press*, June 14, 2020, https://news.yahoo.com/peru-thousands-faces-mass-none-195417788.html

66 Kejal Vyas, "Cow Dung, Garlic and a Prayer: The Fight against Phony Cures for Coronavirus," *Wall Street Journal*, April 7, 2020, www.wsj.com/amp/articles/cow-dung-garlic-and-a-prayer-the-fight-against-phony-cures-for-coronavirus-11586257200

67 Francesca Melandri, "A Letter from Locked Down Italy: This Is What We Know about Your Future," *Portside*, April 8, 2020, https://portside.org/2020-04-08/letter-locked-down-italy-what-we-know-about-your-future

68 John Blake, "Coronavirus Is Bringing a Plague of Dangerous Doomsday Predictions," *CNN*, March 23, 2020, www.cnn.com/2020/03/22/world/doomsday-prophets-coronavirus-blake/index.html

69 Don Miguel Ruiz and Janet Mills, *The Four Agreements (Illustrated Edition): A Practical Guide to Personal Freedom* (Carlsbad, CA: Hay House Inc., 2011), 2.

70 Ibid., 16. Ancient Toltec prophecies foretold a future age defined by all wisdom returning to the people, a state of happiness where sacred traditions around the world are unified across communities, time, nations, and families.

71 FR24 News, "'No One Wanted to Read' His Book on Pandemic Psychology—then Covid Hit," *FR24 News*, August 19, 2021, FR24 News, www.fr24news.com/a/2021/08/no-one-wanted-to-read-his-book-on-pandemic-psychology-then-covid-hit.html

72 Arundhati Roy, "'The Pandemic Is a Portal,'" *Financial Times*, April 3, 2020, www.ft.com/content/10d8f5e8-74eb-11ea-95fe-fcd274e920ca

73 Bil Browning, "Evangelical Christians Are Linking LGBTQ People to the Coronavirus Now," *LGBTQ Nation*, March 6, 2020, www.lgbtqnation.com/2020/03/evangelical-christians-linking-lgbtq-people-coronavirus-now/

74 Brooke Sopelsa, "Trump Cabinet's Bible Teacher Says Gays Cause 'God's Wrath' in COVID-19 Blog Post," *NBC News*, March 25, 2020, www.nbcnews.com/feature/nbc-out/trump-s-bible-teacher-says-gays-among-those-blame-covid-n1168981; Ewan Palmer, "Church Leader Who Blamed Coronavirus on Gay Marriage Contracts COVID-19," *Newsweek*, September 8, 2020, www.newsweek.com/patriarch-filaret-coronavirus-gay-marriage-ukraine-1530261

75 Jessie Hellmann, "Cuomo Reports Another 731 Coronavirus Deaths in NY, Its Largest One-Day Increase," *The Hill*, April 7, 2020, https://thehill.com/policy/healthcare/491553-cuomo-reports-731-coronavirus-deaths-in-the-state-its-largest-one-day

76 Natalia Molina, *How Race Is Made in America: Immigration, Citizenship, and the Historical Power of Racial Scripts* (Berkeley: University of California Press, 2013).

77 Matthew Bell, "This Apocalyptic Korean Christian Group Goes by Different Names. Critics Say It's Just a Cult," *The World*, July 11, 2017, www.pri.org/stories/2017-07-11/apocalyptic-korean-christian-group-goes-different-names-critics-say-its-just-cult?amp

78 Justin McCurry, "How South Korea's Evangelical Churches Found Themselves at the Heart of the Covid Crisis," *The Guardian*, August 23, 2020, www.theguardian.com/world/2020/aug/23/how-south-koreas-evangelical-churches-found-themselves-at-the-heart-of-the-covid-crisis

79 Daniel Villarreal, "South Korea Threatens to Out LGBTQ People after 86 Coronavirus Cases Linked to Gay Clubs," *LGBTQ Nation*, May 11, 2020, www.lgbtqnation.com/2020/05/south-korea-threatens-lgbtq-population-86-coronavirus-cases-linked-gay-clubs/

80 Jason Strother, "South Korea's Coronavirus Contact Tracing Puts LGBTQ Community under Surveillance, Critics Say," *WUNC91.5 North Carolina Public Radio*, May 22, 2020, www.unc.org/post/south-korea-s-coronavirus-contact-tracing-puts-lgbtq-community-under-surveillance-critics-say

81 The Associated Press, "China Bans Effeminate Men from TV," *NPR*, September 2, 2021, www.npr.org/2021/09/02/1033687586/china-ban-effeminate-men-tv-official-morality

82 For a history of these terms as it applies to Asians and race, see Long T. Bui, *Model Machines: A History of the Asian as Automaton* (Philadelphia: Temple University Press, 2022).

83 William Hardy McNeill, *Plagues and Peoples* (Garden City, NY: Anchor, 1998), 62.

84 Ajit Singh, "Hong Kong's 'Pro-Democracy' Movement Allies with Far-Right US Politicians That Seek to Crush Black Lives Matter," *The Gray Zone*, June 9, 2020, https://thegrayzone.com/2020/06/09/hong-kongs-far-right-us-politicians-crush-black-lives-matter

85 Shibani Mahtani, "Boris Johnson Offers Refuge, British Citizenship Path for Nearly 3 Million Hong Kongers," *Washington Post*, June 3, 2020, www.washingtonpost.com/world/asia_pacific/boris-johnson-hong-kong-national-security-law-bno-passport/2020/06/03/3ec6ddf0-a545-11ea-b619-3f9133bbb482_story.html

86 Lisa Lowe, *The Intimacies of Four Continents* (Durham, NC: Duke University Press, 2015).

87 Marco Rubio (@Marcorubio), "#China's Consulate in #Houston Is Not a Diplomatic Facility. It Is the Central Node of the Communist Party's Vast Network of Spies & Influence Operations in the United States. Now That Building Must Close & the Spies Have 72 Hours to Leave or Face Arrest," *Twitter*, July 22, 2020, 5:45 am, https://twitter.com/marcorubio/status/1285909840192315395?

88 Philippine Daily Inquirer, "Knee on the National Neck," *Philippine Daily Inquirer*, June 3, 2020, https://opinion.inquirer.net/130416/knee-on-the-natio nal-neck

89 Yossi Melman, "Coronavirus 'Truce': The Guns Falling Silent across the Middle East," *Haaretz*, March 16, 2020, www.haaretz.com/middle-east-news/.prem ium-coronavirus-truce-the-guns-falling-silent-across-the-middle-east-1.8677993

90 B'Tselem, "During the Coronavirus Crisis, Israel Confiscates Tents Designated for Clinic in the Northern West Bank," *B'Tselem: The Israeli Information Center for Human Rights in the Occupied Territories*, March 26, 2020, www.btselem. org/press_release/20200326_israel_confiscates_clinic_tents_during_coronavirus _crisis

91 Donald Judd, Maegan Vazquez and Donie O'Sullivan, "Biden Says Platforms Like Facebook Are 'Killing People' with Covid Misinformation," *CNN*, July 17, 2021, www.cnn.com/2021/07/16/politics/biden-facebook-covid-19/index.html

92 Ethiopia experienced its words violence in decades with over 200 dead when ethnic Amhara were killed in an attack in the country's Oromia region by rebel groups.

93 United Nations, "COVID-19: UN Chief Calls for Global Ceasefire to Focus on 'the True Fight of Our Lives' " *UN News*, March 23, 2020, https://news.un.org/ en/story/2020/03/1059972

94 William Robinson, *Global Civil War: Capitalism Post-Pandemic* (Oakland: PM Press, 2022).

95 Matthew Chalmers, "Why Hack the World's Largest Meat Company?" *Sentient Media*, June 4, 2021, https://sentientmedia.org/why-hack-the-worlds-largest-meat-company/

96 Facebook did take down Trump's campaign ads that asked people to respond to an official district census linked to his campaign website.

97 Vijay Prashad, "The Great Contest of Our Time Is between Humanity and Imperialism," Thetricontinental.org, July 29, 2021, https://thetricontinental.org/ newsletterissue/30-new-cold-war/?output=pdf

98 Li Yang Hsu and Min-Han Tan, "What Singapore Can Teach the U.S. about Responding to Covid-19," *Stat News*, March 23, 2020, www.statnews.com/ 2020/03/23/singapore-teach-united-states-about-covid-19-response/

99 Álvaro Escalonilla, "The Return of Africa's Strongmen," *Atalayar*, May 27, 2022, https://atalayar.com/en/content/return-africas-strongmen

100 Chauncey Devega, "Pulitzer Winner Chris Hedges: These 'Are the Good Times— Compared to What's Coming Next,' " *Salon*, April 28, 2020, www.salon.com/ 2020/04/28/pulitzer-winner-chris-hedges-these-are-the-good-times--compared-to-whats-coming-next/?fbclid=IwAR01lqVj1dqLtTXIJ--xOdI45D1-N0Q93hsE oTKcesjrDf9A1kqZ0vbwNQY

101 Chris Hedges, *War Is a Force That Gives Us Meaning* (New York: Anchor, 2003).

102 Al-Bulushi, Yousuf. "The Global Threat of Race in the Decomposition of Struggle," *Safundi* 21, no. 2 (2020): 140–165.

103 Sky news, "We've Been Attacked by Another Virus," *Skynews*, March 3, 2022, https://news.sky.com/video/weve-been-attacked-by-another-virus-president-zelenskyy-says-ukraine-will-continue-to-stand-against-russian-aggression-in-address-to-the-nation-12556467

104 Long T. Bui, *Returns of War: South Vietnam and the Price of Refugee Memory* (New York: New York University Press, 2018).

105 CNBC, "Ousted Afghan President Ashraf Ghani Resurfaces in UAE after Fleeing Kabul, Emirati Government says," August 18, 2021, www.cnbc.com/2021/08/18/afghan-president-ashraf-ghani-is-in-uae-after-fleeing-afghanistan.html

106 Patty Berne, "Disability Justice—a Working Draft," *Sins Invalid*, June 9, 2015, www.sinsinvalid.org/blog/disability-justice-a-working-draft-by-patty-berne

107 Sahar Ghumkhor, Anila Daulatzai, "Monsters, Inc: The Taliban as Empire's Bogeyman," *Aljazeera*, August 18, 2021, www.aljazeera.com/opinions/2021/8/18/monsters-inc-the-taliban-as-empires-bogeyman

108 Carlos S. Dimas, *Poisoned Eden: Cholera Epidemics, State-Building, and the Problem of Public Health in Tucumán, Argentina, 1865–1908* (Lincoln, NE: University of Nebraska Press, 2022).

109 Gerald Horne, *The Dawning of the Apocalypse: The Roots of Slavery, White Supremacy, Settler Colonialism, and Capitalism in the Long Sixteenth Century* (New York: Monthly Review Press, 2020), 11.

EPILOGUE

Planet, Poverty, Pedagogy

Like an incredible time machine, COVID-19 tells of worlds fantasized and realized, those dimensions deteriorated and rebuilt. Postmodern diseases, such as this illness, represent global relations which are viral and require us to piece together the different puzzle pieces of information that circulate among persons, groups, and nations. Unbundling the vagaries of a pandemic can explain what the future might hold in a "post-COVID world" or even a "permanent pandemic."[1] Fatalistic types declared humanity would never recover from something like as it marked a descent into the unknown—the onset of the Great Fall of civilization. Others registered the event as the "new normal," something we all must become used to as there is no way to reverse course or change tack. Once the initial crush from this pandemic settled, a corona-struck world found itself uncertain about the future. Many pined for a past that never existed, plugging right back into a naïve state of innocence. To *not* repeat history, AIDS activist Larry Kramer posits that we need more than interventions but inter-visions: "This is always history's greatest failure, its inability to believe what it sees, what, almost always, someone sees."[2]

We can say the pandemic opened new vistas for understanding a viral world by giving groups, nations, and everyday people a chance to converse together at the same time about the state of the world. It asked how to carve out new directions for the planet and how to take action in it, accordingly, with love rather than hate. This pandemic orientation is a politicized form of world-making that allows us to reimagine our place within viral worlds, both real and imagined.

World-building informs the ways our viral humans move through time and space, how we express new sensations and relationships to the social world(s) around us. Feminist scientist Donna Haraway's calls for a worlding

DOI: 10.4324/9781032694535-8

that "stays with the trouble," where people (and nonhuman actors) virally carry "meanings and materials across kinds in order to infect processes and practices that might yet ignite epidemics of multispecies recuperation."[3] As evident with the pandemic, the power of viral truth-telling serves to protect us from the dangerous "virus of transnational politics."[4] The delivery of freedom and liberation to all leads back to the political philosophy of the Zapatistas: *Creemos en un mundo que cabe muchos mundos* (we believe in a world that fits many worlds). This phenomenon fits what I deem as viral worlding and how we are making new worlds on this planet.

This epilogue offers some concluding thoughts about what COVID-19 means for the planet, the increased poverty due to the problem, and the promise of planetary liberation. It provides an example of how the COVID-19 pandemic inspired a student strike at my own university, and how student activists made plans for mutual aid societies. It quotes poetry from writers and words from activists to drive home the paradox that we are part of an emergent viral world that is really old in many ways. To emphasize the virality of the world means returning to the Ebola crisis in West Africa. That health crisis of international concern bore far-reaching implications, one that few noticed until COVID-19 forced social observers to reflect on all the "smaller" signs of a global danger. This epilogue harkens back to all the themes brought up in previous chapters. It concludes with a wish for a better world or new/old worlds, a future dream collectively shared through viral thoughts.

Planet

Viral World centers on the interplay of worldly power, desire, knowledge, and imagination, all which gain force under a snowballing pandemic. The history-making COVID-19 carried the signature of something that would take long to digest—even if people have started to forget it already. It marked a "new" viral moment haunted by remnants of pandemics past. If there is one constant from the conversation about this pandemic and its quicksand moments, it is that this "brave new world" needed to be rid of a craven oppressive one. Earthlings who strike out against impossible odds to restore planetary balance will still find plenty of things wrong, inexorable problems brewing without a magical solution. This critical perspective remains necessary to transcend perpetual crisis mode and pushing full steam against an "invisible enemy." Seeing can lead sometimes to believing, even if privilege of sight relies on maps "printed with the blood of history."[5]

Instead of falling for perverse apocalyptic tales, we can read the written word of Mvskoke (Creek) writer, Joy Harjo. In the poem "Our Map to the Next World," the Native poet writes how we all must take our path together through the "membrane of death" to discover that "we were never perfect."

To eviscerate the monsters of rage and altars of money that have sprung in the modern age, Harjo instructs the soul wanderer to "take your next breath" before entering the road of knowledge. This spiraling place she describes as containing no beginning and exit, a place where "once we knew everything."

We can definitively say and admit COVID-19 changed everything. But little scraps of insight, which can be useful for future planning, are born under a perfidious pandemic. Insofar as COVID-19 made it seem we were all on the same lifeboat together, luxury cruise ships stranded by the pandemic gave reminders that passengers occupied different cabin classes. Pandemic politics of "the armed lifeboat" was predicated on protecting some people to the exclusion of others deemed unworthy of it.[6] Tourism and other industries needed to be "socialized."[7]

COVID-19 exploded myths of a unified humanity or even *humanitas*, the educated ideal of human behavior and decency in public life. Radical claims to democracy and decolonization were held back, but violent clamors for change from below rose from the undercommons. As French-Tunisian critic Albert Memmi (who died in 2020) once observed, "Colonized society is a diseased society … its century-hardened face has become nothing more than a mask under which it slowly smothers and dies."[8] Face masks are a textile extension of "digital viral worlds" composed of ableisms, otherings, and fascist coalitions.[9] Using masks simply then to protect "the public" from disease cannot satisfy the deep craving for political freedom and social transformation, especially when things like the face mask are so thoroughly politicized. The long quest for collective protection feels true to a pandemic-ready axiom from poet Maya Angelou that became popular again with political activists: "Do the best you can until you know better." Improving requires a deconstruction of false thinking that accompanies false universals. It is near impossible to survive a pandemic without an appreciation of the gravitas of it all.

As heavy as it was, COVID-19 was no isolated story in time. It was a sad paean to bad decisions that had done previously, shaking up old human wiring and hubris that we have beheld many a time before. As the pandemic made glaring, the center cannot hold, because there was no middle ground to begin with. No golden age of prosperity came before the novel coronavirus, whose long shadow hung over capitalist militarized societies in terminal decline, especially those countries steeped in structures of domination, denialism, and destruction. Under the pandemic's long haul, fallacies and misdeeds were brought forward to underwrite a tale with surprising contortions, a tragicomedy of errors. Planting the seeds of change can move us forward toward political revolution. In such times, the "viral truth" is preferable to running things into the ground based on viral lies. Without bold action, we shrink caring capacity and our social efficacy. Coronavirus countermeasures enabled some humans to deprogram themselves from greed and nihilism, casting off the fetters of a "survival of the fittest" mindset, even as it emboldens others to kill fellow humans. The viral "world" has to be remade again and again for the sake of justice.

From the pandemic response came the sight of human beings making sense of their viralized environs. Warlords used the pandemic to lord over their fiefdoms and make life even more miserable, but the common people made good use of this time to mobilize. Their collective actions resisted the evil cloud placed over the "coronapocalypse"—a curse that awakened all sorts of incantations and make-believe. From this karmic cycle, humanity seemed to ascend toward another plane of global consciousness, a testament to how the pandemic inverted the narrow purview of living without consequence.

Poor people suffered from a disease that the rich benefitted from and exploited. But from a pandemic ecology of mind, we discovered "what can be studied is always a relationship or an infinite regress of relationships. Never a 'thing'."[10] Rather than just being a thing that merely exists, COVID-19 was a product of global health relations that went viral, both in negative and positive ways. One of the positives is forcing governments to tackle the economic poverty that formed a barrier to vaccination and virus prevention, while the negative is the deepening poverty.

Poverty

Lacking the resources of wealthier nations, smaller countries made do with what they could to deal with the global crisis. So conjoined were they to a viralized world, Zimbabweans declared a national emergency with one case of COVID-19, while Malawi did so with none. A few months after the Ebola announcement, the World Health Organization (WHO) declared COVID-19 an international health emergency before it was declared a pandemic two months later.[11] In February 2020, with other countries obsessing over the new coronavirus, the Democratic Republic of Congo along with Burundi, Ghana, and Zambia licensed an Ebola vaccine in their battle with another pandemic. A health crisis does not need to be of enlarged scope to receive initial consideration as a serious issue. In summer 2019, WHO declared the Ebola outbreak in the Congo a public health emergency of international concern (PHEIC). That it broke out in one country was enough to declare it a problem worth the coordination, funding, and attention of multiple states. A lack of infrastructure and funding gaps in the WHO made this a global fight against Ebola.

Early pandemic predictions arrived from global health experts and philanthrocapitalists like Microsoft founder Bill Gates who believed that COVID-19 would be a total disaster in Africa, due to its poor medical infrastructure and economies. Instead of believing Africans could defy the odds, this troublesome narrative slipped easily into "colonial narratives of Black inferiority and the inability of Black nations to govern themselves at all."[12] But the experience of Uganda, Liberia, and Sierra Leone with contact tracing from Ebola proved invaluable in preventing disaster from happening. These lessons enabled the first contact tracing for COVID-19 in the United States by nonprofits after the African disease-prevention model, one institutionalized by the Africa Medical Supplies Platform (AMSP). Member states took action to buy medical equipment in bulk at a cheap rate. With their tens of millions of people, Ghana and Senegal registered no more than 2,000 COVID-19 deaths each (September 2023). On the score of effective planning, their stellar successes were imperceptible by the so-called West, used to perceiving Africa as a constellation of failing poor states instead of powerhouses that can meet pandemics head-on.

Viral worlds authored by pandemics will continue to take shape. They will do so long as the privileged hold steady in their selfish tendencies, permanently in thrall to well-trod corridors instead of traversing unfamiliar ones. Real solutions for a world on the ropes require feats of imagination. When the next pandemic comes, and it surely will, it will throw up old and new questions. Few people could have predicted or anticipated such a pandemic of this scale, one that could hold leaders to account. The artifice of modern societies cracked open to reveal a viral world(ing) in which the boundaries between subject and environment, persona and placeness (topos) became porous as a matter of viral communication and being.

COVID-19 bore down upon economic systems running on market-based rationales. Whole industries like education or medicine needed to be rebooted, and professionals transformed into tele-workers overnight. There was never any backup plan to these episodic moments of pandemic disorientation. The global relations that emerged from the pandemic provided more than a smokescreen to cover up the senescent moments of fraying global orders that did not work (and never did work) for everyone. There was no coming back "on track" when "this thing is over." In a system designed to benefit a privileged few, most people flailed in the uncharted territory of a viral storm and the dawning of a new viral age.[13] *Who* works and *where* does work fall? Why do "functioning" societies fall out-of-sync? What worked or did nothing appear to be "working" before COVID-19? When all facets of society burst wide open, leaving a trail of death, how does one retrace lost steps to avert disaster?

A time with no disease where everyone is protected from illness appears almost like a distant dream. What is not yet possible comes out of disenchantment with modern lifestyles and an awakening to a viral world and its worldings. Viruses are timeless, but the *political antibodies* developed in response allow for enduring an "all-living" reality. An opportunity to pool together "funds of knowledge" and develop communities of learned care can make a world of difference. COVID-19 was the world-altering event that will change all of us, both exploding and reinforcing existing social divides. Connecting people who were "worlds apart," it gave a roadmap to (other) worldly justice and new global futurities.[14] Beyond the pessimistic idea that people cannot adapt to the times since our days are numbered, the COVID-19 story (or stories) retread the familiar question of who gets protected first, who is best to solve the problem, and who is ultimately in charge of this world?

Apart from the gambit to sacrifice a few to save the rest, human pandemic responses strayed far from the usual health crisis to consider how the ends justify the means. One perennial question throughout the pandemic pivoted around who could access social services and medical treatment. Modern societies erected on economic unfairness and contentious power plays totter on shaky bearings that a new entrant like COVID-19 can exploit. In the media, feats of heroism by the working classes or "frontliners" weighed against the pusillanimity of capitalist elites. The latter fled to opulent safe houses and decamping in remote "disaster bunkers"—while still being served by service workers.

The pandemic touched those most burdened by caste or station in life. Poverty shall trouble these solutions for the foreseeable future, but not eradicating it will spell disaster on the order of a full-blown pandemic. With commodity chains working in sync with supply-side "coronavirus chains," poverty reduction and communion with animals will bring some solutions to a non-singular crisis.

The pandemic's vertical integration of global inequalities provoked a series of cascading *poly-crises*. This moment-to-moment crisis touched on a "multiscalar toxicity."[15] On the same day as the electoral college voted to decisively pick Joe Biden for President and the COVID-19 death count blew past 300,000, Sandra Lindsay took the first vaccine jab in the arm to proclaim,

> I would like to thank all the frontline workers, all my colleagues who have been doing a yeoman's job to fight this pandemic all over the world … I hope this marks the beginning of the end of a very painful time in our history.[16]

This quote from a Black woman medical worker speaks volumes about the kind of vulnerable people who are at the frontlines of a sick planet.

As big as it was, the pandemic pointed to something bigger. When in spring 2021, states began lifting quarantine restrictions, the United States fell under a national terrorist alert, warning that civilians could be targets for extremists. In 2020, the compensation fund set up to pay survivors of 9/11 terrorist attacks was amended to include COVID-related deaths. A whole sense of terror, alongside new bodily knowledge, and other ways of being arrived with death on the horizon.

Global relations are at a proverbial crossroads. Even more so under the scythe of a novel coronavirus and a "viral world" swept in its path. The tattered remains of human civilization are built on imperial ruins and corporate spoils that have reaped so much misery, but there remains hope for change. Despite the temporary sight of vacant city streets and closed schools as well as empty malls, overrun hospitals, refugee camps, and crowded prisons never lacked for signs of a better world. Half-baked pandemic measures that put the environment and social justice as secondary to "the economy" or politics will never do. How will future generations remember this pandemic? A critical pedagogy is in order for this remembrance.

Pedagogy

The *force majeure* of COVID-19 shattered any fantasy of boundless human mastery. Cobbling together creative genius and collective wisdom, people began to write their "coronavirus diaries." Whether in fictional form or social media *testimonios*, this living archive comprised a story about futurity, but one built on precarity—viral worldings based on the practice of "spiral retelling."[17] Futurists and economists attempted to predict the future, publishing rush-to-print books and tracts in record speed. Fortune-telling scribes could probably have predicated the political fall of New York's governor Andrew Cuomo, who fought hard against Trump over ventilators for COVID-19 patients. The "Prince of Darkness," as he was called, stepped down from power after sexual harassment allegations, ushering in the state's first female executive. Political heroes proved to be false gods fell by their own sword.

Doomscrolling on social media became ceaseless given the bombardment of COVID-19-related information. Jolted by 24-hour news and conspiracy yarns, people told their own stories through microblogging, vlogging, crowdsourcing, and creative writing. Pandemic memes went viral with messages of solidarity, while wrong information about the virus disorienting consumers. Dogged by "COVID is fake" memes, these false murmurs became grist for the mill of corona-conspiracies that said we reached the end of the world. Jair Bolsonaro claimed his athletic past meant he himself would not be adversely affected. In a national address, the president of Brazil boasted how Brazilians are granted natural immunity by virtue of being Brazilian. Using race-purity language not dissimilar from Burma's leaders claiming their people's fine fitness and diet could deter COVID-19, the president claimed, "90 percent of us will have no symptoms if contaminated" since the Brazilian "doesn't catch anything … Nothing happens to him. I think a lot of people were already infected in Brazil, weeks or months ago, and they already have the antibodies that help it not proliferate."[18] In a hard time which necessitated hard data and science, the old language of anti-communism, nationalism, and the pseudoscience of race once again resurfaced.

But everything returns to form in a rebounding of time as when in 2023 Luiz Inácio "Lula" Da Silva overcame a second round of tight elections to defeat Bolsonaro to win the presidency again. While one might attribute the success to another "pink wave" boomerang in Brazil, it shows how the mishandling of a pandemic by leaders brought consequences. COVID-19 was the teacher, and we were its students. The velocity of human activity and the Anthropocene found its coefficient in the pandemic's volition and the voraciousness of a virus.

With college students scattered over the earthly plane, education shifted over to remote online learning. From Costa Rica to Iran, college student protesters and professors fought university policies that clamped down on free speech and academic freedom. With the footprints of the novel coronavirus everywhere, the "distributed university" where learning and protest can happen anywhere was now in full effect. At my home university, the status of international and poor unsheltered students was left in the lurch. On pace with other school closures, the school found it wise to shutter its doors against COVID-19, but it did so scarcely a week after graduate students agitated for cost-of-living adjustment through wildcat strikers.

The shutdown and immediate move to online classes threw a curveball to student strikes that were already in full swing. With plans afoot to withhold grades and hurt the status quo, student activists altered the course of plan as campuses sought to close for the rest of the year. Student researchers decided to unionize and strike. The pandemic did not put a stop to the political work of college students, who initiated a social welfare strike. Catapulted into quick action, they took care of one another, while funneling aid for campus workers and centering community needs. Pandemic pedagogy and real education in social justice involve fighting for and maintaining human relations in a viral world.

A prompt shift by universities toward "distance teaching" led worried educators to speculate if this pandemic was the excuse to digitize all classes and hire more adjunct part-time professors. Fears of casualization of labor are not without merit. The administration of University of Illinois—while everyone was away observing social distancing protocols—surreptitiously passed policies that upped student health premiums by one-third, hiked up the president's salary, and refused sick days to employees testing positive for COVID-19. In January 2020, service union workers at the University of California, like food service, parking attendants, custodial workers, landscapers, received a not-so-great contract after a long dispute with administrators over jobs from being outsourced to part-time private contractors. The University approved tuition hikes at a time when people were losing their jobs.

Students initiated a class action lawsuit against universities for their epic failure to teach in a fungible, humane manner without contingent labor and high student fees. Agitation against "death-by-debt" matched the fury of "die-in" protests at reopened universities experiencing high infection rates. From the pandemic's rubble, student activists staked out a viral spirit of protest. Despite the pandemic's twisting global relations, these protests were making our worlds breathable and livable again.

Viral World: Global Relations during the COVID-19 Pandemic diagnosed the compulsive actions and relations that accompanied a debilitating disease and its accompanying pandemic. COVID-19's winding pathways were the capillaries of viral "co-presence," dragging communities, nations, and governments into accountability. Global lockdown held people in place to be fully present, while hurling them toward the next stage of life development.

Viral World makes evident the ways people have pushed against the closure of their lifeworlds by states and corporations, offering examples that bespeak the infectious viral energy of people power: Workers mobilizing strikes to push for a post-pandemic socialist world, citizens under state lockdown putting out songs to the world to fight the communist government, or promoting theories that COVID-19 was a Western disease to critique colonialism. Ours was a viral worlding, where information about the novel coronavirus fell into a web of lies and deceit as well as imaginative agendas for minoritized groups. As a portent to collective futurities built on trust, the COVID-19 crisis is what happens to societies caught up in the rapture of denial and destruction as well as love and solidarity. It is not hard to fathom what seemed implausible when we shake off commitment to our loved ones, our bodies, our neighbors, because to do so would mean killing ourselves and the world(s) we live in. Released from the rigid jaws and politics of COVID-19 death-making, we as worldmakers can finally deal with this pandemic and the many more to come on our terms.

Notes

1 Justi E.H. Smith, "Permanent Pandemic," *Harpers*, September 2023, https://harpers.org

2 Larry Kramer, *The American People: Volume 1: Search for My Heart: A Novel* (New York: Macmillan, 2015), 341.

3 See Donna J. Haraway, *Staying with the Trouble: Making Kin in the Chthulucene* (Durham, NC: Duke University Press, 2016), 29.

4 Ibid., 268.

5 Joy Harjo, *How We Became Human: New and Selected Poems: 1975–2001* (New York: W.W. Norton and Company, 2002), 129–132.

6 Ajay Singh Chaudhary, "We're Not in This Together," *The Baffler*, April 2020, https://thebaffler.com/salvos/were-not-in-this-together-chaudhary

7 Freya Higgins-Desbiolles, *Socialising Tourism for Social and Ecological Justice after COVID-19* (London: Routledge, 2021).

8 Albert Memmi, *The Colonizer and the Colonized* (London: Routledge, 2013), 143–144.

9 Pinar Tuzcu and Loren Britton, "Witnessing Fabrics: How Face Masks Change Social Perceptions during the Covid-19 Pandemic in Digital Times," in *Covid, Crisis, Care, and Change?: International Gender Perspectives on Re/Production, State and Feminist Transitions*, eds. Antonia Kupfer and Constanze Stutz (Toronto: Verlag Barbara Budrich. 2022), 180.

10 Gregory Bateson, *Steps to an Ecology of Mind* (New York: Ballantine, 1972), 249.

11 With a near 90% mortality rate, Ebola, also known as Ebola hemorrhagic fever (EHF), portents a gruesome end to its victims.

12 Karen Attiah, "Africa Has Defied the Covid-19 Nightmare Scenarios. We Shouldn't Be Surprised," *Washington Post*, September 22, 2020, www.washingtonpost.com/opinions/2020/09/22/africa-has-defied-covid-19-nightmare-scenarios-we-shouldnt-be-surprised/

13 Nathan Wolfe, *The Viral Storm: The Dawn of a New Pandemic Age* (New York: Macmillan, 2011).

14 Long T. Bui, "Global Futurities: Articulating the Collective Struggle for (Other) worldly Justice," *New Global Studies* (2024).

15 Olmos, Daniel. "Unsung Heroes or Exploited Workers? Latino Migrant Day Laborers in Post-Harvey Houston and Critical Environmental Justice," *Resilience: A Journal of the Environmental Humanities* 9, no. 2 (2022): 46–62.

16 ABC News, "NY Nurse Sandra Lindsay Is First in US to Get COVID-19 Vaccine after FDA Authorization," *ABC News*, December 14, 2020, https://abc7.com/covid-vaccine-pfizer-sandra-lindsay-first/8768796/

17 Édouard Glissant, *Poetics of Relation* (Ann Arbor: University of Michigan Press, 1997), 16.

18 Morgan Phillips, "Bolsonaro Calls Brazilian Cities' Coronavirus Lockdowns a 'Crime,'" *Fox News*, March 25, 2020, www.foxnews.com/world/bolsonaro-calls-brazilian-cities-coronavirus-lockdowns-a-crime

BIBLIOGRAPHY

ABC7.com Staff. "NY Nurse Sandra Lindsay Is First in US to Get COVID-19 Vaccine after FDA Authorization." *ABC News*, December 14, 2020. https://abc7.com/covid-vaccine-pfizer-sandra-lindsay-first/8768796/

Abromaviciute, Jurgita and Emily K. Carian. "The COVID-19 Pandemic and the Gender Gap in Newly Created Domains of Household Labor." *Sociological Perspectives* 65, no. 6 (2022): 1169–1187.

Ackerman, Edwin F. "The Mainstream Media versus Andrés Manuel López Obrador." *Jacobin*, March 31, 2020. https://jacobinmag.com/2020/03/amlo-coronavirus-mexico-covid-19-response

Acosta, Nelson. "Cuban Doctors Head to Italy to Battle Coronavirus." *Reuters*, March 21, 2020. www.reuters.com/article/us-health-coronavirus-cuba/cuban-doctors-head-to-italy-battle-coronavirus-idUSKBN219051

Adey, Peter, Kevin Hannam, Mimi Sheller, and David Tyfield. "Pandemic (Im)mobilities." *Mobilities* 16, no. 2 (2021): 1–19.

Agren, David. "Coronavirus Advice from Mexico's President: 'Live Life as Usual.'" *The Guardian*, March 25, 2020. www.theguardian.com/world/2020/mar/25/coronavirus-advice-from-mexicos-president-live-life-as-usual

Ahlquist, John S. and Margaret Levi. *The Interest of Others: Organizations and Social Activism*. Princeton: Princeton University Press, 2013.

Ahmed, Abiy. "If Covid-19 Is Not Beaten in Africa It Will Return to Haunt Us All: Only a Global Victory Can End This Pandemic, Not a Temporary Rich Countries' Win." *The Guardian*, March 25, 2020. www.ft.com/content/c12a09c8-6db6-11ea-89df-41bea055720b

Alberti, Mia and Vasco Cotovio. "Portugal Gives Migrants and Asylum-Seekers Full Citizenship Rights during Coronavirus Outbreak." *CNN*, March 30, 2020. www.cnn.com/2020/03/30/europe/portugal-migrants-citizenship-rights-coronavirus-intl/index.html

Al-Bulushi, Yousuf. "The Global Threat of Race in the Decomposition of Struggle." *Safundi* 21, no. 2 (2020): 140–165.

Aljazeera. "Iran Leader Refuses US Help; Cites Coronavirus Conspiracy Theory." *Aljazeera*, March 23, 2020. www.aljazeera.com/news/2020/03/iran-leader-refuses-cites-coronavirus-conspiracy-theory-200322145122752.html

Allen-Ebrahimian, Bethany. "Chinese Coronavirus Test Maker Agreed to Build a Xinjiang Gene Bank." *Axios*, June 3, 2020. www.axios.com/chinese-coronavirus-test-maker-agreed-to-build-a-xinjiang-gene-bank-f82b6918-d6c5-45f9-90b8-dad3341d6a6e.html

Amante, Angelo, Parisa Hafezi, and Hayoung Choi. "'There Are No Funerals:' Death in Quarantine Leaves Nowhere to Grieve." *Reuters*, March 19, 2020. www.reuters.com/article/us-health-coronavirus-rites-insight-idUSKBN2161ZM

Amar, Paul. "Turning the Gendered Politics of the Security State Inside Out?" *International Feminist Journal of Politics* 13, no. 3 (2011): 299–328.

———. "Military Capitalism: In Egypt and Brazil, the Foundations of a Terrifying New 'Para-populism' Are Taking Shape at the Intersection of International Finance, Mega-Construction, and Military Rule." *NACLA Report on the Americas* 50, no. 1 (2018): 82–89.

———. "Insurgent African Intimacies in Pandemic Times: Deimperial Queer Logics of China's New Global Family in Wolf Warrior 2." *Feminist Studies* 47, no. 2 (2021): 427.

Amaro, Silvia. "Italy's Death Toll Surpasses 10,000 as Prime Minister Warns of Rising 'Nationalist Instincts.'" *CNBC*, March 30, 2020. www.cnbc.com/2020/03/30/italy-coronavirus-deaths-above-10000-conte-warns-against-anti-eu-sentiment.html

American Internet Broadcasting Corporation. "Native Americans Ignored amid Coronavirus." *American Internet Broadcasting Corporation*, April 1, 2020. https://amibc.com/clear-lens/coronavirus/native-americans-ignored-amid-coronavirus

Amrith, Megha. "Ageing Bodies, Precarious Futures: The (Im)Mobilities of 'Temporary' Migrant Domestic Workers Over Time." *Mobilities* 16, no. 2 (2021): 249–261.

Apoorvanand. "How the Coronavirus Outbreak in India Was Blamed on Muslims." *Al Jazeera*, April 18, 2020. www.aljazeera.com/indepth/opinion/coronavirus-outbreak-india-blamed-muslims

Appadurai, Arjun. "Disjuncture and Difference in the Global Cultural Economy." *Theory, Culture & Society* 7, no. 2–3 (1990): 295–310.

Apparasu, Srinivasa Rao. "Fearing He Had Contracted Coronavirus, Man Locks Family, Kills Himself: No Coronavirus Case Has Been Reported in Andhra Pradesh and Telangana." *Hindustani Times*, February 12, 2020. www.hindustantimes.com/india-news/man-suffering-from-cold-and-fever-commits-suicide-in-andhra-pradesh-feared-he-had-contracted-coronavirus-says-family/story-nECI2mhrvB5FiX2vHruFcK.html

Aratani, Lauren. "'Coughing while Asian': Living in Fear as Racism Feeds Off Coronavirus Panic." *The Guardian*, March 24, 2020. www.theguardian.com/world/2020/mar/24/coronavirus-us-asian-americans-racism

Arraf, Jane. "Jordan Keeps Coronavirus in Check with One of the World's Strictest Lockdowns." *NPR*, March 25, 2020. www.npr.org/sections/coronavirus-live-updates/2020/03/25/821349297/jordan-keeps-coronavirus-in-check-with-one-of-world-s-strictest-lockdowns

Asher Hamilton, Isobel. "11 Countries Are Now Using People's Phones to Track the Coronavirus Pandemic, and It Heralds a Massive Increase in Surveillance." *Business Insider*, March 26, 2020. www.businessinsider.com/countries-tracking-citizens-phones-coronavirus-2020-3

Associated Press. "China Bans Effeminate Men from TV." *NPR*, September 2, 2021. www.npr.org/2021/09/02/1033687586/china-ban-effeminate-men-tv-official-morality

Attiah, Karen. "Africa Has Defied the Covid-19 Nightmare Scenarios. We Shouldn't Be Surprised." *Washington Post*, September 22, 2020. www.washingtonpost.com/opinions/2020/09/22/africa-has-defied-covid-19-nightmare-scenarios-we-shouldnt-be-surprised/

Atwood, Haleigh. "The End of Ice." *Lion's Roar*, October 2, 2019. www.lionsroar.com/the-end-of-ice/

Bacon, David. "America's Farmworkers—Now 'Essential,' but Denied the Just-Enacted Benefits." *The American Prospect*, April 1, 2020. https://prospect.org/coronavirus/american-farmworkers-essential-but-unprotected/

Barbaro, Michael. "The Great Pandemic Theft." *New York Times*, September 27, 2022. www.nytimes.com/2022/09/27/podcasts/the-daily/pandemic-fraud.html

Barron, Laignee. "What We Can Learn from Singapore, Taiwan and Hong Kong about Handling Coronavirus." *Time*, March 13, 2020. https://time.com/5802293/coronavirus-covid19-singapore-hong-kong-taiwan/

Bateson, Gregory. *Steps to an Ecology of Mind*. New York: Ballantine, 1972.

Baudrillard, Jean. *L'illusion De La Fin*. Stanford, CA: Stanford University Press, 1994.

Baume, Matt. "Pope Francis Sends Money to Struggling Trans Sex Workers in Italy." *Them*, May 1, 2020. www.them.us/story/pope-francis-makes-emergency-gift-to-trans-sex-workers-in-italy

BBC Africa. "Africa Live: African Leaders Back WHO Head against Trump Attacks." *BBC World Service Africa*, April 8, 2020. www.bbc.com/news/live/world-africa-47639452

Beech, Hannah. "Tracking the Coronavirus: How Crowded Asian Cities Tackled an Epidemic." *New York Times*, March 17, 2020. www.nytimes.com/2020/03/17/world/asia/coronavirus-singapore-hong-kong-taiwan.html

Begay, Jade. "Decolonizing Community Care in Response to Covid-19." *NDN Collective*, March 13, 2020. https://ndncollective.org/indigenizing-and-decolonizing-community-care-in-response-to-covid-19/

Bélanger, Danièle and Rachel Silvey. "An Im/mobility Turn: Power Geometries of Care and Migration." *Journal of Ethnic and Migration Studies* 46, no. 16 (2020): 3423–3440.

Bell, Matthew. "This Apocalyptic Korean Christian Group Goes by Different Names. Critics Say It's Just a Cult." *The World*, July 11, 2017. www.pri.org/stories/2017-07-11/apocalyptic-korean-christian-group-goes-different-names-critics-say-its-just-cult?amp

Bengali, Shashank. "From 'Gold Standard' To a Coronavirus 'Explosion': Singapore Battles New Outbreak." *Los Angeles Times*, April 14, 2020. www.latimes.com/world-nation/story/2020-04-14/coronavirus-surges-migrant-workers-in-singapore

Benjamin, Ruha. *Race after Technology: Abolitionist Tools for the New Jim Code*. Hoboken, NJ: John Wiley & Sons, 2019.

———. *Viral Justice: How We Grow the World We Want*. *Princeton*: Princeton University Press, 2022.

Berman, Carol W. and Xi Chen. "COVID Threatens to Bring a Wave of Hikikomori to America." *Scientific American*, January 19, 2022. www.scientificamerican.com/article/covid-threatens-to-bring-a-wave-of-hikikomori-to-america/

Berne, Patty. "Disability Justice—a Working Draft." *Sins Invalid*, June 9, 2015. www.sinsinvalid.org/blog/disability-justice-a-working-draft-by-patty-berne

———— and Vanessa Raditz. "To Survive Climate Catastrophe, Look to Queer and Disabled Folk." *Yes! Magazine*, July 31, 2019. www.yesmagazine.org/opinion/2019/07/31/climate-change-queer-disabled-organizers

Bernini, Lorenzo. *Queer Apocalypses: Elements of Antisocial Theory*. New York: Springer, 2016.

Bhaskar, Anurag. "When It Comes to Dalit and Tribal Rights, the Judiciary in India Just Does Not Get It." *The Wire*, May 3, 2020. https://thewire.in/law/when-it-comes-to-dalit-and-tribal-rights-the-judiciary-in-india-just-does-not-get-it

Biddle, Sam. "Facebook Contractors Must Work in Offices during Coronavirus Pandemic—while Staff Stay Home." *The Intercept*, March 12, 2020. https://theintercept.com/2020/03/12/coronavirus-facebook-contractors/

Biller, David. "Brazil's Bolsonaro Makes Life-or-Death Coronavirus Gamble." *Associated Press*, March 28, 2020. https://apnews.com/b21a2963694c6726d03e027134dafl

Bishnupriya Ghosh, *The Virus Touch: Theorizing Epidemic Media*. Durham, NC: Duke University Press, 2023.

Biswas, Soutik. "Coronavirus: India's Pandemic Lockdown Turns into a Human Tragedy." *BBC News*, March 30, 2020. www.bbc.com/news/world-asia-india-52086274

Blake, John. "Coronavirus Is Bringing a Plague of Dangerous Doomsday Predictions." *CNN*, March 23, 2020. www.cnn.com/2020/03/22/world/doomsday-prophets-coronavirus-blake/index.html

Borell, Josep. "The Coronavirus Pandemic and the New World It Is Creating." *European External Action Service*, March 23, 2020. https://eeas.europa.eu/headquarters/headquarters-homepage/76379/coronavirus-pandemic-and-new-world-it-creating_en

Borowiec, Steven. "How South Korea's Coronavirus Outbreak Got So Quickly Out of Control." *Time*, February 24, 2020. https://time.com/5789596/south-korea-coronavirus-outbreak/

Borowitz, Andy. "Michigan Governor Arrogantly Forcing Residents to Remain Alive." *The New Yorker*, May 1, 2020. www.newyorker.com/humor/borowitz-report/michigan-governor-arrogantly-forcing-residents-to-remain-alive

Boswell, Rose. "If Men Want to Be Heroes, They Should Do the Dirty Work." *Corona Times*, April 2, 2020. www.coronatimes.net/if-men-want-to-be-heroes-they-should-do-the-dirty-work/

Boxwell, Robert. "How China's Fake News Machine Is Rewriting the History of Covid-19, Even as the Pandemic Unfolds," *Politico*, April 4, 2020. www.politico.com/news/magazine/2020/04/04/china-fake-news-coronavirus-164652

Branford, Sue. "Spreading the Word of God and Coronavirus: Outrage Over Evangelical Group Trying to Contact Isolated Amazon Tribes amid Pandemic." *Common Dreams*, March 18, 2020. www.commondreams.org/views/2020/03/18/spreading-word-god-and-coronavirus-outrage-over-evangelical-group-trying-contact

Brenegar, Dr. Ed. *All Crises Are Local: Understanding the Covid-19 Global Pandemic*. New York: Circle of Impact Institute, Llc, 2020.

Briceño, Franklin. "In Peru, Thousands of Faces at Mass—None Now Alive." *Associated Press*, June 14, 2020. https://news.yahoo.com/peru-thousands-faces-mass-none-195417788.html

Browning, Bil. "Evangelical Christians Are Linking LGBTQ People to the Coronavirus Now." *LGBTQ Nation*, March 6, 2020. www.lgbtqnation.com/2020/03/evangeli cal-christians-linking-lgbtq-people-coronavirus-now/

Brown-Vincent, Layla. "The Pandemic of Racial Capitalism: Another World Is Possible." *From the European South 7* (2020): 61–74.

Brueck, Hilary. "Sweden's Gamble on Coronavirus Herd Immunity Couldn't Work in the US—and It May Not Work in Sweden." *Business Insider*, May 2, 2020. www.businessinsider.com/sweden-coronavirus-strategy-explained-culture-of-trust-and-obedience-2020-4

———. "The WHO Made a Thinly Veiled Dig at Sweden's Loose Coronavirus Lockdown, Saying 'Humans Are Not Herds' and Old People Are Not Disposable." *Business Insider*, May 11, 2020. www.businessinsider.com/herd-immunity-few-people-have-had-the-coronavirus-who-2020-5

Brunnstrom, David and Daphne Psaledakis. "Pompeo Urges More Assertive Approach to 'Frankenstein' China." *Reuters*, July 23, 2020. www.usnews.com/news/world/articles/2020-07-23/pompeo-calls-for-more-assertive-response-to-frankenstein-china

B'Tselem. "During the Coronavirus Crisis, Israel Confiscates Tents Designated for Clinic in the Northern West Bank." *B'Tselem—The Israeli Information Center for Human Rights in the Occupied Territories*, March 26, 2020. www.btselem.org/press_release/20200326_israel_confiscates_clinic_tents_during_coronavirus_crisis

Buckley, Chris. "Chinese Doctor, Silenced after Warning of Outbreak, Dies from Coronavirus." *New York Times*, February 6, 2020. www.nytimes.com/2020/02/06/world/asia/chinese-doctor-Li-Wenliang-coronavirus.html

Bui, Long T. "The Debts of Memory: Historical Amnesia and Refugee Knowledge in *the Reeducation of Cherry Truong*." *Journal of Asian American Studies* 18, no. 1 (2015): 73–97.

———. *Returns of War: South Vietnam and the Price of Refugee Memory*. New York: New York University Press, 2018.

———. "Global Futurities: Articulating the Collective Struggle for (Other)worldly Justice," *New Global Studies*, forthcoming.

Burrows, Dan. "China's Evergrande Crisis: A Real Threat to U.S. Stocks?" *Kiplinger*, September 20, 2021. www.kiplinger.com/investing/stocks/603465/china-evergra nde-crisis-us-stock-market

Butler, Judith. *What World Is This? A Pandemic Phenomenology*. New York: Columbia University Press, 2022.

Byler, Darren. *Terror Capitalism: Uyghur Dispossession and Masculinity in a Chinese City*. Durham, NC: Duke University Press, 2021, 37.

Cacho, Lisa Marie. *Social Death: Racialized Rightlessness and the Criminalization of the Unprotected*. New York: New York University Press, 2012.

Caduff, Carlo. "The Semiotics of Security: Infectious Disease Research and the Biopolitics of Informational Bodies in the United States." *Cultural Anthropology* 27, no. 2 (May 2012): 333–357.

Campbell, Monica. "US Deportation Flights Risk Spreading Coronavirus Globally." *PRI*, April 14, 2020. www.pri.org/stories/2020-04-14/us-deportation-flights-risk-spreading-coronavirus-globally

Capatides, Christina. "Doctors without Borders Dispatches Team to the Navajo Nation." *CBS News*, May 11, 2020. www.cbsnews.com/news/doctors-without-borders-navajo-nation-coronavirus/

Caputi, Jane. *Gossips, Gorgons and Crones: The Fates of the Earth*. Vermont: Inner Traditions/Bear and Company, 1993.

Carleton, Sean. "Coronavirus Colonialism: How the COVID-19 Crisis Is Catalyzing Dispossession." *Canadian Dimension*, March 23, 2020. https://canadiandimension.com/articles/view/coronavirus-colonialism-how-crisis-is-catalyzing-dispossession

CBS News. "'Shoot Them Dead': Philippine President Orders Police, Military to Kill Citizens Who Defy Coronavirus Lockdown." *CBS News*, April 2, 2020. www.news9.com /story/41967605/shoot-them-dead-philippine-president-orders-police-military-to-kill-citizens-who-defy-coronavirus-lockdown

Cervantes, Maria. "Peru Indigenous Warn of 'Ethnocide by Inaction' as Coronavirus Hits Amazon Tribes." *Reuters*, April 24, 2020. www.reuters.com/article/us-health-coronavirus-peru-indigenous/peru-indigenous-warn-of-ethnocide-by-inaction-as-coronavirus-hits-amazon-tribes-idUSKCN22639A

Chalmers, Matthew. "Why Hack the World's Largest Meat Company?" *Sentient Media*, June 4, 2021. https://sentientmedia.org/why-hack-the-worlds-largest-meat-company/

Chang, Rachel. "Racism against Asian Americans Isn't Unique to the Coronavirus Pandemic—Everyone Else Is Just Becoming More Aware Now." *Hello Giggles*, April 29, 2020. https://hellogiggles.com/lifestyle/racism-asian-americans-coronavirus/

Chappell, Bill. "'We Alerted the World' to Coronavirus on Jan. 5, WHO Says in Response to U.S." *NPR*, April 15, 2020. www.npr.org/sections/goatsandsoda/2020/04/15/835179442/we-alerted-the-world-to-coronavirus-on-jan-5-who-says-in-response-to-u-s

Chari, Sharad. "Detritus in Durban: Polluted Environs and the Biopolitics of Refusal." *Imperial Debris*, 131–161. Durham, NC: Duke University Press, 2013.

Chatterjee, Elizabeth. "The Asian Anthropocene: Electricity and Fossil Developmentalism." *The Journal of Asian Studies* 79, no. 1 (2020): 3–24.

Chaudhary, Ajay Singh. "We're Not in This Together." *The Baffler*, April 2020. https://thebaffler.com/salvos/were-not-in-this-together-chaudhary

Chen, Mel Y. *Animacies: Biopolitics, Racial Mattering, and Queer Affect*. Durham, NC: Duke University Press, 2012.

CNA. "COVID-19: Singapore Concerned as Some Countries Have Given Up on Containment, Says Minister," *CNA*, March 15, 2020. www.youtube.com/watch?v=AxAuMEo5XTs&feature=youtu.be

CNBC. "Ousted Afghan President Ashraf Ghani Resurfaces in UAE after Fleeing Kabul, Emirati Government Says." *CNBC*, August 18, 2021. www.cnbc.com/2021/08/18/afghan-president-ashraf-ghani-is-in-uae-after-fleeing-afghanistan.html

CNN. "READ: Trump's Oval Office Speech on the Coronavirus Outbreak." *CNN*, March 11, 2020. www.cnn.com/2020/03/11/politics/read-trump-coronavirus-address/index.html

Cole, Brendan. "Brazil Government Aide Says COVID-19's Toll on Elderly Will Reduce Pension Deficit as Country's Outbreak Escalates." *Newsweek*, May 27, 2020. www.newsweek.com/brazil-government-aide-says-covid-19s-toll-elderly-will-reduce-pension-deficit-countrys-1506830

Cole, Leonard A. *Clouds of Secrecy: The Army's Germ Warfare Tests over Populated Areas*. Louisville, KY: Rowman & Littlefield, 1990.

Collins, Ben. "How QAnon Rode the Pandemic to New Heights—and Fueled the Viral Anti-Mask Phenomenon." *NBC News*, August 14, 2020. www.nbcnews.com/tech/tech-news/how-qanon-rode-pandemic-new-heights-fueled-viral-anti-mask-n1236695

Concha, Joe. "Glenn Beck: 'I'd Rather Die' from Coronavirus 'than Kill the Country' from Economic Shutdown." *The Hill*, March 25, 2020. https://thehill.com/homenews/media/489472-glenn-beck-id-rather-die-from-coronavirus-than-kill-the-country-from-economic

Conley, Julia. "'The Strike Wave Is in Full Swing': Amazon, Whole Foods Workers Walk Off Job to Protest Unjust and Unsafe Labor Practices." *Common Dreams*, March 30, 2020. www.commondreams.org/news/2020/03/30/strike-wave-full-swing-amazon-whole-foods-workers-walk-job-protest-unjust-and-unsafe

Constant, Paul. "Coronavirus Didn't Bring the Economy Down—40 Years of Greed and Corporate Malfeasance Did." *Insider*, April 10, 2020. www.businessinsider.com/pitchfork-economics-coronavirus-not-hurting-economy-corporate-greed-is-2020-4

Cox, Alicia Marie. "Autobiographical Indiscipline: Queering American Indian Life Narratives." PhD. diss., University of California, Riverside, 2014, 112.

Cuevas, Ofelia. "400 Years of Resistance: Race, Policing, and Abolition." *UC Davis Humanities Institute*, July 6, 2020. www.youtube.com/watch?v=M38dX4gnyqk

Cyranoski, David. "Bat Cave Solves Mystery of Deadly SARS Virus—and Suggests New Outbreak Could Occur." *Nature*, December 2017. www.nature.com/articles/d41586-017-07766-9

Dados, Nour and Lucy Taksa. "Pandemic's Economic Blow Hits Women Hard." *The Lighthouse*, April 14, 2020. https://lighthouse.mq.edu.au/article/april-2020/Pandemics-economic-blow-hits-women-hard

Daily Monitor. "Uganda's Coronavirus Cases Rise to 53." *Daily Monitor*, April 8, 2020. www.monitor.co.ug/News/National/Uganda-s-coronavirus-cases-rise-53/688334-5518396-76ms9dz/index.html

Dajose, Lori. "The Tip of the Iceberg: Virologist David Ho (BS '74) Speaks about COVID-19." *Caltech*, March 20, 2020. www.caltech.edu/about/news/tip-iceberg-virologist-david-ho-bs-74-speaks-about-covid-19

Daniyal, Shoaib. "Not China, Not Italy: India's Coronavirus Lockdown Is the Harshest in the World." *Scroll.in*, March 29, 2020. https://scroll.in/article/957564/not-china-not-italy-indias-coronavirus-lockdown-is-the-harshest-in-the-world

Darian-Smith, Eve. *Global Burning: Rising Antidemocracy and the Climate Crisis*. Stanford, CA: Stanford University Press, 2022.

Darian-Smith, Eve, and Philip C. McCarty. *The Global Turn: Theories, Research Designs, and Methods for Global Studies*. Berkeley: University of California Press, 2017.

Da Silva, Chantal. "Coronavirus in the Age of Protest: How the Pandemic Could Change the Way We Organize." *Newsweek*, April 8, 2020. www.newsweek.com/coronavirus-age-protest-how-pandemic-could-change-way-we-organize-1496701

Da Silva, Denise Ferreira. *Toward a Global Idea of Race*. Minneapolis: University of Minnesota Press, 2007.

———. "Toward a Black Feminist Poethics: The Quest (ion) of Blackness toward the End of the World." *The Black Scholar* 44, no. 2 (2014): 81–97.

Davidson, Helen. "China Calls Hong Kong Protesters a 'Political Virus'." *The Guardian*, May 6, 2020. www.theguardian.com/world/2020/may/06/china-calls-hong-kong-protesters-a-political-virus

Davis, Angela Y. *Women, Race, & Class*. New York: Vintage, 2011, 232.

Davis, Mike. "The Coronavirus Crisis Is a Monster Fueled by Capitalism." *In These Times*, March 20, 2020. http://inthesetimes.com/article/22394/coronavirus-crisis-capitalism-covid-19-monster-mike-davis

Day, Iyko. *Alien Capital: Asian Racialization and the Logic of Settler Colonial Capitalism*. Durham, NC: Duke University Press, 2016.

De Bengy Puyvallee, Antoine and Sonja Kittelsen. "'Disease Knows No Borders': Pandemics and the Politics of Global Health Security." In *Pandemics, Publics, and Politics: Staging Responses to Public Health Crises*, edited by Kristen Bjørkdahl and Benedicte Carlsen, 59–73. New York: Palgrave MacMillan, 2019.

Deerinwater, Jen. "I'm Native and Disabled. The US Government Is Sacrificing My People." *Truth Out*, April 26, 2020. https://truthout.org/articles/im-native-and-disabled-the-government-is-sacrificing-my-people/

Delanty, Gerard, ed. *Pandemics, Politics, and Society: Critical Perspectives on the Covid-19 Crisis*. Berlin: Walter de Gruyter GmbH & Co KG, 2021.

Democracy Now. "Standoff in South Dakota: Cheyenne River Sioux Refuse Governor's Demand to Remove COVID Checkpoints." *Democracy Now*, May 12, 2020. www.democracynow.org/2020/5/12/cheyenne_river_sioux_coronavirus_checkpoints_south

Derham, Tristan and Freya Mathews. "Elephants as Refugees." *People and Nature* (2020): 103–110.

Devega, Chauncey. "Pulitzer Winner Chris Hedges: These 'Are the Good Times—Compared to What's Coming Next.'" *Salon*, April 28, 2020. www.salon.com/2020/04/28/pulitzer-winner-chris-hedges-these-are-the-good-times--compared-to-whats-coming-next/?

Devereaux, Ryan. "'Burials Are Cheaper than Deportations': Virus Unleashes Terror in a Troubled ICE Detention Center." *The Intercept*, April 12, 2020. https://theintercept.com/2020/04/12/coronavirus-ice-detention-jail-alabama/

Dimas, Carlos S. *Poisoned Eden: Cholera Epidemics, State-Building, and the Problem of Public Health in Tucumán, Argentina, 1865-1908*. Lincoln: University of Nebraska Press, 2022.

Dougé-Prosper, Mamyrah. "Solidarity Economy Praxis in Limonade." *Women's Studies Quarterly* 47, no. 3/4 (2019): 190–211.

———. "An Island in the Chain: The Geopolitical Fallout of the U.S. Wars on Drugs and Terror Reveal How the United States Continues to Exploit Haiti as a Tool for Guarding Global Power." *NACLA Report on the Americas* 53, no. 1 (2021): 32–38.

Dougé-Prosper, Mamyrah, and Mark Schuller. "After Moïse Assassination, Popular Sectors Must Lead the Way." *NACLA*, July 8, 2021. https://nacla.org/haiti-jovenel-moise-assassination-social-movements

Dowdy, David and Gypsyamber D'Souza. 2020. "Early Herd Immunity against COVID-19: A Dangerous Misconception." *Johns Hopkins Research University & Medicine, Coronavirus Resource Center*. Accessed December 17, 2020. https://coronavirus.jhu.edu/from-our-experts/early-herd-immunity-against-covid-19-a-dangerous-misconception

Duarte, Marisa Elena. *Network Sovereignty: Building the Internet across Indian Country*. Seattle: University of Washington Press, 2017.

DuBois, William Edward Burghardt. "Worlds of Color." *Foreign Affairs* 3, no. 3 (1925): 423–444.

Duenes, Jorge. "Mexico Closes U.S.-Owned Plant for Alleged Refusal to Sell Ventilators to Mexican Hospitals." *The Globe and Mail*, April 10, 2020. www.theglobeandmail.com/world/article-mexico-closes-us-owned-plant-for-alleged-refusal-to-sell-ventilators/

Duhaime-Ross, Arielle. "The Tiny Nation of Kiribati Will Soon Be Underwater—Here's the Plan to Save Its People." *Vice*, September 22, 2016. www.vice.com/en_us/article/a39m7k/doomed-by-climate-change-kiribati-wants-migration-with-dignity

Dukes, Kevin. "Transgender Woman Shot to Death in Ambulance while Being Treated in South Charlotte." *Lovelyti*, March 19, 2020. https://lovelyti.com/2020/03/19/transgender-woman-shot-to-death-in-ambulance-while-being-treated-in-south-charlotte/

Dunmore, Royce. "Gov. Brian Kemp Is Slammed as Committing 'Genocide' after COVID-19 Stats on Black People Are Released." *Newsone*, April 30, 2020. https://newsone.com/playlist/brian-kemp-slammed-genocide-covid-19-stats-black-people/

Elbe, Stefan and Nadine Voelkner. "Viral Sovereignty: The Downside Risk of Securitizing Infectious Disease." In *The Handbook of Global Health Policy*, edited by Garrett W. Wallace Brown, Gavin Yamey, and Sarah Wamala, 305–317. Hoboken, NJ: Wiley-Blackwell, 2014.

Elks, Sonia. "Carrot or Stick? How Countries Are Tackling COVID-19 Vaccine Hesitancy." *Thomson Reuters Foundation*, July 6, 2021. https://news.trust.org/item/20210601155421-gr1fs/

Escalonilla, Álvaro. "The Return of Africa's Strongmen." *Atalayar*, May 27, 2022. https://atalayar.com/en/content/return-africas-strongmen

Escobar, Martha D. *Captivity Beyond Prisons: Criminalization Experiences of Latina (Im)migrants*. Austin: University of Texas Press, 2016.

Fabian, Jordan. "Trump Told Governors to Buy Own Virus Supplies, Then Outbid Them." *Bloomberg*, March 19, 2020. www.bloomberg.com/news/articles/2020-03-19/trump-told-governors-to-buy-own-virus-supplies-then-outbid-them

Faddis, Charles "Sam". "Bioterror: We Aren't Ready." *The Hill*, February 19, 2020. https://thehill.com/opinion/national-security/483506-bioterror-we-arent-ready

Fassin, Didier. "Another Politics of Life Is Possible." *Theory, Culture & Society* 26, no. 5 (2009): 44–60.

Filipovic, Jill. "Trump's Malicious Use of 'Chinese Virus.'" *CNN*, March 18, 2020. www.cnn.com/2020/03/18/opinions/trumps-malicious-use-of-chinese-virus-filipovic/index.html

Flores, Glenda M. "Latina Physicians as 'Essential' Workers." *Contexts* 19, no. 4 (2020): 62–64.

Foust, Jeff. "White House Looks for International Support for Space Resource Rights." *Space News*, April 6, 2020. https://spacenews.com/

FR24 News. "'No One Wanted to Read' His Book on Pandemic Psychology—Then Covid Hit." *FR24 News*, August 19, 2021. www.fr24news.com/a/2021/08/no-one-wanted-to-read-his-book-on-pandemic-psychology-then-covid-hit.html

Fries, Lauren. "UC Berkeley Had to Apologize for Saying Anti-Chinese Xenophobia Is a 'Normal Reaction' to the Coronavirus." *Business Insider*, January 31, 2020. www.businessinsider.com/uc-berkeley-called-out-anti-chinese-xenophobia-normal-reaction-coronavirus-2020-1

Funes, Katherine. "El Salvador's State of Exception Turns One." *NACLA*, March 27, 2023. https://nacla.org/el-salvadors-state-exception-turns-one.

Furlow, Bryant. "A Hospital's Secret Coronavirus Policy Separated Native American Mothers from Their Newborns." *ProPublica*, June 13, 2020. www.propublica.org/article/a-hospitals-secret-coronavirus-policy-separated-native-american-mothers-from-their-newborns

Gadarian, Shana Kushner, Sara Wallace Goodman, and Thomas B. Pepinsky. *Pandemic Politics: The Deadly Toll of Partisanship in the Age of COVID.* Princeton, NJ: Princeton University Press, 2022.

Galeano, Eduardo. "Upside Down." *Salon*, October 12, 2000. www.salon.com/2000/10/12/galeano/

Gamboa, Suzanne. "Julián Castro: Latinos Grapple with 'the Worst of All Worlds' amid Coronavirus Pandemic." *NBC News*, April 27, 2020. www.nbcnews.com/news/latino/juli-n-castro-latinos-grapple-worst-all-worlds-amid-coronavirus-n1193666

Gane, Mike and Michael Gane. *Jean Baudrillard: In Radical Uncertainty.* London: Pluto Press, 2000.

Garcia, Sierra. "'We're the Virus': The Pandemic Is Bringing Out Environmentalism's Dark Side." *Grist*, March 30, 2020. https://grist.org/climate/were-the-virus-the-pandemic-is-bringing-out-environmentalisms-dark-side/

Garofoli, Joe. "Gavin Newsom Wants California to Be Its Own Nation-State in the Trump Era." *San Francisco Chronicle*, February 12, 2019. www.sfchronicle.com/politics/article/Gavin-Newsom-wants-California-to-be-its-own-13611747.php

Garrett, Laurie. *The Coming Plague: Newly Emerging Diseases in a World Out of Balance.* New York: Macmillan, 1994.

Gasviani, Gvantsa. "Inner Martyrdom: Deconstructing the Sacrificial Female Subject in Post-Soviet Georgia." *Journal of Feminist Scholarship* 20, no. 20 (2022): 19–32.

Gay, Roxane. "On the Death of Sandra Bland and Our Vulnerable Bodies." *New York Times*, July 24, 2015. www.nytimes.com/2015/07/25/opinion/on-the-death-of-sandra-bland-and-our-vulnerable-bodies.html

Germanos, Andrea. "Coronavirus Pandemic Triggered 'One of the Greatest Wealth Transfers in History.'" *Salon*, June 7, 2020. www.salon.com/2020/06/07/coronavirus-pandemic-triggered-one-of-the-greatest-wealth-transfers-in-history_partner/

Gessen, Masha. "What Lessons Does the AIDS Crisis Offer for the Coronavirus Pandemic?." *The New Yorker*, April 8, 2020. www.newyorker.com/news/our-col umnists/what-lessons-does-the-aids-crisis-offer-for-the-coronavirus-pandemic

Ghumkhor, Sahar and Anila Daulatzai. "Monsters, Inc: The Taliban as Empire's Bogeyman." *Aljazeera*, August 18, 2021. www.aljazeera.com/opinions/2021/8/18/ monsters-inc-the-taliban-as-empires-bogeyman

Gies, Heather and John Washington. "'Maybe If I Had Papers, It Would Have Been Different': Undocumented during a Pandemic." *The Nation*, March 25, 2020. www.thenation.com/article/politics/undocumented-coronavirus/

Gilmore, Ruth Wilson. "Fatal Couplings of Power and Difference: Notes on Racism and Geography." *The Professional Geographer* 54, no. 1 (2002): 15–24.

———. *Abolition Geography: Essays towards Liberation*. New York: Verso Books, 2022.

Gilpin, Emilee. "COVID-19 Crisis Tells World What Indigenous Peoples Have Been Saying for Thousands of Years." *National Observer*. Accessed March 24, 2020. www.nationalobserver.com/2020/03/24/news/covid-19-crisis-tells-world-what-ind igenous-peoples-have-been-saying-thousands-years

Glissant, Édouard. *Poetics of Relation*. Ann Arbor, MI: University of Michigan Press, 1997.

Goldberg, David Theo. "Dread: The Politics of Our Time." *University of California Humanities Research Institute*, June 2018. https://uchri.org/foundry/dread-the-politics-of-our-time/

Goldstein, Ruth. "Ayahuasca and Arabidopsis: The Philosopher Plant and the Scientist's Specimen." *Ethnos* 86, no. 2 (2021): 245–272.

Gomez-Temesio, Veronica. "Outliving Death: Ebola, Zombies, and the Politics of Saving Lives." *American Anthropologist* 120, no. 4 (2018): 745–748.

Górska, Magdalena. *Breathing Matters: Feminist Intersectional Politics of Vulnerability, Vol. 683*. Linköping: Linköping University, 2016, 298.

Green, Toby and Thomas Fazi. *The Covid Consensus: The Global Assault on Democracy and the Poor? A Critique from the Left*. Oxford: Oxford University Press, 2023.

Greenfield, Patrick and Erin McCormick. "'No One Comes': The Cruise Ship Crews Cast Adrift by Coronavirus." *The Guardian*, May 1, 2020. www.theguardian. com/environment/2020/may/01/no-one-comes-the-cruise-ship-crews-cast-adrift-by-coronavirus

Grusin, Richard, ed. *Anthropocene Feminism*. Minneapolis: University of Minnesota Press, 2017.

Gunter, Sabrina. "Under Trump, Undocumented Immigrants with COVID-19 Are Being Denied Care." *In These Times*, April 6, 2020. http://inthesetimes.com/arti cle/22434/trump-undocumented-immigrants-covid-19-coronavirus

Hafezi, Parisa. "Iran's Khamenei Rejects U.S. Help Offer, Vows to Defeat Coronavirus." *Reuters*, March 22, 2020. www.reuters.com/article/us-health-coro navirus-iran/irans-khamenei-rejects-us-help-offer-vows-to-defeat-coronavirus-idUSKBN21909Y

Hall, Porsha and Mary Anne Adams. "Creating Havens for Black Lesbian Elders during COVID-19." *Journal of Lesbian Studies* 40 (2023): 1–13.

Hamdy, Sherine. *Our Bodies Belong to God: Organ Transplants, Islam, and the Struggle for Human Dignity in Egypt*. Berkeley: University of California Press, 2012.

Hamilton, Isobel Asher. "11 Countries Are Now Using People's Phones to Track the Coronavirus Pandemic, and It Heralds a Massive Increase in Surveillance." *Business Insider*, March 26, 2020. www.businessinsider.com/countries-tracking-citizens-phones-coronavirus-2020-3

Hanauer, Nick. "Our Uniquely American Virus." *The Prospect*, April 14, 2020. https://prospect.org/coronavirus/our-uniquely-american-virus/

Haraway, Donna. *Simians, Cyborgs and Women: The Reinvention of Nature.* New York: Routledge, 1991.

———. *When Species Meet.* Minneapolis: University of Minnesota Press, 2013.

———. *Staying with the Trouble: Making Kin in the Chthulucene.* Durham, NC: Duke University Press, 2016.

Harjo, Joy. How *We Became Human: New and Selected Poems: 1975-2001.* New York: W.W. Norton and Company, 2002.

Hartman, Saidiya. "The End of White Supremacy, An American Romance." *Bomb*, June 5, 2020. https://bombmagazine.org/articles/the-end-of-white-supremacy-an-american-romance/

Hassanin, Alexandre. "Coronavirus Could Be a 'Chimera' of Two Different Viruses, Genome Analysis Suggests." *Science Alert*, March 24, 2020. www.scienceal ert.com/genome-analysis-of-the-coronavirus-suggests-two-viruses-may-have-combined

Haynes, Douglas. "Policing the Air Out of Us." *Orange County Register*, June 14, 2020. www.ocregister.com/2020/06/13/policing-the-air-out-of-us-douglas-haynes/

Hazel Biana, Hazel T. and Rosallia Domingo. "Lesbian Single Parents: Reviewing Philippine COVID-19 Policies." *Journal of International Women's Studies* 22, no. 12 (2021): 135–147.

Hearse, Phil and Neil Faulkner. "The Coming Social Collapse." *Mutiny*, April 3, 2020. www.timetomutiny.org/post/the-coming-social-collapse

Hedges, Chris. *War Is a Force That Gives Us Meaning.* New York: Anchor, 2003.

Heer, Jeet. "Meatpacking Plants Are a Front in the Covid-19 Class War." *The Nation*, April 29, 2020. www.thenation.com/article/politics/meatpacking-coro navirus-class-war/

Hellmann, Jessie. "Cuomo Reports Another 731 Coronavirus Deaths in NY, Its Largest One-Day Increase." *The Hill*, April 7, 2020. https://thehill.com/policy/healthcare/491553-cuomo-reports-731-coronavirus-deaths-in-the-state-its-larg est-one-day

Henley, Jon. "Sweden's Covid-19 Strategist under Fire Over Herd Immunity Emails." *The Guardian*, August 17, 2020. www.theguardian.com/world/2020/aug/17/swed ens-covid-19-strategist-under-fire-over-herd-immunity-emails

———. "Culled Mink Rise from the Dead to Denmark's Horror." *The Guardian*, November 25, 2020. www.theguardian.com/world/2020/nov/25/culled-mink-rise-from-the-dead-denmark-coronavirus

Hersher, Rebecca. "U.S. Formally Begins to Leave the Paris Climate Agreement." *National Public Radio*, November 4, 2019. www.npr.org/2019/11/04/773474657/u-s-formally-begins-to-leave-the-paris-climate-agreement

Hickok, Kimberly. "How Does the COVID-19 Pandemic Compare to the Last Pandemic?" *Live Science*, March 19, 2020. www.livescience.com/covid-19-pande mic-vs-swine-flu.html

Higgins-Desbiolles, Freya. *Socializing Tourism for Social and Ecological Justice after COVID-19.* London: Routledge, 2021.

Hirsch, Afua. "Why Are Africa's Coronavirus Successes Being Overlooked?" *Microsoft News*, May 21, 2020. www.msn.com/en-ie/news/coronavirus/why-are-africas-coronavirus-successes-being-overlooked/ar-BB14pbLy

Hjelmgaard, Kim. " 'What about COVID-20?' U.S. Cuts Funding to Group Studying Bat Coronaviruses in China." *USA Today*, May 9, 2020. www.usatoday.com/story/news/world/2020/05/09/coronavirus-us-cuts-funding-group-studying-bat-viruses-china/3088205001/

Holman, E. Alison, Nickolas M. Jones, Dana Rose Garfin, and Roxane Cohen Silver. "Distortions in Time Perception during Collective Trauma: Insights from a National Longitudinal Study during the COVID-19 Pandemic." *Psychological Trauma: Theory, Research, Practice, and Policy*, August 8, 2022.

Hong, Mai-Linh K., ed. *The Auntie Sewing Squad Guide to Mask Making, Radical Care, and Racial Justice*. Berkeley: University of California Press, 2021.

Hooks, Bell. *Sisters of the Yam: Black Women and Self-Recovery*. London: Routledge, 2014.

Hornblum, Allen M., Newman, Judith L., and Dober, Gregory J. *Against Their Will: The Secret History of Medical Experimentation on Children in Cold War America*. New York: Macmillan, 2013.

Horne, Gerald. *The Dawning of the Apocalypse: The Roots of Slavery, White Supremacy, Settler Colonialism, and Capitalism in the Long Sixteenth Century*. New York: Monthly Review Press, 2020.

Hsu, Li Yang and Min-Han Tan. "What Singapore Can Teach the U.S. about Responding to Covid-19." *Stat News*, March 23, 2020. www.statnews.com/2020/03/23/singapore-teach-united-states-about-covid-19-response/

Huang, Chaolin MD, Wang, Yeming MD, and Li, Xingwang MD. "Infected with 2019 Novel Coronavirus in Wuhan, China." *The Lancet* 395, no. 10223 (February 2020): 497–506.

Huang, Josie. "In LA County, Pacific Islanders Are Dying from Coronavirus at a Rate 12 Times Higher than Whites. These Leaders Are Fighting Back." *LAist*, April 30, 2020. https://laist.com/news/pacific-islanders-coronavirus-death-rate-california

Huber, Makenzie. " 'Essential Worker Just Means You're on the Death Track': John Deranamie Is a 50-Year-Old Liberian Man Whose Dream Led Him to a Meatpacking Plant in South Dakota. He Contracted COVID-19 as Part of His Job." *USA Today*, May 5, 2020. www.usatoday.com/in-depth/news/2020/05/04/meat-packing-essent ial-worker-hogs-south-dakota-smithfield-food-chain-covid-19-coronavirus-inside/3064329001/

Human Rights Watch. "India: Protests, Attacks over New Citizenship Law." *Human Rights Watch*, April 9, 2020. www.hrw.org/news/2020/04/09/india-protests-atta cks-over-new-citizenship-law

———. "Covid-19 Fueling Anti-Asian Racism and Xenophobia Worldwide." *Human Rights Watch*, May 12, 2020. www.hrw.org/news/2020/05/12/covid-19-fueling-anti-asian-racism-and-xenophobia-worldwide#

Humphrey, Olivia. "Is Coronavirus China's Chernobyl?" *China Channel*, March 24, 2020. https://chinachannel.org/2020/03/24/corona-chernobyl/

Hung, Lee Shiu. "The SARS Epidemic in Hong Kong: What Lessons Have We Learned?." *Journal of the Royal Society of Medicine* 96, no. 8 (2003): 374–378.

Iling, Sean. " 'Flood the Zone with Shit': How Misinformation Overwhelmed Our Democracy." *Vox*, February 6, 2020. www.vox.com/policy-and-politics/2020/1/16/20991816/impeachment-trial-trump-bannon-misinformation

Imbert, Fred. "Bank of America CEO Moynihan Says 'We're in a War to Contain This Virus.'" CNBC.com, March 15, 2020. www.cnbc.com/2020/03/15/bank-of-amer ica-ceo-moynihan-says-were-in-a-war-to-contain-this-virus.html

Indigenous Action group. "Rethinking the Apocalypse: An Indigenous Anti-Futurist Manifesto." *Indigenous Action*, March 19, 2020. www.indigenousaction.org/ret hinking-the-apocalypse-an-indigenous-anti-futurist-manifesto/

INF News. "A Zombie Speaks." Pompeo Intervened in Venezuela's Internal Affairs and Was Mercilessly Taunted by the Venezuelan Minister of Foreign Affairs." *iNews*, July 28, 2021 HKT. https://inf.news/en/world/f6f3fd211c642e90af2e3 4ab68ffe2fa.html#:~:text=%22dying%20to%20struggle.%22

Isaacs, David. "Apocalypse Perhaps." *Journal of Paediatrics and Child Health* 56, no. 8 (2020): 1169.

Jackson, George. *Soledad Brother: The Prison Letters of George Jackson*. Chicago: Lawrence Hill Books, 1994.

Jackson, Janine. "'Our Food System Is Very Much Modeled on Plantation Economics.'" *Fair*, May 13, 2020. https://fair.org/home/our-food-system-is-very-much-modeled-on-plantation-economics/

Jackson, Zakiyyah Iman. *Becoming Human: Matter and Meaning in an Antiblack World*. New York: New York University Press, 2020.

Jankowicz, Mia. "A 39-Year-Old Coronavirus Patient Who Could Hardly Breathe Posted a Video from the ICU to Warn People Who Think It Won't Happen to Them." *Business Insider*, March 20, 2020. www.businessinsider.com/coronavirus-woman-hospital-warns-people-who-doubt-will-affect-them-2020-3

JCB. "Pinay Nurse in California Shares Struggles in Battling COVID-19: 'We Are the Guinea Pigs.'" *GMA News*, May 2, 2020. www.gmanetwork.com/news/lifestyle/ content/736543/pinay-nurse-in-california-shares-struggles-in-battling-covid-19-we-are-the-guinea-pigs/story/

Jenkins, David and Lipin Ram. "Kerala's Pandemic Response Owes Its Success to Participatory Politics." *Novara Media*, August 7, 2020. https://novaramedia.com/ 2020/08/07/keralas-pandemic-response-owes-its-success-to-participatory-politics/

Jerng, Mark C. *Racial Worldmaking: The Power of Popular Fiction*. New York: Fordham University Press, 2017.

Jones Sam. "'Arrogance' Blinded Big Countries to Virus Risk, Says Austria Adviser." *Financial Times*, May 3, 2020. www.ft.com/content/87495a18-f7a1-4657-a517-ba2b16c146dc

Judd, Donald, Vazquez, Maegan, and O'Sullivan, Donie. "Biden Says Platforms Like Facebook Are 'Killing People' with Covid Misinformation." *CNN*, July 17, 2021. www.cnn.com/2021/07/16/politics/biden-facebook-covid-19/index.html

Juhasz, Alexandra, Nishant Shahani, and Jih-Fei Cheng, eds. "Foreword, Preface, and Introduction." *AIDS and the Distribution of Crises*. Durham, NC: Duke University, 2020. 4, 16.

Kahl, Colin and Thomas Wright. *Aftershocks: Pandemic Politics and the End of the Old International Order*. New York: St. Martin's Press, 2021.

Kahura, Dauti. "The Unforeseen Threat." *Africa Is a Country*, April 2, 2021. https:// africasacountry.com/2021/04/the-unforeseen-threat?fbclid=IwAR2P7T2idwd oh3KPB_q_NUKXppx_aB-wAIu4vyCugRuWmBVoZNmZmE9jAaw

Kakissis, Joanna. "Turkmenistan Has Banned Use of the Word 'Coronavirus'." *NPR*, March 31, 2020. www.npr.org/sections/coronavirus-live-updates/2020/03/31/ 824611607/turkmenistan-has-banned-use-of-the-word-coronavirus

Karlidag, Ilgin. "Turkey Feeds Stray Animals during Covid-19 Outbreak." *BBC*, April 7, 2020. www.bbc.com/news/blogs-news-from-elsewhere-52199691

Kashkett, Steven. "Czech Republic Has Lifesaving COVID-19 Lesson for America: Wear a Face Mask." *USA Today*, July 14, 2020. www.usatoday.com/story/opinion/2020/07/14/how-czech-republic-beat-covid-require-everyone-wear-face-masks-column/5426602002/

Kelley, Robin D.G. *Freedom Dreams: The Black Radical Imagination*. Boston: Beacon Press, 2002.

———. "From the River to the Sea to Every Mountain Top: Solidarity as Worldmaking," *Journal of Palestine Studies* 48, no. 4 (2019): 69–91.

Kelloway, Claire. "Food Workers Are on the Frontlines of Coronavirus. They Need Our Support." *Civil Eats*, March 20, 2020. https://civileats.com/2020/03/20/op-ed-food-workers-are-on-the-frontlines-of-coronavirus-they-need-our-support

Kendi, Ibram X. "We're Still Living and Dying in the Slaveholder's Republic." *The Atlantic*, May 4, 2020. www.theatlantic.com/ideas/archive/2020/05/what-freedom-means-trump/611083/

Kennedy, Paul. *Vampire Capitalism: Fractured Societies and Alternative Futures*. New York: Springer, 2016.

Kertscher, Tom. "Melanin Doesn't Protect against Coronavirus." *Politifact*, March 10, 2020. www.politifact.com/factchecks/2020/mar/10/facebook-posts/melanin-doesnt-protect-against-coronavirus/

———. "People of Color May Be Immune to the Coronavirus Because of Melanin." *Politifact*, March 10, 2020. www.politifact.com/factchecks/2020/mar/10/facebook-posts/melanin-doesnt-protect-against-coronavirus/

Kestler-D'Amours, Jillian. "Why Are Muslim Women Living 'in Fear' in This Canadian City?" *Aljazeera*, July 13, 2021. www.aljazeera.com/news/2021/7/13/why-are-muslim-women-living-in-fear-in-this-canadian-city

Kettley, Sebastian. "Coronavirus in the Bible: Preacher Warns of 'Apocalyptic Signs' as 'End of World Nears.'" *Express*, March 17, 2020. www.express.co.uk/news/weird/1256517/Coronavirus-bible-end-of-the-world-warning-COVID19-apocalypse-latest-coronavirus-news

Kim, Claire Jean. *Dangerous Crossings*. Cambridge: Cambridge University Press, 2015.

Kim, Jeong-Min et al. "Identification of Coronavirus Isolated from a Patient in Korea with COVID-19." *Osong Public Health and Research Perspectives* 11, no. 1 (2020): 3.

Kirby, Jen. "George Floyd Protests Go Global: Foreign Leaders Are Also Reacting to the Turmoil in the United States." *Vox*, May 31, 2020. www.vox.com/2020/5/31/21276031/george-floyd-protests-london-berlin

Klein, Naomi. *The Shock Doctrine: The Rise of Disaster Capitalism*. New York: Macmillan, 2007.

Klinenberg, Eric. *Heat Wave: A Social Autopsy of Disaster in Chicago*. Chicago: University of Chicago Press, 2015.

Knickmeyer, Ellen. "Citing Outbreak, EPA Has Stopped Enforcing Environmental Laws." *Associated Press*, March 27, 2020. www.pbs.org/newshour/economy/citing-outbreak-epa-has-stopped-enforcing-environmental-laws

Kolb, Anjuli Fatima Raza. *Epidemic Empire: Colonialism, Contagion, and Terror, 1817–2020*. Chicago: University of Chicago Press, 2021.

Koran, Mario and Sam Levin. "All Californians Ordered to Shelter in Place as Governor Estimates More than 25m Will Get Virus." *The Guardian*, March 19, 2020. www.theguardian.com/world/2020/mar/19/coronavirus-california-more-than-half-gavin-newsom

Kossoff, Julian. "2 Top French Doctors Said on Live TV that Coronavirus Vaccines Should Be Tested on Poor Africans, Leaving Viewers Horrified." *Business Insider*, April 3, 2020. www.businessinsider.com/coronavirus-vaccines-france-doctors-say-test-poor-africans-outrage-2020-4

Kovac, Carl. "Nigerians to Sue US Drug Company over Meningitis Treatment." *BMJ* 323, no. 7313 (2001): 592.

Kramer, Larry. *The American People: Volume 1: Search for My Heart: A Novel.* New York: Macmillan, 2015.

Krause-Jensen, Jakob and Keir Martin. "Trickster's Triumph: Donald Trump and the New Spirit of Capitalism." In *Magical Capitalism: Enchantment, Spells, and Occult Practices in Contemporary Economies*, edited by Brian Moeran and Dewaal Malefyt Timothy, 89–113. New York: Palgrave Macmillan, 2018.

Krishna, Shyam A. "How the Spanish Flu Changed the Course of Indian History." *Gulf News*, March 15, 2020. https://gulfnews.com/opinion/op-eds/how-the-spanish-flu-changed-the-course-of-indian-history-1.1584285312898/

Kuo, Lily. "Coronavirus: Wuhan Doctor Speaks Out against Authorities." *The Guardian*, March 11, 2020. https://amp.theguardian.com/world/2020/mar/11/coronavirus-wuhan-doctor-ai-fen-speaks-out-against-authorities

Kwon, Peter Banseok. "Building Bombs, Building a Nation: The State, Chaeböl, and the Militarized Industrialization of South Korea, 1973–1979." *The Journal of Asian Studies* 79, no.1 (2020): 51–75.

LaDuke, Winona. "Traditional Ecological Knowledge and Environmental Futures." *Colorado Journal of International Environmental Law & Policy* 5 (1994): 127–148.

LaDuke, Winona, and Sean Aaron Cruz. *The Militarization of Indian Country.* East Lansing: Michigan State University Press, 2013.

La Izquierda Diario Argentina. "Italy Calls General Strike: 'Our Lives Are Worth More than Your Profits.'" *Left Voice*, March 25, 2020. www.leftvoice.org/italy-calls-general-strike-our-lives-are-worth-more-than-your-profits

Langreth, Robert and Susan Berfield. "Famed AIDS Researcher is Racing to Find a Coronavirus Treatment." *Bloomberg*, March 20, 2020. www.bloomberg.com/news/features/2020-03-19/this-famous-aids-researcher-wants-to-find-a-coronavirus-cure

Laterza, Vito and Louis Philippe Römer. "COVID-19, the Freedom to Die, and the Necropolitics of the Market." *Somatosphere*, May 12, 2020. http://somatosphere.net/2020/necropolitics-of-the-market.html/

Laud, Georgina. "Coronavirus Explained: Why Is It Called Coronavirus? What Does Corona Mean?" *Express*, March 20, 2020. www.express.co.uk/life-style/health/1241302/Coronavirus-named-COVID-19-meaning-WHO-coronavirus-latest-update

Laughland, Oliver and Amanda Holpuch. "'We're Modern Slaves': How Meat Plant Workers Became the New Frontline in Covid-19 War." *The Guardian*, May 2, 2020. www.theguardian.com/world/2020/may/02/meat-plant-workers-us-coronavirus-war

Lawtoo, Nidesh. *Conrad's Shadow: Catastrophe, Mimesis, Theory*. Lansing: Michigan State University Press, 2016.

Lee, Seulki. "South Korea's First Feminist Party Launches on International Women's Day." *The Jakarta Post*, March 3, 2020. www.thejakartapost.com/news/2020/03/03/south-koreas-first-feminist-party-launches-on-international-womens-day.html

Levitz, Eric. "Meatpacking Crisis Shows Limits of Human Sacrifice as Recovery Plan." *New York Magazine*, May 6, 2020. https://nymag.com/intelligencer/2020/05/coronavirus-meat-packing-plants-trump-reopen-economy-workers.html

Li, Jane. "China Writer Fang Closes Wuhan Coronavirus Lockdown Diary." *Quartz*, March 26, 2020. https://qz.com/1825896/china-writer-fang-fang-closes-wuhan-coronavirus-lockdown-diary

Lin, Shiqi. "CUT! Community, Immunity, Vulnerability in the Time of Coronavirus." *University of California Humanities Research Institute*, March 2020. https://uchri.org/foundry/cut-community-immunity-vulnerability-in-the-time-of-coronavirus/

Liu, Andrew. " 'Chinese Virus,' World Market." *N+1 Magazine*, March 20, 2020. https://nplusonemag.com/online-only/online-only/chinese-virus-world-market/

Liu, Joyce C.H. "Irregular Population and the Aporia of Communities." *University of California Humanities Research Institute*, May 2019. https://uchri.org/foundry/irregular-population-and-the-aporia-of-communities-toward-a-critique-of-internal-coloniality-in-the-age-of-neoliberal-capitalism/

Liu, Melinda. "Is China Ground Zero for a Future Pandemic?" *Smithsonian Magazine*, November 2017. www.smithsonianmag.com/science-nature/china-ground-zero-future-pandemic-180965213/

Livingston, Julie. *Self-Devouring Growth: A Planetary Parable as Told from Southern Africa*. Durham, NC: Duke University Press, 2019.

Locke, Taylor. "Barack Obama: 'If Every Nation on Earth Was Run by Women' for 2 Years, Things Would Be Better." *CNBC*, December 17, 2019. www.cnbc.com/2019/12/16/barack-obama-how-women-are-better-leaders-than-men.html

London, Eric. "Hundreds of Mexican Maquiladora Workers Dying after Back-To-Work Orders Take Effect." *World Socialist Website*, May 19, 2020. www.wsws.org/en/articles/2020/05/19/mexi-m19.html

Lorde, Audre. *A Litany for Survival: The Life and Work of Audre Lorde*, directed by Ada G. Griffin and Michelle Parkerson. New York: Third World Newsreel, 1996.

———. *A Burst of Light: And Other Essays*. Mineola, NY: Courier Dover Publications, 2017.

Los Angeles Times. "Editorial: Coronavirus Makes Jails and Prisons Potential Death Traps. That Puts Us All in Danger." *The Los Angeles Times*, March 18, 2020. www.latimes.com/opinion/story/2020-03-18/coronavirus-prisons-releases

Lowe, Celia. "Viral Clouds: Becoming H5N1 in Indonesia." *Cultural Anthropology* 25, no. 4 (2010): 625–649.

Lowe, Lisa. *The Intimacies of Four Continents*. Durham, NC: Duke University Press, 2015.

———. "Afterword." In *Revolutionary Feminisms: Conversations on Collective Action and Radical Thought*, edited by Brenna Bhandar and Rafeef Ziadah, 210, 217–227. New York: Verso, 2020.

Lugones, Maria. "Toward a Decolonial Feminism." *Hypatia* 25, no. 4 (2010): 742–759.

Lyons, Kat. "Anger in Guam at 'Dangerous' Plan to Offload US Sailors from Virus-Hit Aircraft Carrier." *The Guardian*, April 1, 2020. www.theguardian.com/world/2020/apr/02/anger-in-guam-at-dangerous-plan-to-offload-us-sailors-from-virus-hit-aircraft-carrier

MacPhail, Theresa. *The Viral Network: A Pathography of the H1N1 Influenza Pandemic*. Ithaca, NY: Cornell University Press, 2015.

Mahtani, Shibani. "Boris Johnson Offers Refuge, British Citizenship Path for Nearly 3 Million Hong Kongers." *Washington Post*, June 3, 2020. www.washingtonpost.com/world/asia_pacific/boris-johnson-hong-kong-national-security-law-bno-passport/2020/06/03/3ec6ddf0-a545-11ea-b619-3f9133bbb482_story.html

Maiden, Samantha. "Chinese State Media Labels Australia 'The Dog of the United States.'" *News.Com.Au*, May 20, 2020. www.news.com.au/world/coronavirus/global/chinese-state-media-labels-australia-the-dog-of-the-united-states/news-story/fb1464c8a04b61e8863038c7d0dada84

Malik, Ayesha Mahmood. "We Had Always Been 'Socially Distant' from the Destitute and Vulnerable—Only Now It Is Worse." *The Review of Religions*, April 28, 2020. www.reviewofreligions.org/21768/we-had-always-been-socially-distant-from-the-destitute-and-vulnerable-only-now-it-is-worse/

Manganyi, Chabani N. *Being Black in the World*. Johannesburg: Wits University Press, 2019.

Manjoo, Farhad. "Republicans Want Medicare for All, But Just for This One Disease: Everyone's a Socialist in a Pandemic." *New York Times*, March 11, 2020. www.nytimes.com/2020/03/11/opinion/coronavirus-socialism.html

Mankeker, Purnima and Akhil Gupta. "Future Tense: Capital, Labor, and Technology in a Service Industry: The 2017 Lewis Henry Morgan Lecture." *Journal of Ethnographic Theory* 7, no. 3 (2017): 67–87.

Marr, Bernard. "Robots and Drones Are Now Used to Fight COVID-19." *Forbes*, March 18, 2020. www.forbes.com/sites/bernardmarr/2020/03/18/how-robots-and-drones-are-helping-to-fight-coronavirus/#799a5c212a12

Marsh, Jenni, Shawn Deng, and Nectar Gan. "Africans in Guangzhou Are on Edge, after Many Are Left Homeless amid Rising Xenophobia as China Fights a Second Wave of Coronavirus." *CNN*, April 12, 2020. www.cnn.com/2020/04/10/china/africans-guangzhou-china-coronavirus-hnk-intl/index.html

Marsh, Sarah. "Cuba Credits Two Drugs with Slashing Coronavirus Death Toll." *Reuters*, May 22, 2020. www.reuters.com/article/us-health-coronavirus-cuba/cuba-credits-two-drugs-with-slashing-coronavirus-death-toll-idUSKBN22Y2Y4?feedType=mktg&feedName=healthNews&WT.mc_id=Partner-Google&fbclid=IwAR34b9eelnNjXTIFTsSPv9hwzqpBkotwZzNtu4l9AD2AVfHtwlcgzU86lkc

Martin, Nick. "Against Productivity in a Pandemic." *New Republic*, March 17, 2020. https://newrepublic.com/article/156929/work-home-productivity-coronavirus-pandemic

———. "This Is Crisis Colonization." *The New Republic*, March 30, 2020. https://newrepublic.com/article/157091/crisis-colonization

Massey, Doreen. *Space, Place and Gender*. Minneapolis: University of Minnesota Press, 1994.

Maxouris, Christina, Holly Yan, and Ralph Ellis. "Cities Extend Curfews for Another Night in an Attempt to Avoid Violent Protests over George Floyd's Death." *CNN*,

May 31, 2020. www.cnn.com/2020/05/31/us/george-floyd-protests-sunday/index.html

Mbembe, Achille and Diogo Bercito. "The Pandemic Democratizes the Power to Kill: An Interview." *European Journal of Psychoanalysis*, March 31, 2020. www.journal-psychoanalysis.eu/the-pandemic-democratizes-the-power-to-kill-an-interview/

McCurry, Justin. "How South Korea's Evangelical Churches Found Themselves at the Heart of The Covid Crisis." *The Guardian*, August 23, 2020. www.theguardian.com/world/2020/aug/23/how-south-koreas-evangelical-churches-found-themselves-at-the-heart-of-the-covid-crisis

McKittrick, Katherine. "Mathematics Black Life." *The Black Scholar* 44, no. 2 (2014): 16–28.

McNally, David. *Monsters of the Market: Zombies, Vampires and Global Capitalism.* Leiden: Brill, 2011.

McNeill, William Hardy. *Plagues and Peoples.* Garden City, NY: Anchor, 1998.

Mead, Walter Russell. "China Is the Real Sick Man of Asia." *Wall Street Journal*, February 3, 2020. www.wsj.com/articles/china-is-the-real-sick-man-of-asia-11580773677

Melandri, Francesca. "A Letter from Locked Down Italy: This Is What We Know about Your Future." *Portside*, April 8, 2020. https://portside.org/2020-04-08/letter-locked-down-italy-what-we-know-about-your-future

Melman, Yossi. "Coronavirus 'Truce': The Guns Falling Silent across the Middle East." *Haaretz*, March 16, 2020. www.haaretz.com/middle-east-news/.premium-coronavirus-truce-the-guns-falling-silent-across-the-middle-east-1.8677993

Memmi, Albert. *The Colonizer and the Colonized.* London: Routledge, 2013.

Merriam-Webster. "Apocalypse." Merriam-Webster, accessed June 12, 2020. www.merriam-webster.com

Michener, Jamila. *Fragmented Democracy: Medicaid, Federalism, and Unequal Politics.* Cambridge: Cambridge University Press, 2018.

Migrant Rights. "The COVID-19 Crisis Is Fueling More Racist Discourse towards Migrant Workers in the Gulf." *Migrant Rights*, April 5, 2020. www.migrant-rights.org/2020/04/the-covid-19-crisis-is-fueling-more-racist-discourse-towards-migrant-workers-in-the-gulf/

Millhiser, Ian. "The Fake Text Message about the 'Stafford Act' and a National Quarantine, Explained: Don't Believe Everything You Read Online." *Vox*, March 16, 2020. www.vox.com/2020/3/16/21181486/stafford-act-text-message-hoax-coronavirus-national-quarantine-trump

Mirchandani, Maya, Shoba Suri, and Laetitia Bruce Warjri, eds. *The Viral World.* New Delhi: ORF and Global Policy Journal, 2020.

Molina, Natalia. *How Race Is Made in America: Immigration, Citizenship, and the Historical Power of Racial Scripts.* Berkeley: University of California Press, 2013.

Molteni, Megan. "Snakes?! The Slippery Truth of a Flawed Wuhan Virus Theory." *Wired*, January 23, 2020. www.wired.com/story/wuhan-coronavirus-snake-flu-theory/

Monella, Lillo Montalto and Rita Palfi. "Orban Uses Coronavirus as Excuse to Suspend Asylum Rights in Hungary." *Euronews*, March 3, 2020. www.euronews.com/2020/03/03/orban-uses-coronavirus-as-excuse-to-suspend-asylum-rights-in-hungary

Montaigne, Michel De. *Complete Essays*. Stanford: Stanford University Press, 1965.

Montgomery, Marc. "2020 World Democracy Index: Worrisome Decline." *RCI*, January 27, 2020. www.rcinet.ca/en/2020/01/27/2020-world-democracy-index-worrisome-decline/

Moore, Lorrie. "Experiencing the Coronavirus Pandemic as a Kind of Zombie Apocalypse." *The New Yorker*, April 6, 2020. www.newyorker.com/magazine/2020/04/13/the-nurses-office

Moraga, Cherríe. "Preface." In *This Bridge Called My Back: Writings by Radical Women of Color, XV–XVII*, edited by Gloría Anzaldúa and Toni Cade Bambara, xv–xxxiii. Watertown, MA: Persephone Press, 1981.

Moreno, Jonathan D. *Undue Risk: Secret State Experiments on Humans*. Philadelphia: Routledge, 2013.

Mormina, Maru and Ifeanyi M. Nosofor. "What Developing Countries Can Teach Rich Countries about How to Respond to a Pandemic." *Quartz Africa*, October 19, 2020. https://qz.com/africa/1919785/what-africa-and-asia-teach-rich-countries-on-handling-a-pandemic

Morrison, Patt. "What the Deadly 1918 Flu Epidemic Can Teach Us about Our Coronavirus Reaction." *Gulf News*, March 15, 2020. https://gulfnews.com/opinion/op-eds/what-the-deadly-1918-flu-epidemic-can-teach-us-about-our-coronavirus-reaction-1.70313751

Morrissey, Kate. "San Diego Fund to Help Unauthorized Immigrants Out of Work due to Coronavirus Pandemic." *San Diego Union Tribune*, March 27, 2020. www.sandiegouniontribune.com/news/immigration/story/2020-03-27/san-diego-fund-to-help-unauthorized-immigrants-out-of-work-due-to-coronavirus-pandemic

Murphy, Michelle. *The Economization of Life*. Durham, NC: Duke University Press, 2017.

Nadurata, Edward. "Who Cares?: Ability and the Elderly Question in Filipinx Studies." In *Filipinx American Critique: An Interdisciplinary Reckoning*, edited by Rick Bonus and Antonio Tiongson, 341–353. New York: Fordham University Press, 2022.

Na'puti, Tiara R. "Archipelagic Rhetoric: Remapping the Marianas and Challenging Militarization from 'A Stirring Place.'" *Communication and Critical/Cultural Studies* 16, no. 1 (2019): 4–25.

Newcomb, Alyssa. "173 years, $170: Why Irish People Are Donating to Help Native Americans Hit by Coronavirus." *NBC News*, May 6, 2020. www.nbcnews.com/news/us-news/173-years-170-why-irish-people-are-donating-help-native-n1200811

Nguyen, Frances. "This State Says It Has a 'Feminist Economic Recovery Plan.' Here's What That Looks Like." *The Lily*, April 22, 2020. www.thelily.com/this-state-says-they-have-a-feminist-economic-recovery-plan-heres-what-that-looks-like/

Nguyen, Vinh-Kim. *The Republic of Therapy: Triage and Sovereignty in West Africa's Time of AIDS*. Durham, NC: Duke University Press, 2010.

Nixon, Rob. *Slow Violence and the Environmentalism of the Poor*. Cambridge: Harvard University Press, 2011.

Nortajuddin, Athira. "Suicide: Thailand's Epidemic in a Pandemic." *The ASEAN Post*, March 18, 2021. https://theaseanpost.com/article/suicide-thailands-epidemic-pandemic

Oh, David C. "Ethical (Re)Positioning: Asian American Doctors and the Struggle against Structural Racism and Covid-19." *Texas A&M University*, https://oaktrust.library.tamu.edu/bitstream/handle/1969.1/188225/David%20C.%20Oh%20%28QAB%20Entry%20%235%29.pdf?sequence=1&isAllowed=y

Olmos, Daniel. "Unsung Heroes or Exploited Workers? Latino Migrant Day Laborers in Post-Harvey Houston and Critical Environmental Justice." *Resilience: A Journal of the Environmental Humanities* 9, no. 2 (2022): 46–62.

Oppenheim, Maya. "Mexico Sees Almost 1,000 Women Murdered in Three Months as Domestic Abuse Concerns Rise amid Coronavirus." *Yahoo*, April 28, 2020. https://news.yahoo.com/mexico-sees-almost-1-000-135946687.html

Ossei-Owusu, Shaun. "Coronavirus and the Politics of Disposability." *Boston Review*, April 8, 2020. http://bostonreview.net/class-inequality-race-politics/shaun-ossei-owusu-coronavirus-and-politics-disposability/

Palmer, Ewan. "Church Leader Who Blamed Coronavirus on Gay Marriage Contracts COVID-19." *Newsweek*, September 8, 2020. www.newsweek.com/patriarch-filaret-coronavirus-gay-marriage-ukraine-1530261

Papenfuss, Mary. "Norway College Urges Students to Return from 'Poorly Developed' U.S. amid Pandemic." *HuffPost*, March 15, 2020. www.huffpost.com/entry/norway-students-us-collectiveinfrastructure_n_5e6ec485c5b6dda30fcbba2a

———. "Trump Reportedly Weighed Letting COVID-19 'Wash Over' U.S., But Was Warned of Grim Toll." *HuffPost*, April 4, 2020. www.huffpost.com/entry/trump-free-range-covid-19-death-toll_n_5e925a48c5b6f7b1ea82dcd7

Park, Lisa Sun-Hee. *Entitled to Nothing.* New York: New York University Press, 2011.

Park, S. Nathan. "Confucianism Isn't Helping Beat the Coronavirus." *Foreign Policy*, April 2, 2020. https://foreignpolicy.com/2020/04/02/confucianism-south-korea-coronavirus-testing-cultural-trope-orientalism/

Patterson, Orlando. *Slavery and Social Death: A Comparative Study.* Cambridge, MA: Harvard University Press, 2018.

Penney, Joe. "African Nations Turn the Tables, Imposing Travel Restrictions against U.S., Europe, and China to Stave Off Coronavirus." *The Intercept*, March 15, 2020. https://theintercept.com/2020/03/15/african-nations-turn-the-tables-imposing-travel-restrictions-against-u-s-europe-and-china-to-stave-off-coronavirus/

Peter, Zsombor. "Malaysia Rounds up Hundreds of Undocumented Migrants amid Coronavirus Fears." *Voanews*, May 3, 2020. www.voanews.com/east-asia-pacific/malaysia-rounds-hundreds-undocumented-migrants-amid-coronavirus-fears

Peters, Michael A. and Tina Besley. *Pandemic Education and Viral Politics.* Abingdon, Oxon; New York, NY: Routledge, 2021.

Pettypiece, Shannon and Peter Alexander. "Trump Says He Wants Country 'Opened Up' by Easter, despite Caution from Health Experts." *NBC News*, March 24, 2020. www.nbcnews.com/politics/white-house/trump-says-he-wants-country-open-back-april-12-easter-n1167721

Philippine Daily Inquirer. "Knee on the National Neck." *Philippine Daily Inquirer*, June 3, 2020. https://opinion.inquirer.net/130416/knee-on-the-national-neck

Phillips, Dom. "Brazil Using Coronavirus to Cover Up Assaults on Amazon, Warn Activists." *The Guardian*, May 6, 2020. www.theguardian.com/world/2020/may/06/brazil-using-coronavirus-to-cover-up-assaults-on-amazon-warn-activists

Phillips, Kristine. " 'They Look at Me and Think I'm Some Kind of Virus': What It's Like to Be Asian during the Coronavirus Pandemic." *The Daytona Beach*

News-Journal, March 30, 2020. www.news-journalonline.com/zz/news/20200
330/they-look-at-me-and-think-im-some-kind-of-virus-what-its-like-to-be-asian-
during-coronavirus-pandemic

Phillips, Morgan. "Bolsonaro Calls Brazilian Cities' Coronavirus Lockdowns a
'Crime.'" *Fox News*, March 25, 2020. www.foxnews.com/world/bolsonaro-calls-
brazilian-cities-coronavirus-lockdowns-a-crime

Phillips, Tom. "Brazil's Jair Bolsonaro Says Coronavirus Crisis Is a Media Trick."
The Guardian, March 23, 2020. www.theguardian.com/world/2020/mar/23/braz
ils-jair-bolsonaro-says-coronavirus-crisis-is-a-media-trick

Phoenix, Davin L. *The Anger Gap: How Race Shapes Emotion in Politics.*
Cambridge: Cambridge University Press, 2019.

Phu, Thy. *Picturing Model Citizens: Civility in Asian American Visual Culture.*
Philadelphia: Temple University Press, 2011.

Piela, Anna. "COVID-19 Is Increasing Religious Tolerance. Here's Why." *Fast
Company*, February 8, 2021. www.fastcompany.com/90602111/covid-19-is-inc
reasing-religious-tolerance-heres-why

Piña, D. Alex. "White Supremacy in Rainbow: Global Pride and Black Lives
Matter in the Era of COVID. *New Sociology: Journal of Critical Praxis*, 3, no. 1
(2022): 136–146.

Pirtle, Whitney N. Laster. "Racial Capitalism: A Fundamental Cause of Novel
Coronavirus (COVID-19) Pandemic Inequities in the United States." *Health
Education and Behavior* 47, no. 4 (August 2020): 504–08.

Porterfield, Carlie. "Two-Thirds of Religious Americans Believe Coronavirus Is a
Message from God." *Forbes*, May 15, 2020. www.forbes.com/sites/carlieporterfi
eld/2020/05/15/two-thirds-of-religious-americans-believe-coronavirus-is-a-mess
age-from-god/#446e7cbea2ae

Prashad, Vijay. "The Great Contest of Our Time Is between Humanity and
Imperialism: The Thirtieth Newsletter." Thetricontinental.org, July 29, 2021.
https://thetricontinental.org/newsletterissue/30-new-cold-war/?output=pdf

Prashad, Vijay, and Subin Dennis. "An Often Overlooked Region of India Is a Beacon
to the World for Taking on the Coronavirus." *People's Dispatch*, March 24, 2020.
https://peoplesdispatch.org/2020/03/24/an-often-overlooked-region-of-india-is-a-
beacon-to-the-world-for-taking-on-the-coronavirus/

Prieur, Jacques. "Critical Warning! Preventing the Multidimensional Apocalypse on
Planet Earth." *Ecosystem Services* 45 (2020): 101161.

Prison Pandemic Project, *University of California*, Irvine. https://prisonpandemic.uci.
edu/, accessed June 12, 2020.

Puar, Jasbir K. *The Right to Maim: Debility, Capacity, Disability.* Durham, NC: Duke
University Press, 2017.

Quammen, David. *Spillover: Animal Infections and the Next Human Pandemic.*
New York: W.W. Norton & Company, 2012.

Rautray, Samanwaya. "SC Wonders How Its Two-Judge Bench Usurped Powers of
CJI." *Times of India*, November 10, 2017. https://timesofindia.indiatimes.com/
india/sc-wonders-how-its-two-judge-bench-usurped-powers-of-cji/articleshow/
61597707.cms

Reeves, Jay. "In Clamor to Reopen, Many Black People Feel Overlooked." *AP News*,
May 5, 2020. https://apnews.com/5a70d53a228265269c07a59764382273

Regencia, Ted. "'Kill Them': Duterte Wants to 'Finish Off' Communist Rebels." *Aljazeera*, March 6, 2021. www.aljazeera.com/news/2021/3/6/kill-them-all-dute rte-wants-communist-rebels-finished

Ren, Li-Li et al. "Identification of a Novel Coronavirus Causing Severe Pneumonia in Human: A Descriptive Study." *Chinese Medical Journal* 133, no. 9 (2019): 1015–1024. doi: 10.1097/CM9.0000000000000722

Robinson, William. *Global Civil War: Capitalism Post-Pandemic*. Oakland: PM Press, 2022.

Reuters. "MSF Urges Greece to Evacuate Migrant Camps due to Coronavirus Risk." *Reuters*, March 13, 2020. www.reuters.com/article/us-health-coronavirus-greece-migrants/msf-urges-greece-to-evacuate-migrant-camps-due-to-coronavirus-risk-idUSKBN2102M1

———. "Taking COVID-19 Vaccine Will Not Alter Your DNA, Ghana President Says." *Reuters*, February 28, 2021. www.reuters.com/article/uk-health-coronavi rus-ghana-president/taking-covid-19-vaccine-will-not-alter-your-dna-ghana-president-says-idUSKCN2AT1L3

Reyes, Victoria. *Global Borderlands: Fantasy, Violence, and Empire in Subic Bay, Philippines*. Stanford: Stanford University Press, 2020.

Rich, Motoko. "Why Asia's New Wave of Virus Cases Should Worry the World." *New York Times*, March 31, 2020. www.nytimes.com/2020/03/31/world/asia/coronavirus-china-hong-kong-singapore-south-korea.html

Ripple, William J., Christopher Wolf, Thomas M. Newsome, Phoebe Barnard, and William R. Moomaw. "World Scientists' Warning of a Climate Emergency." *BioScience* 70, no. 1 (2020): 8–12.

Rivlin-Nadler, Max. "'Remain-in-Mexico' Paused as Asylum-Seekers Stranded in Crowded Shelters during Pandemic." *KPBS*, March 24, 2020. www.kpbs.org/news/2020/mar/24/remain-mexico-program-paused-asylum-seekers-are-st/

Roberts, Samuel. *Infectious Fear: Politics, Disease, and the Health Effects of Segregation*. Chapel Hill: University of North Carolina Press, 2009.

Romero Tenario, José Manuel, and William Andres Alvarez. "La Máquina De Guerra Nómada Del COVID-19: Paisajes Estéticos Del Epidemiocapitalismo." *Trans/Form/Ação* 44 (2021): 267–284.

Rosario, Isabella. "Jesus Was Divisive: A Black Pastor's Message to White Christians." *NPR*, June 12, 2020. www.npr.org/sections/codeswitch/2020/06/12/699611293/jesus-was-divisive-a-black-pastors-message-to-white-christians

Roy, Arundhati. "'The Pandemic Is a Portal.'" *Financial Times*, April 3, 2020. www.ft.com/content/10d8f5e8-74eb-11ea-95fe-fcd274e920ca

Rozsa, Matthew. "QAnon Is the Conspiracy Theory that Won't Die: Here's What They Believe, and Why They're Wrong." *Salon*, August 18, 2019. www.salon.com/2019/08/18/qanon-is-the-conspiracy-theory-that-wont-die-heres-what-they-believe-and-why-theyre-wrong/

Rubin, Joel. "Coronavirus Misinformation and Hoax Text Messages Are Making the Rounds. Here's How to Spot Them." *Los Angeles Times*, March 18, 2020. www.latimes.com/california/story/2020-03-18/coronavirus-martial-law-email-message-hoax

Rubin, Vera. Facebook, April 24, 2023. www.facebook.com/FleshPrisonBreak/timel ine?lst=1171484871%3A575001312%3A1589154462

Rubio, Marco (@Marcorubio). "#China's Consulate in #Houston Is Not a Diplomatic Facility. It Is the Central Node of the Communist Party's Vast Network of Spies & Influence Operations in the United States. Now That Building Must Close & the Spies Have 72 Hours to Leave or Face Arrest." *Twitter*, July 22, 2020, 5:45 am. https://twitter.com/marcorubio/status/1285909840192315395?

Ruiz, Don Miguel and Janet Mills. *The Four Agreements (Illustrated Edition): A Practical Guide to Personal Freedom.* Carlsbad, CA: Hay House Inc., 2011.

Ruiz, Sandra. *Ricanness: Enduring Time in Anticolonial Performance.* New York: New York University Press, 2019, 171.

Ruiz, Stevie. *Earth Stewards: Reclaiming Hidden Labor Practices in Environmental Spaces.* Chapel Hill, N.C.: University of North Carolina Press, 2025.

———. "Contesting Legal Borderlands: Policing Insubordinate Spaces in Imperial County's Farm Worker Communities, 1933–1940." *Kalfou* 7, no. 2 (2020).

Rummler, Orion. "Brazil and Ecuador Emerge as Latin America's Coronavirus Epicenters." *Axios*, April 23, 2020. www.axios.com/2020/04/23/coronavirus-latin-america-brazil-ecuador

Ryan, J. Michael. "The Blessings of COVID-19 for Neoliberalism, Nationalism, and Neoconservative Ideologies." In *COVID-19: Volume II: Social Consequences and Cultural Adaptations*, edited by J. Michael Ryan, 80–93. London: Routledge, 2020.

———. "The SARS-CoV-2 Virus and the COVID-19 Pandemic." In *COVID-19: Volume II: Social Consequences and Cultural Adaptations*, edited by J. Michael Ryan, n.p. London: Routledge, 2020.

Sabarini, Prodita. "Coronavirus: Migrants in Frontline Jobs Not Entitled to Any Financial Help If They Get Sick." *The Conversation*, April 2, 2020. https://theconversation.com/coronavirus-migrants-in-frontline-jobs-not-entitled-to-any-financial-help-if-they-get-sick-134970

Salomón, Amrah. "Decolonizing the Disaster: Defending Land & Life during Covid-19." *Political Theology*, October 24, 2020. https://politicaltheology.com/decolonizing-the-disaster-defending-land-life-during-covid-19/

Samilton, Tracy. "Detroit Unveils Water Restart Plan Because of Coronavirus Threat." *Michigan Radio*, March 9, 2020. www.michiganradio.org/post/detroit-unveils-water-restart-plan-because-of-coronavirus-threat

Sang-Hun, Choe. "South Korean Leader Said Coronavirus Would 'Disappear.' It Was a Costly Error." *New York Times*, February 27, 2020. www.nytimes.com/2020/02/27/world/asia/coronavirus-south-korea.html?searchResultPosition=2

Saskia Sassen, "Global Cities and Survival Circuits." In *Woman: Nannies, Maids, and Sex Workers in the New Economy*, edited by Saskia Sassen, Barbara Ehrenreich, and Arlie Russell Hochschild, 254–247. New York: Metropolitan, 2002.

Scarr, Lanai and Peter Law. "Ban Trips from Indian Hell." *The West Australia*, April 28, 2021.

Schama, Simon. Foreign Bodies: *Pandemics, Vaccines, and the Health of Nations.* New York: Ecco, 2023.

Schuller, Kyla. "Losing Paradise." *The Rumpus*, June 2, 2020. https://therumpus.net/2020/06/losingparadise/

Schultz, Eric. "Belgians Target Some Royal Monuments in Black Lives Matter Protest." *NPR*, June 5, 2020. www.npr.org/sections/live-updates-protests-for-racial-justice/2020/06/05/871278150/belgians-target-some-royal-monuments-in-black-lives-matter-protest

Schultz, Katherine and Russell Hsiao. "Why Taiwan's Coronavirus Response Shows Europe It Should Join the World Health Organization." *The National Interest*, March 31, 2020. https://nationalinterest.org/feature/why-taiwans-coronavirus-response-shows-europe-it-should-join-world-health-organization/

Schwab, Klaus and Thierry Malleret. *COVID-19: The Great Reset*. Geneva: Forum Publishing, 2020.

Schwartz, Ian. "Eddie Glaude: 'I Overestimated White People,' I Didn't Think They Would Put Trump in Office." *Real Clear Politics*, October 31, 2018. www.realcl earpolitics.com/video/2018/10/31/msnbc_eddie_glaude_i_overestimated_white_ people_i_didnt_think_they_would_put_trump_in_office.html

Sen, Amartya. "Human Rights and Capabilities." *Journal of Human Development* 6, no. 2 (2005): 151–166.

Shah, Nayan. *Contagious Divides: Epidemics and Race in San Francisco's Chinatown*. Berkeley: University of California Press, 2001.

Shah, Sonia. "Think Exotic Animals Are to Blame for the Coronavirus? Think Again." *The Nation*, February 18, 2020. www.thenation.com/article/environm ent/coronavirus-habitat-loss/

Sharpe, Christina. *In the Wake: On Blackness and Being*. Durham, NC: Duke University Press, 2016.

Shesgreen, Deirdre. "'Gross Misjudgment': Experts Say Trump's Decision to Disband Pandemic Team Hindered Coronavirus Response." *USA Today*, March 18, 2020. www.usatoday.com/story/news/world/2020/03/18/coronavirus-did-president-tru mps-decision-disband-global-pandemic-office-hinder-response/5064881002/

Shesgreen, Deirdre, and Tom Vanden Brook. "Navy Says It Can't Empty Roosevelt amid Coronavirus Because of Its Weapons, Nuclear Reactor." *USA Today*, April 1, 2020. www.usatoday.com/story/news/politics/2020/04/01/coronavirus-navy-sail ors-roosevelt-guard-weapons-more-sick/5104785002/

Shin, Hyonhee and Sangmi Cha. "'Like a Zombie Apocalypse': Residents on Edge as Coronavirus Cases Surge in South Korea." *Reuters*, February 19, 2020. www.reut ers.com/article/us-china-health-southkorea-cases/like-a-zombie-apocalypse-reside nts-on-edge-as-coronavirus-cases-surge-in-south-korea-idUSKBN20E04F

Shinozuka, Jeannie N. "Deadly Perils: Japanese Beetles and the Pestilential Immigrant, 1920s-1930s." *American Quarterly* 65, no. 4 (2013): 831–852.

Silbergeld, Ellen K. *Chickenizing Farms and Food: How Industrial Meat Production Endangers Workers, Animals, and Consumers*. Baltimore: Johns Hopkins University Press, 2016.

Simmons, Kristen. "Settler Atmospherics." *Society for Cultural Anthropology*, November 20, 2017. https://culanth.org/fieldsights/settler-atmospherics

Simpson, Leanne Betasamosake. *As We Have Always Done: Indigenous Freedom through Radical Resistance*. Minneapolis: University of Minnesota Press, 2017.

Singh, Ajit. "Hong Kong's 'Pro-Democracy' Movement Allies with Far-Right US Politicians that Seek to Crush Black Lives Matter." *The Gray Zone*, June 9, 2020. https://thegrayzone.com/2020/06/09/hong-kongs-far-right-us-politicians-crush-black-lives-matter

Sky News. "We've Been Attacked by Another Virus." *Skynews*, March 3, 2022. https://news.sky.com/video/weve-been-attacked-by-another-virus-president-zelens kyy-says-ukraine-will-continue-to-stand-against-russian-aggression-in-address-to-the-nation-12556467

Slattery, G. and R. Moraes. "In Violent Rio, U.S. Protests Stoke Backlash against Deadly Cops." *Reuters*, June 7, 2020. www.reuters.com/article/us-brazil-prote sts-race-feature/in-violent-rio-u-s-protests-stoke-backlash-against-deadly-cops-idUSKBN23E0QF

Smith, David. "Trump Claims 99% of US Covid-19 Cases Are 'Totally Harmless' as Infections Surge." *The Guardian*, July 4, 2020. https://amp.theguardian.com/world/2020/jul/05/trump-claims-99-of-us-covid-19-cases-are-totally-harmless-as-infections-surge

Smith, Justi E.H. "Permanent Pandemic." *Harpers*, June 2022. https://harpers.org/archive/2022/06/permanent-pandemic-will-covid-controls-keep-controlling-us/

Smith, Nicola. "Taiwan Builds 'Nerd Immunity' to Resist Chinese Disinformation Campaigns." *The Telegraph*, June 2020. www.telegraph.co.uk/news/2020/06/13/taiwan-builds-nerd-immunity-resist-chinese-disinformation-campaigns/

Smith, Oli. "Coronavirus Horror: Social Media Footage Shows Infected Wuhan Residents 'Act Like Zombies': Disturbing Footage Emerged Overnight Showing People Collapsing in the Street in Wuhan, China, as They Quickly Succumb to the Deadly Coronavirus." *Express*, January 24, 2020. www.express.co.uk/news/world/1232814/Coronavirus-horror-China-virus-Wuhan-zombies-epidemic-video

Sopelsa, Brooke. "Trump Cabinet's Bible Teacher Says Gays Cause 'God's Wrath' in COVID-19 Blog Post." *NBC News*, March 25, 2020. www.nbcnews.com/feat ure/nbc-out/trump-s-bible-teacher-says-gays-among-those-blame-covid-n1168981

Sottek, T.C. "The Coronavirus Is Now the American Virus." *The Verge*, March 26, 2020. www.theverge.com/2020/3/26/21196267/coronavirus-usa-cases-covid-19-pandemic-china-number-positive-trump

Sottile, Chiara and Erik Ortiz. "Coronavirus Hits Indian Country Hard, Exposing Infrastructure Disparities." *NBC News*, April 19, 2020. www.nbcnews.com/news/us-news/coronavirus-hits-indian-country-hard-exposing-infrastructure-disparit ies-n1186976

Sparke, Matt and Dimitar Anguelov. "Contextualizing Coronavirus Geographically." *Royal Geographical Society*, April 30, 2020, 498–508. https://rgs ibg.onlinelibrary. wiley.com/journal/14755661

Spinney, Laura. *Pale Rider: The Spanish Flu of 1918 and How It Changed the World*. New York: Public Affairs, 2017.

Spivak, Gayatri Chakravorty. "Three Women's Texts and a Critique of Imperialism." *Critical Inquiry* 12, no. 1 (1985): 243–261.

Steger, Manfred and Paul James. "Disjunctive Globalization in the Era of the Great Unsettling." *Theory, Culture & Society* 37, no. 7–8 (2020): 187–203.

Stodulka, Thomas. "Emotive Banners and Billboards: Worlding Covid-19 and Orders of Feeling in Kupang, Indonesia." *European Journal of East Asian Studies* 1, no. 2 (2022): 1–28.

Stone, Jon. "Scottish Parliament Votes for Immediate Suspension of Tear Gas, Rubber Bullet and Riot Shield Exports to US." *Independent*, June 11, 2020. www.inde pendent.co.uk/news/uk/politics/scotland-us-exports-tear-gas-rubber-bullets-riot-shields-blm-protests-a9560586.html.

Stone, Michael. "Christian Group Defends '2 God Fearing Men' Who Killed Ahmaud Arbery." *Patheos*, May 8, 2020. www.patheos.com/blogs/progressivesecularh umanist/2020/05/christian-group-defends-2-god-fearing-men-who-killed-ahm aud-arbery/

Strother, Jason. "South Korea's Coronavirus Contact Tracing Puts LGBTQ Community under Surveillance, Critics Say." *WUNC 91.5 North Carolina Public Radio*, May 22, 2020. www.wunc.org/post/south-korea-s-coronavirus-contact-tracing-puts-lgbtq-community-under-surveillance-critics-say

Sullivan, Michael. "Don't Nag Your Husband during Lockdown, Malaysia's Government Advises Women." *NPR*, April 1, 2020. www.npr.org/2020/04/01/825051317/dont-nag-your-husband-during-lock-down-malaysias-government-advises-women

Syedullah, Jasmine. "Who Are We to Make Diamonds of Coal? Or, to Reorient to Disorient Democratic Progress with 'Confrontation Teaching'" and Harris, Christopher. "(Caring for) the World that Must Be Undone." *Contemporary Political Theory Critical Exchange*, August 24, 2021. https://doi.org/10.1057/s41296-021-00515-8

Sweeney, Steve. "US Blocks Sale of Ventilators to Cuba after Acquiring Medical Companies." *Morning Star*, April 14, 2020. https://morningstaronline.co.uk/article/w/us-blocks-sale-ventilators-cuba-after-acquiring-medical-companies

Takei, George (@GeorgeTakei). "I Didn't Spend My Childhood in Barbed Wire Enclose Internment Camps So I Could Listen To Grown Adults Today Cry Oppression Because They Have to Wear a Mask at Costco." *Twitter*, May 9, 2020, 7:00pm. https://twitter.com/GeorgeTakei/status/1258939947723169792

Taylor, Chloe. "Brazil's President Attacks Amazon Rainforest 'Lies' and Thanks Trump for Support." *CNBC*, September 24, 2019. www.cnbc.com/2019/09/24/brazils-president-attacks-amazon-rainforest-lies-thanks-trump.html

Teague, Matthew. " 'He Wears the Armor of God': Evangelicals Hail Trump's Church Photo Op." *The Guardian*, June 3, 2020. www.theguardian.com/us-news/2020/jun/03/donald-trump-church-photo-op-evangelicals

Teresa. "Chinese Doctors Confirmed African Blood Genetic Composition Resist Coronavirus after Student Cured." *Af.FeedNews*, February 14, 2020. https://news-af.feednews.com/news/detail/223e120f939f8d0a06b7ce3cee65318c?client=news

Terhune, Chad, Dan Levine, Hyunjoo Jin, and Jane Lanhee Lee. "Special Report: How Korea Trounced U.S. in Race to Test People for Coronavirus." *Reuters*, March 18, 2020. www.reuters.com/article/us-health-coronavirus-testing-specialrep/special-report-how-korea-trounced-u-s-in-race-to-test-people-for-coronavirus-idUSKBN2153BW

Terry, Jennifer. *Attachments to War: Biomedical Logics and Violence in Twenty-First-Century America*. Durham, NC: Duke University Press, 2017.

Tharoor, Ishaan. "Coronavirus Kills Its First Democracy." *Washington Post*, March 30, 2020. www.washingtonpost.com/world/2020/03/31/coronavirus-kills-its-first-democracy/

The Guardian. " 'Tip of the Iceberg': Is Our Destruction of Nature Responsible for Covid-19?" *The Guardian*, March 18, 2020. www.theguardian.com/environment/2020/Mar/18/Tip-Of-The-Iceberg-Is-Our-Destruction-Of-Nature-Responsible-For-Covid-19-Aoe.

———. "Guatemala Calls US 'Wuhan of Americas' in Battle Over Deportees." *The Guardian*, April 15, 2020. www.theguardian.com/world/2020/apr/15/us-deportation-flights-guatemala-coronavirus

The White House. "Remarks by President Trump, Vice President Pence, and Members of the Coronavirus Task Force in Press Briefing." *The White House*, April 10,

2020. www.whitehouse.gov/briefings-statements/remarks-president-trump-vice-president-pence-members-coronavirus-task-force-press-briefing-24/

Thomas, Ebony Elizabeth. *The Dark Fantastic: Race and the Imagination from Harry Potter to the Hunger Games*. New York: New York University Press, 2019.

Thompson, Derek. "Mass Shootings in America Are Spreading Like a Disease." *The Atlantic*, November 6, 2017. www.theatlantic.com/health/archive/2017/11/ameri cas-mass-shooting-epidemic-contagious/545078/

Tian, Ian Liujia. "Vampiric Affect: The Afterlife of a Metaphor in a Global Pandemic." *Social Text Online*, June 17, 2020. https://socialtextjournal.org/periscope_article/vampiric-affect-the-afterlife-of-a-metaphor-in-a-global-pandemic/

Tilley, Lisa. "Saying the Quiet Part Out Loud: Eugenics and the 'Aging Population' in Conservative Pandemic Governance." *Discover Society*, April 6, 2020. https://discoversociety.org/2020/04/06/saying-the-quiet-part-out-loud-eugenics-and-the-aging-population-in-conservative-pandemic-governance/

Times of Israel. "Indian Immigrant Beaten in Tiberias in Apparent Coronavirus-Linked Hate Crime." *Times of Israel*, March 16, 2020. www.timesofisr ael.com/indian-immigrant-beaten-in-tiberias-in-apparent-coronavirus-lin ked-hate-crime/

Tinoco, Robert. Facebook. August 19, 2020. www.facebook.com/roberto.tinoco.92

Tobar, Héctor. "Letter from Los Angeles: On a Generational Uprising." *Literary Hub*, June 5, 2020. https://lithub.com/letter-from-los-angeles-on-a-generational-uprising/

Tu, Jessie. "Taiwan's First Female President Is Delivering a Stunning COVID-19 Response." *Women's Agenda*, April 3, 2020. https://womensagenda.com.au/latest/taiwans-first-female-president-is-delivering-a-stunning-covid-19-response/

Turner, Bryan S. "Theodicies of the COVID-19 Catastrophe." In *COVID-19: Volume I: Global Pandemic, Societal Responses, Ideological Solutions*, edited by Michael J. Ryan, 29–42. London: Routledge, 2020.

Tuzcu, Pinar and Loren Britton. "Witnessing Fabrics: How Face Masks Change Social Perceptions during the Covid-19 Pandemic in Digital Times." In *Covid, Crisis, Care, and Change?: International Gender Perspectives on Re/Production, State and Feminist Transitions*, edited by Antonia Kupfer and Constanze Stutz, 179–194. Toronto: Verlag Barbara Budrich. 2022.

UCI Office of Inclusive Excellence. "The Fire Next Time: Anti-Black Racism and the Struggle to Live in the United States." *UCI Office of Inclusive Excellence*, June 4, 2020. https://inclusion.uci.edu/2020/06/04/the-fire-next-time/

United Nations. "COVID-19: UN Chief Calls for Global Ceasefire to Focus on 'The True Fight of Our Lives'." *UN News*, March 23, 2020. https://news.un.org/en/story/2020/03/1059972

University of Alberta Faculty of Medicine and Dentistry. "Drug Meant for Ebola May Also Work against Coronaviruses." *Science Daily*, February 27, 2020. www.scien cedaily.com/releases/2020/02/200227122123.htm

Vagianos, Alanna. "Legal Sex Workers and Others in Adult Industry Denied Coronavirus Aid." *HuffPost*, April 2, 2020. www.huffpost.com/entry/legal-sex-workers-denied-coronavirus-aid_n_5e86287ac5b6d302366ca912

Valencia, Jorge. "'Die, Bacteria, Die': Mexican Nurses Croon in Hand-Washing PSA Video." *PRI*, March 6, 2020. www.pri.org/stories/2020-03-06/die-bacteria-die-mexican-nurses-croon-hand-washing-psa-video

Varlik, Nükhet. *Plague and Empire in the Early Modern Mediterranean World.* Cambridge: Cambridge University Press, 2015, 95–96.

VICE. "The Netherlands Is Letting People Get Sick to Beat Coronavirus." *VICE*, March 23, 2020. www.youtube.com/watch?v=ozmh40wwAGc&feature=youtu.be

Villarreal, Daniel. "South Korea Threatens to Out LGBTQ People after 86 Coronavirus Cases Linked to Gay Clubs." *LGBTQ Nation*, May 11, 2020. www.lgbtqnation.com/2020/05/south-korea-threatens-lgbtq-population-86-coronavirus-cases-linked-gay-clubs/

Voelkner, Nadine. "Viral Becomings: From Mechanical Viruses to Viral (Dis) Entanglements in Preventing Global Disease." *Global Studies Quarterly* 2, no. 3 (2022): 1–12.

Von Oech, Roger. *Expect the Unexpected or You Won't Find It: A Creativity Tool Based on the Ancient Wisdom of Heraclitus.* Oakland: Berrett-Koehler Publishers, 2002.

Vyas, Kejal. "Cow Dung, Garlic and a Prayer: The Fight against Phony Cures for Coronavirus." *Wall Street Journal*, April 7, 2020. www.wsj.com/amp/articles/cow-dung-garlic-and-a-prayer-the-fight-against-phony-cures-for-coronavirus-11586257200

Wade, Peter. "Just When You Thought Things Couldn't Get Worse, Neo-Nazis Are Trying to Weaponize Coronavirus." *Rolling Stone*, March 22, 2020. www.rollingstone.com/politics/politics-news/neo-nazis-are-trying-to-weaponize-the-coronavirus-971002/

———. "California Official Ousted after Saying Herd Immunity Killing Elderly and Homeless Would Fix 'Burden on Society.'" *Rolling Stone*, May 3, 2020. Accessed April 30, 2023. www.yahoo.com/entertainment/calif-official-ousted-saying-herd-000143108.html

Walker, Alissa. "Coronavirus Is Not Fuel for Urbanist Fantasies: This Moment Should Be about Reassessing Our Broken Cities." *Curbed*, May 20, 2020. www.curbed.com/2020/5/20/21263319/coronavirus-future-city-urban-covid-19

Walker, Sam. "In the Coronavirus Crisis, Deputies Are the Leaders We Turn to." *The Watertown Works*, April 4, 2020. www.watertownworks.com/in-the-coronavirus-crisis-deputies-are-the-leaders-we-turn-to/

Wallace, Rob. *Big Farms Make Big Flu: Dispatches on Influenza, Agribusiness, and the Nature of Science.* New York: New York University Press, 2016.

———. "Notes on a Novel Coronavirus." *New York University Press*, March 24, 2020. www.fromthesquare.org/notes-on-a-novel-coronavirus/#.Xn2LBKhKhPY

Wallace, Rob, Alex Liebman, Luis Fernando Chaves, and Rodrick Wallace. "COVID-19 and Circuits of Capital." *Monthly Review*, May 1, 2020. https://monthlyreview.org/2020/05/01/covid-19-and-circuits-of-capital/

Wamsted, Jay. "ZIP Code May Not Be Destiny, but It's as Hard to Fight as Gravity." *Education Post*, May 15, 2020. https://educationpost.org/zip-code-may-not-be-destiny-but-its-as-hard-to-fight-as-gravity/

Wang, Vivian. "China-Writer-Fang-Fang-Closes-Wuhan-Coronavirus-Lockdown-Diary." *MSN*, April 8, 2020. www.msn.com/en-us/news/world/china-writer-fang-fang-closes-wuhan-coronavirus-lockdown-diary/ar-BB11JB7L

Wasserstrom, Jeffrey. "What to Do and Not to Do amidst a Crisis If You Are a Public Representative." *The Wire*, April 13, 2020. https://thewire.in/world/california-hong-kong-leaders

————. "Four Masks and a Funeral: On the Loss of Freedoms in Hong Kong." *The American Scholar*, April 10, 2021. https://theamericanscholar.org/four-masks-and-a-funeral/

Watts, Jonathan. "Bruno Latour: 'This Is a Global Catastrophe that Has Come from Within'." *The Guardian*, June 6, 2020. www.theguardian.com/world/2020/jun/06/bruno-latour-coronavirus-gaia-hypothesis-climate-crisis

Waxman, Olivia B. "The Surprisingly Deep—and Often Troubling—History of 'Social Distancing.'" *Time*, June 30, 2020. https://time.com/5856800/social-distancing-history/

WBUR Newsroom. "Secretary of Interior Orders Mashpee Wampanoag Reservation 'Disestablished,' Tribe Says." *WBUR*, March 28, 2020. www.wbur.org/news/2020/03/28/mashpee-wampanoag-reservation-secretary-interior-land-trust

Weatherby, Leif. "Delete Your Account: On the Theory of Platform Capitalism." *Los Angeles Review of Books*, April 24, 2018. https://lareviewofbooks.org/article/delete-your-account-on-the-theory-of-platform-capitalism/#!

Weir, Alison. "Minneapolis Cops Trained by Israeli Police, Who Often Use Knee-on-Neck Restraint." *Israel-Palestine News*, June 2, 2020. https://israelpalestinenews.org/minn-cops-trained-by-israeli-police-who-often-use-knee-on-neck-restraint/

Whitney Jr., W.T. "Cuba Develops COVID-19 Vaccines, Takes Socialist Approach." *People's World*, February 4, 2021. www.peoplesworld.org/article/cuba-develops-covid-19-vaccines-takes-socialist-approach/#:~:text=Cuba's%20socialist%20approach%20to%20developing,Cubans%2C%20and%20in%20international%20solidarity

Williams, Devin. "The Time to Dismantle the Racial Structures that Pervade Global Science Is Now." *Scientific American*, June 23, 2021. www.scientificamerican.com/article/the-time-to-dismantle-the-racial-structures-that-pervade-global-science-is-now/

Willouby-Herard, Tiffany. *Waste of a White Skin: The Carnegie Corporation and the Racial Logic of White Vulnerability*. Berkeley: University of California Press, 2015.

————. "(Political) Anesthesia or (Political) Memory: The Combahee River Collective and the Death of Black Women in Custody." *Theory & Event* 21, no. 1 (2018): 259–281.

————. Facebook. March 19, 2020. Accessed March 19, 2020. www.facebook.com/tiffany.herard

Willsher, Kim, Julian Borger, and Oliver Holmes. "US Accused of 'Modern Piracy' after Diversion of Masks Meant for Europe." *The Guardian*, April 3, 2020. www.theguardian.com/world/2020/apr/03/mask-wars-coronavirus-outbidding-demand

Wilson, Joseph and Alicia León. "Spain's Far-Right Holds Car Protest against Virus Lockdown." *ABC News*, May 23, 2020. https://abcnews.go.com/amp/Health/wireStory/spains-holds-car-protest-virus-lockdown-70847709

Wise, Justin. "Fauci on Trump Coronavirus Comments: 'I Can't Jump in Front of the Microphone and Push Him Down.'" *The Hill*, March 23, 2020. https://thehill.com/homenews/administration/488961-fauci-on-trump-coronavirus-comments-i-cant-jump-in-front-of-the

Wolfe, Nathan. *The Viral storm: The Dawn of a New Pandemic Age*. New York: Macmillan, 2011.

Wong, Alvin K. "Thinking Hong Kong's Freedom in Multiplicity." *Hong Kong Protesting*, September 21, 2019. https://hkprotesting.com/2020/07/16/multiplicity/

Wood, Trina J. "Can Pets Contract Coronavirus from Humans or vice versa?" *UC Davis Veterinary Medicine*, February 6, 2020. www.vetmed.ucdavis.edu/news/can-pets-contract-coronavirus-humans-or-vice-versa

World Health Organization. *Report of the WHO-China Joint Mission on Coronavirus Disease 2019 (COVID-19)*, February 16-24, 2020. www.who.int/docs/default-source/coronaviruse/who-china-joint-mission-on-covid-19-final-report.pdf

Yaffe, Helen. "Cuba's Contribution to Combating Covid-19." *URPE: Union for Radical Political Economics*, March 20, 2020. https://urpe.org/2020/03/20/cubas-contribution-to-combating-covid-19/

Yam, Kimmy. "Black, Asian and Hispanic House Caucus Chairs Unite in 'No Tolerance' for Coronavirus Racism." *MSN*, March 31, 2020. www.msn.com/en-us/news/politics/black-asian-and-hispanic-house-caucus-chairs-unite-in-no-tolerance-for-coronavirus-racism/ar-BB11YZqf

Yang, Andrew (@Andrew Yang). "Apparently I Should Have Been Talking about a Pandemic Instead of Automation." *Twitter*, March 12, 2020, 6:30 am. https://twitter.com/AndrewYang/status/1238095725721944065?lang=ar

Yeung, Jessie, Helen Regan, Adam Renton, Emma Reynolds, and Fernando Alfonso III. "March 19 Coronavirus News." *CNN*, March 19, 2020. www.cnn.com/world/live-news/coronavirus-outbreak-03-19-20-intl-hnk/h_21c623966aa148dbeed242de4e94943e

Yip, Ka-che. "Segregation, Isolation, and Quarantine: Protecting Hong Kong from Diseases in the Pre-War Period." *Journal of Comparative Asian Development* 11, no. 1 (2012): 93–116.

Yusoff, Kathryn. *A Billion Black Anthropocenes or None*. Minneapolis: University of Minnesota Press, 2018.

Yves Engler, "Racial Capitalism and the Betrayal of Haiti," *Canadian Dimension*, February 26, 2021. https://canadiandimension.com/articles/view/racial-capitalism-and-the-betrayal-of-haiti

Zárate, Salvador Elias. "Invisible Bodies, Devalued Labor: Contract, Reproductive Labor, and the US Sunbelt, 1900–1963." PhD. diss., University of California San Diego, 2017.

———. "Migrant Labor and a Life under Fire: A Triptych." *Foundry*, June 2021. https://uchri.org/foundry/migrant-labor-and-a-life-under-fire-a-triptych/

Zauzmer, Julie and Sarah Pulliam Bailey. "This Is Not the End of The World, According to Christians Who Study the End of the World." *Washington Post,* March 17, 2020. www.washingtonpost.com/religion/2020/03/17/not-end-of-the-world-coronavirus-bible-prophecy/

Zhan, Mei. "Civet Cats, Fried Grasshoppers, and David Beckham's Pajamas: Unruly Bodies after SARS." *American Anthropologist* 107, no. 1 (2005): 31–42.

Zhang, Li. "Coronavirus Leaked from a Lab? Blame Capitalism, Not China." *Al Jazeera*, May 20, 2020. www.aljazeera.com/indepth/opinion/coronavirus-leaked-lab-blame-capitalism-china200519133348487.html

———. *The Origins of Covid-19: China and Global Capitalism*. Stanford, CA: Stanford University Press, 2021.

Zhou, Xiaodan, et al. "Excess of COVID-19 Cases and Deaths due to Fine Particulate Matter Exposure during the 2020 Wildfires in the United States." *Science Advances* 7, no. 33 (2021).

Zizek, Slavoj. *Pandemic!: COVID-19 Shakes the World.* New York: OR Books LLC, 2020.

Zuboff, Shoshana. *The Age of Surveillance Capitalism: The Fight for a Human Future at the New Frontier of Power.* London: Profile Books, 2019.

Zylinska, Joanna. *The End of Man: A Feminist Counterapocalypse.* Minneapolis: University of Minnesota Press, 2018.

INDEX